Donated by

to EAPMC

October 2002 -

D1756798

Progress in Pain Research and Management
Volume 21

Neuropathic Pain: Pathophysiology and Treatment

Mission Statement of IASP Press®

The International Association for the Study of Pain (IASP) is a nonprofit, interdisciplinary organization devoted to understanding the mechanisms of pain and improving the care of patients with pain through research, education, and communication. The organization includes scientists and health care professionals dedicated to these goals. The IASP sponsors scientific meetings and publishes newsletters, technical bulletins, the journal *Pain,* and books.

The goal of IASP Press is to provide the IASP membership with timely, high-quality, attractive, low-cost publications relevant to the problem of pain. These publications are also intended to appeal to a wider audience of scientists and clinicians interested in the problem of pain.

Progress in Pain Research and Management Series

Pharmacological Approaches to the Treatment of Chronic Pain: New Concepts and Critical Issues, edited by Howard L. Fields and John C. Liebeskind

Proceedings of the 7th World Congress on Pain, edited by Gerald F. Gebhart, Donna L. Hammond, and Troels S. Jensen

Touch, Temperature, and Pain in Health and Disease: Mechanisms and Assessments, edited by Jörgen Boivie, Per Hansson, and Ulf Lindblom

Temporomandibular Disorders and Related Pain Conditions, edited by Barry J. Sessle, Patricia S. Bryant, and Raymond A. Dionne

Visceral Pain, edited by Gerald F. Gebhart

Reflex Sympathetic Dystrophy: A Reappraisal, edited by Wilfrid Jänig and Michael Stanton-Hicks

Pain Treatment Centers at a Crossroads: A Practical and Conceptual Reappraisal, edited by Mitchell J.M. Cohen and James N. Campbell

Proceedings of the 8th World Congress on Pain, edited by Troels S. Jensen, Judith A. Turner, and Zsuzsanna Wiesenfeld-Hallin

Molecular Neurobiology of Pain, edited by David Borsook

Measurement of Pain in Infants and Children, edited by G. Allen Finley and Patrick J. McGrath

Sickle Cell Pain, by Samir K. Ballas

Assessment and Treatment of Cancer Pain, edited by Richard Payne, Richard B. Patt, and C. Stratton Hill

Chronic and Recurrent Pain in Children and Adolescents, edited by Patrick J. McGrath and G. Allen Finley

Opioid Sensitivity of Chronic Noncancer Pain, edited by Eija Kalso, Henry J. McQuay, and Zsuzsanna Wiesenfeld-Hallin

Psychological Mechanisms of Pain and Analgesia, by Donald D. Price

Proceedings of the 9th World Congress on Pain, edited by Marshall Devor, Michael C. Rowbotham, and Zsuzsanna Wiesenfeld-Hallin

Sex, Gender, and Pain, edited by Roger B. Fillingim

Pain Imaging, edited by Kenneth L. Casey and M. Catherine Bushnell

The Child with Headache: Diagnosis and Treatment, edited by Patricia A. McGrath and Loretta M. Hillier

Acute and Procedure Pain in Infants and Children, edited by G. Allen Finley and Patrick J. McGrath

Progress in Pain Research and Management
Volume 21

Neuropathic Pain: Pathophysiology and Treatment

Editors

Per T. Hansson, MD, PhD, DDS

Neurogenic Pain Unit, Multidisciplinary Pain Center,
Department of Rehabilitation Medicine,
Karolinska Hospital, Stockholm, Sweden

Howard L. Fields, MD, PhD

Department of Neurology, University of California,
San Francisco, California, USA

Raymond G. Hill, PhD

The Neuroscience Research Centre, Merck Sharp and Dohme,
Terlings Park, Essex, United Kingdom

Paolo Marchettini, MD

Pain Medicine Center, Scientific Institute
and Hospital San Raffaele, Milan, Italy

IASP PRESS® • SEATTLE

Library of Congress Cataloging-in-Publication Data

Neuropathic pain : pathophysiology and treatment / editors, Per T. Hansson ... [et al.].
    p. ; cm. -- (Progress in pain research and management ; v. 21)
  Includes bibliographical references and index.
  ISBN 0-931092-38-8 (alk. paper)
   1. Nervous system--Pathophysiology. 2. Neuralgia. 3. Central pain. I. Hansson, Per, 1955- II Series.
   [DNLM: 1. Neuralgia--physiopathology. 2. Neuralgia--therapy. WL 544 N4946 2001]
  RC347.N4797 2001
  616.8'047--dc21

                                                                    2001026397

Published by:

IASP Press
International Association for the Study of Pain
909 NE 43rd St., Suite 306
Seattle, WA 98105 USA
Fax: 206-547-1703
www.painbooks.org

Printed in the United States of America

Contents

Contributing Authors

Miroslav Backonja, MD *Department of Neurology, University of Wisconsin, Madison, Wisconsin, USA*

Mark Baker, PhD *Department of Biology, University College London, London, United Kingdom*

Ralf Baron, Dr med *Neurology Clinic, University of Kiel, Kiel, Germany*

Joel A. Black, PhD *Department of Neurology and PVA-EPVA Neuroscience Research Center, Yale University School of Medicine, New Haven, Connecticut; and Rehabilitation Research Center, Veterans Affairs Hospital, West Haven, Connecticut, USA*

Mario Campero, MD *Department of Neurology, University of Chile, Santiago, Chile*

Theodore R. Cummins, PhD *Department of Neurology and PVA-EPVA Neuroscience Research Center, Yale University School of Medicine, New Haven, Connecticut; and Rehabilitation Research Center, Veterans Affairs Hospital, West Haven, Connecticut, USA*

Sulayman Dib-Hajj, PhD *Department of Neurology and PVA-EPVA Neuroscience Research Center, Yale University School of Medicine, New Haven, Connecticut; and Rehabilitation Research Center, Veterans Affairs Hospital, West Haven, Connecticut, USA*

Anthony H. Dickenson, PhD *Department of Pharmacology, University College London, London, United Kingdom*

Howard L. Fields, MD, PhD *Department of Neurology, University of California, San Francisco, California, USA*

Per T. Hansson, MD, PhD, DDS *Neurogenic Pain Unit, Multidisciplinary Pain Center, Department of Rehabilitation Medicine, Karolinska Hospital/Institute, Stockholm, Sweden*

Raymond G. Hill, PhD *The Neuroscience Research Centre, Merck Sharp and Dohme, Terlings Park, Essex, United Kingdom*

Wilfrid Jänig, Dr med *Institute of Physiology, University of Kiel, Kiel, Germany*

Troels S. Jensen, MD *Department of Neurology, Aarhus University Hospital, Aarhus, Denmark*

Marco Lacerenza, MD *Pain Medicine Center, Scientific Institute and Hospital San Raffaele, Milan, Italy*

Josephine Lai, PhD *Department of Pharmacology, Health Sciences Center, University of Arizona, Tucson, Arizona, USA*

Bengt Linderoth, MD, PhD *Department of Neurosurgery, Karolinska Hospital/Institute, Stockholm, Sweden*

T. Philip Malan, Jr., MD, PhD *Departments of Pharmacology and Anesthesiology, Health Sciences Center, University of Arizona, Tucson, Arizona, USA*

Paolo Marchettini, MD *Pain Medicine Center, Scientific Institute and Hospital San Raffaele, Milan, Italy*

Elizabeth A. Matthews, BSc *Department of Pharmacology, University College London, London, United Kingdom*

Björn A. Meyerson, MD, PhD *Department of Neurosurgery, Karolinska Hospital/Institute, Stockholm, Sweden*

Turo J. Nurmikko, MD, PhD *Pain Research Institute, Department of Neurological Science, University of Liverpool, Liverpool, United Kingdom*

José Ochoa, MD, PhD *Neuromuscular Unit, Good Samaritan Hospital and Medical Center, and Oregon Health Sciences University, Portland, Oregon, USA*

Kenji Okuse, PhD *Department of Biology, University College London, London, United Kingdom*

Michael H. Ossipov, PhD *Department of Pharmacology, Health Sciences Center, University of Arizona, Tucson, Arizona, USA*

Frank Porreca, PhD *Departments of Pharmacology and Anesthesiology, Health Sciences Center, University of Arizona, Tucson, Arizona, USA*

Michael C. Rowbotham, MD *Pain Clinical Research Center, University of California, San Francisco, California, USA*

Jordi Serra, MD *Neuropathic Pain Unit, Sagrada Familia Clinic, Barcelona, Spain*

Søren H. Sindrup, MD *Department of Neurology, Odense University Hospital, and Department of Clinical Pharmacology, University of Southern Denmark, Odense, Denmark*

Claudia Sommer, MD *Department of Neurology, University of Würzburg, Würzburg, Germany*

Rie Suzuki, PhD *Department of Pharmacology, University College London, London, United Kingdom*

Todd W. Vanderah, PhD *Departments of Pharmacology and Anesthesiology, Health Sciences Center, University of Arizona, Tucson, Arizona, USA*

C. Peter N. Watson, MD, FRCPC *Department of Medicine, University of Toronto, Toronto, Ontario, Canada*

Stephen G. Waxman, MD, PhD *Department of Neurology and PVA-EPVA Neuroscience Research Center, Yale University School of Medicine, New Haven, Connecticut; and Rehabilitation Research Center, Veterans Affairs Hospital, West Haven, Connecticut, USA*

John N. Wood, DSc *Department of Biology, University College London, London, United Kingdom*

Preface

Pain in neuropathy has been extensively studied, both clinically and experimentally. Despite this multifaceted research approach we still face significant shortcomings in our ability to successfully treat patients with neuropathic pain, partly due to our inadequate knowledge of pathophysiological mechanisms related to its initiation and maintenance. Several animal models of neuropathic pain have been developed to facilitate the study of such mechanisms. To be able to apply what we have learned from these models to clinical neuropathic pain, we must address significant limitations of animal research related to painful neuropathy. For example, we can certainly accept the relevance of the various ways to induce neuropathy, but we are left with uncertainty regarding the presence of spontaneous or stimulus-evoked pain. Behavioral studies in animal models of neuropathy rely heavily on stimulus-induced reflex abnormalities such as extremity withdrawal latency or duration, and these may or may not reflect the conscious perception of stimulus-evoked pain in humans. An open discussion between clinicians/clinical scientists and animal researchers on the clinical relevance of animal models and sensory testing techniques in such models may aid in defining to what extent animal models mimic clinical neuropathic pain.

Initial inspiration for this book came from the attractive content of two symposia on neuropathic pain held in conjunction with the International Association for the Study of Pain's 9th World Congress in Vienna. In Como, Italy, symposium contributors focused on pharmacological treatment of ongoing and stimulus-evoked neuropathic pain, and in Seeon, Germany, participants addressed mechanism-based approaches to the treatment of neuropathic pain. These meetings suggested the timeliness of a cohesive volume summarizing the latest knowledge within crucial areas of neuropathic pain. Chapter authors were invited to concentrate on key issues regarding diagnosis and treatment as well as research related to pathophysiology, whether clinical or experimental. Most importantly, we chose to present a state-of-the-art review of research and clinical practice in the field, rather than simply to create a proceedings book of the symposia.

With this volume, editors and authors hope to provide the reader with a fundamental background as well as recently emerging information within the area of neuropathic pain. The book should assist health care professionals in providing high-quality patient care, including a more rational application of possible pain mechanisms and the latest information about effective treatments. The content illustrates the potential value of current and future research efforts directed toward increased understanding of the pathophysiology of pain in neuropathy. Better understanding of the mechanisms underlying the different aspects of neuropathic pains holds the promise of treatment strategies that selectively target each mechanism. We hope this book will provide a ray of hope to the thousands of people suffering from the relentless assaults on their lives from neuropathic pain.

Per T. Hansson, MD, PhD, DDS
Howard L. Fields, MD, PhD
Raymond G. Hill, PhD
Paolo Marchettini, MD

Neuropathic Pain: Pathophysiology and Treatment,
Progress in Pain Research and Management, Vol. 21,
edited by Per T. Hansson, Howard L. Fields, Raymond G.
Hill, and Paolo Marchettini, IASP Press, Seattle, © 2001.

1

Aspects of Clinical and Experimental Neuropathic Pain: The Clinical Perspective

Per Hansson,[a] Marco Lacerenza,[b] and Paolo Marchettini[b]

[a]Neurogenic Pain Unit, Multidisciplinary Pain Center and Department of Rehabilitation Medicine, Karolinska Hospital/Institute, Stockholm, Sweden; [b]Pain Medicine Center, Scientific Institute and Hospital San Raffaele, Milan, Italy

Painful neuropathic conditions may accompany a lesion of the peripheral or central nervous system. Table I summarizes conditions that may be associated with pain. All types of neuropathic pain are projected to the innervation territory of the damaged nerve or pathway, according to the somatotopic organization of the primary somatosensory cortex. Examples of projected pain are pain localized to the amputated area in phantom pain or pain perceived in the ulnar part of the hand in ulnar nerve entrapment in the elbow. Nerve root compression from a herniated disk usually involves a combination of nociceptive pain in the area of the ruptured disk and neuropathic pain projected within the dermatome corresponding to the affected root(s). When the nociceptors innervating the perineurium (the endings of the nervi nervorum) are activated during inflammation or compression, the resulting pain is nociceptive and is mainly localized to the site of disturbance.

Painful neuropathies are characterized by spontaneous and/or abnormal stimulus-evoked pain. Evoked pain is defined as *allodynia* when caused by normally innocuous stimuli, usually light mechanical stimuli (Merskey and Bogduk 1994). Pain caused by normally innocuous stimuli is not unique to neuropathic pain; it may also occur in non-neuropathic conditions such as skin injury (e.g., sunburn), joint inflammation, and hysterical pain conditions. The mechanisms underlying allodynia in various clinical conditions are different, and a thorough medical history and examination will point to

Table I
Conditions in which neuropathic/neurogenic pain may appear

Peripheral

Traumatic (including iatrogenic) nerve injury

Ischemic neuropathy

Nerve compression/entrapment

Polyneuropathy (hereditary, metabolic, toxic, inflammatory, infectious,
     paraneoplastic, nutritional, in amyloidosis and vasculitis)

Plexus injury

Root compression

Stump and phantom pain after amputation

Herpes zoster/postherpetic neuralgia

Trigeminal and glossopharyngeal neuralgia

Cancer-related neuropathy (due to neural invasion of the tumor,
     surgical nerve damage, radiation-induced nerve damage,
     chemotherapy-induced neuropathy)

Central

Stroke (infarct or hemorrhage)

Multiple sclerosis

Spinal cord injury

Syringomyelia/syringobulbia

Epilepsy

Space-occupying lesions

the underlying cause. From a quality of life point of view, allodynia, especially dynamic mechanical allodynia, is highly disabling to affected subgroups of neuropathic pain patients.

In contrast to allodynia, *hyperalgesia* is defined as increased pain intensity evoked by normally painful stimuli (Merskey and Bogduk 1994). Neuropathic pain states are also often associated with nonpainful abnormal spontaneous and evoked sensory phenomena such as paresthesia and dysesthesia.

For the vast majority of neuropathic diagnostic entities the percentage of subjects reporting neuropathic pain is not precisely known. However, an estimated 5% of patients with traumatic nerve injury suffer from pain (Sunderland 1993). Further, about 8% of stroke patients suffer from central neuropathic pain (Andersen et al. 1995), as do 28% of patients with multiple sclerosis and 75% of patients with syringomyelia (Boivie 1999). Detailed studies in patients with central pain due to stroke (Boivie et al. 1989; Leijon et al. 1989) or multiple sclerosis (Boivie et al. 1989; Osterberg et al. 1994) have identified a common denominator in central pain: somatosensory examination typically reveals signs of involvement of the spino- (trigemino-) thalamocortical system, resulting in altered sensitivity to temperature and/or pain stimuli. The painful condition is not consistently related to alterations in other somatosensory channels or in the motor system (Leijon et al. 1989). No common denominator has been identified in peripheral neuropathic pain states, although small myelinated and unmyelinated fibers are probably involved in most cases because neuropathies with predominant involvement of large myelinated fibers often are not painful (Asbury 1990). We still do not know why seemingly similar nerve injuries can be painful in some cases and painless in others. In addition, no systematic studies in neuropathic pain patients have investigated the correlation between the intensity of symptoms and the nature and severity of the nerve injury. In highly specialized units for neuropathic pain, patients with pain in areas with partial nerve injury greatly outnumber patients with complete deafferentation and pain. This finding could imply a lower incidence of painful sequelae in total deafferentation or may simply reflect the lower frequency of total deafferentation in the population of neuropathic pain patients.

Current drug and nondrug therapies for chronic neuropathic pain, based on observations from clinical studies, clinical anecdotes, and experimental findings, offer substantial pain relief to no more than half of the affected patients (Hansson 1994b). In the vast majority of cases, chronic neuropathic pain cannot be successfully treated using conventional analgesics and is resistant to oral opioids. Opioid sensitivity in neuropathic pain is a controversial issue within the scientific community (Arnér and Meyerson 1988; Kupers et al. 1991; Rowbotham et al. 1991). The array of therapeutic agents is multifaceted (Table II), but is efficacious, to some extent, in only about half of the patients. No systematic studies have evaluated drug combinations in different neuropathic pain conditions. In clinical practice it is important to inform the patient and relatives, early on, about the difficulties related to treatment, without creating despair, explaining that most patients who benefit from treatment achieve only partial relief of pain. Unrealistic expectations regarding treatment outcome may deprive the patient of enjoying partial relief. There is no predictor for the response of an individual patient to a specific intervention, and the treatment strategy is based on trial and error. Effective new treatment strategies are desperately needed.

DEFINITION OF NEUROGENIC/NEUROPATHIC PAIN

The International Association for the Study of Pain (Merskey and Bogduk 1994) defines neurogenic pain as "Pain initiated or caused by a primary lesion or dysfunction or transitory perturbation in the peripheral or central nervous system." Neuropathic pain is a subentity where "transitory perturbation" is

Table II
Proposed therapies for neuropathic pain

Pharmacological Therapies

Antidepressants (amitriptyline, maprotiline, selective
    serotonin reuptake inhibitors)

Antiepileptics (gabapentin, carbamazepine, clonazepam,
    lamotrigine, topiramate, phenytoin)

Local anesthetics and mexiletine

Baclofen

Clonidine

Ketamine

Dextrorphan

Tramadol

Guanethidine

Opioids (morphine, methadone, ketobemidone, fentanyl)

Neurostimulation Techniques

Transcutaneous electrical nerve stimulation

Spinal cord stimulation

Motor cortex stimulation

Deep brain stimulation

Surgical Interventions

Decompression

Neuroma removal

Neurotomy

Glycerol injection

Radiofrequency nerve/root lesion

Dorsal root entry zone lesion

Cordotomy

Stereotactic radiosurgery

omitted. The inclusion of "dysfunction" in the definition may be a source of confusion because it allows nociceptive and psychogenic conditions to be improperly diagnosed as neurogenic/neuropathic. A neurobiological response to nerve injury, such as alteration of sodium channel expression or peripheral and central sensitization, might be considered "dysfunctions" of the nervous system. There is evidence for sensitization of primary afferents in some neuropathic pain patients, such as subgroups of patients with postherpetic neuralgia (Rowbotham and Fields 1996; Petersen et al. 2000), but also in nociceptive pain states such as rheumatoid arthritis. Central sensitization, expressing itself as allodynia to mechanical and/or thermal stimuli, is a prominent sign of both clinical neurogenic/neuropathic and nociceptive pain conditions. Thus, if such alterations are accepted as "dysfunctions" of the nervous system, the term is too broad to be part of the definition of neurogenic/neuropathic pain. Therefore, and for the sake of simplicity, we suggest amending the definition of neuropathic pain to: "pain due to a primary lesion of the peripheral or central nervous system." The use of "neurogenic pain" could be confined to classical neurological painful conditions such as trigeminal and glossopharyngeal neuralgia where neuropathy may be difficult to demonstrate. Symptom irreversibility is not critical because in long-standing conditions pain may subside over time.

Clinical neurologists commonly encounter patients with pain and other symptoms and signs suggesting abnormalities within the somatosensory system that cannot be linked to an identifiable structural lesion of the nervous system. Such symptoms are commonly labeled as "nonorganic," based on the assumption that symptoms and signs are "psychogenic" in nature. Psychogenicity is clearly an expression of brain function, and symptoms most likely result from biochemical and/or physiological alterations. Abnormal modification of inhibitory or facilitatory systems might be responsible for the loss or amplification of somatosensory or other functions. Modulatory systems may also contribute to complex regional pain syndrome type I and chronic pain localized to musculoskeletal structures. In addition, processing of nociceptive inputs is attenuated across sleep stages (Lavigne et al. 2000). Clinical conditions with spontaneous and abnormal induced pain may result from altered central modulation within the somatosensory system. This phenomenon has been suggested to occur in conditions such as fibromyalgia (Kosek et al. 1996) and osteoarthritis (Kosek and Ordeberg 2000). While we emphasize that these sensory dysfunctions are not due to structural lesions of classical neurological pathways, we propose that they are organic and may be due to abnormal activation of facilitatory or inhibitory systems or pain projection pathways. Abnormal frontal lobe activity has so far been described in only a few patients with neurological symptoms from hysteria (Tiihonen et al. 1995; Marshall et al. 1997). Patients with this kind of sensory disorder require meticulous neurological and psychological assessment and possibly pharmacological testing to determine appropriate treatments aimed at recovering inhibition or erasing abnormal facilitation. Careful diagnosis is necessary to differentiate between traditional "organic" neurological disorders and "functional-organic" conditions and to prevent invasive, potentially harmful interventions in the latter category (Ron 1994). Somatization in depression is known to be a condition at high risk for iatrogenesis (Kouyanou et al. 1998; Marchettini et al. 2000), as is Munchausen's syndrome (Wallace and Fitzmorris 1978). The category of "functional-organic" conditions should include patients diagnosed with hysteria or with psychosomatic or somatoform disorders that are considered unconscious dysfunctions. Malingering subjects should not be included in this category.

DIAGNOSTIC WORK-UP

Neuropathic pain is part of the neurological disease spectrum, and classical diagnostic criteria apply. The first step in the diagnostic work-up is taking a meticulous medical history, exploring the onset of pain and its possible association with current diseases, trauma, and surgery. The physician should explore the temporal aspects of the painful condition, which can lead to a specific diagnosis in a few neurogenic pain conditions, i.e., trigeminal and glossopharyngeal neuralgia. Other neuropathic pain conditions have no distinctive temporal profile but are continuous, sometimes with superimposed intermittent or paroxysmal painful or nonpainful symptoms. The presence of stimulus-evoked pain, often as disabling for the patient as spontaneous pain, should be carefully identified. Neuropathic pain conditions are often associated with unfamiliar symptom qualities that can be difficult for the patient to communicate. To enhance communication, the examining physician should reassure the patient that the symptoms are common expressions of such conditions.

The literature does not report consistent pathognomonic pain descriptors in peripheral or central neuropathic pain, and each patient may use several sensory-discriminative descriptors. Leijon and coworkers (1989) reported no common denominators from their series of patients with central pain. However, burning, sometimes shock-like or electrical pain in conjunction with numbness, tingling, and pins and needles projected to a cutaneous area is highly indicative of a neuropathic condition. Importantly, aching pain does not rule out the possibility of a neuropathic basis and may be a frequent complaint in patients with central pain due to multiple sclerosis (Osterberg et al. 1994) or syringomyelia (Boivie 1999). The pain distribution, with few exceptions (see below), matches the level of the lesion. A neuroanatomical distribution correlating with the site of the lesion supports the diagnosis of neuropathic pain and should be explored thoroughly using a pain drawing completed by the patient (Fig. 1a–e).

Physicians examining neuropathic pain patients should evaluate sensory, motor, and autonomic signs to confirm or reject the suspected anatomical localization of the lesion extracted from a careful history. Because pain is part of the somatosensory system, the diagnosis of painful neuropathy rests heavily on the demonstration of sensory abnormalities in the area corresponding to the innervation territory of the damaged nerve, plexus, root, or central pathway. A careful bedside examination of somatosensory functions, using an array of instruments (Hansson 1994a) to explore the entire spectrum of fibers/pathways, is crucial because sensory aberrations may be confined to a single or few sensory modalities. The examination of somatosensory function should be the final part of the diagnostic work-up, and should be guided by a tentative diagnosis based on the information collected up to that point. The outcome of the bedside examination is often a sufficient basis for diagnosis. Since the distribution of sensory abnormalities matches the innervation territory of the damaged nervous structure, the borders of the area of sensory dysfunction should be carefully mapped using different modalities. If the sensory examination is started within the area of dysfunction and is directed toward the normal areas around it, the area of abnormality will appear larger than when testing from the outside in. The reason for this discrepancy is the inherent reaction time that it takes for the patient to perceive and report alterations in sensations. In clinical practice, we recommend testing from the inside out to explore an area of sensory deficit, but from the outside in to explore a territory with positive sensory phenomena, such as mechanical or thermal allodynia or hyperalgesia, so as to minimize the duration of painful stimulation.

Extraterritorial spread of pain and/or sensory dysfunction should be accepted as evidence of central sensitization only after careful differential diagnosis to rule out non-neurological conditions. Extraterritorial spread, seen only occasionally, usually develops after a period of proper distribution of signs and symptoms and may in some cases be interpreted as variations in the innervation territories of nerves or roots (Tal and Bennett 1994; Sotgiu and Biella 1995; Lacerenza et al. 1996) (Fig. 1e). The extension of the extraterritorial spread varies over time, is arbitrary, and cannot be quantified. Sound clinical reasoning should be the basis for diagnosis.

Regarding the somatosensory examination, specific characteristics apply to true neuropathic conditions, i.e., the modality profile and borders of abnormalities are reproducible during one examination. To further explore the somatosensory status, psychophysical quantitative somatosensory testing techniques (Hansson 1994a) may be added to assess perception threshold, so as to complement standard clinical neurophysiological methods, which fall short in demonstrating pathology of the small fiber system and in revealing positive phenomena such as dynamic mechanical allodynia (Verdugo and Ochoa 1992).

Motor dysfunction, such as tremor and weakness, in the absence of damage to the motor system, is either a somatomotor reflex, a protective behavior, or a psychologically conditioned overlay. Autonomic signs may be a direct consequence of the nerve injury, or a spinal/supraspinal reflex to

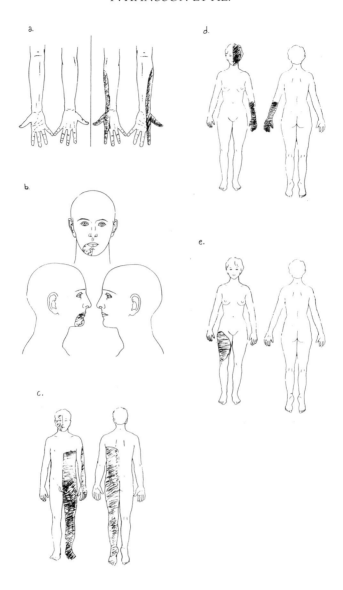

Fig. 1. Drawings from five different patients with neuropathic pain, emphasizing their usefulness in defining the neuroanatomically correlated distribution of projected pain and other sensory symptoms. Symptomatic areas are shaded. (a) A 30-year-old male patient with a herniated disk at the C5–C6 level and a painful rhizopathy distributed in the C6 dermatome of the left arm. On the whole-body drawing (not shown), the patient also indicated pain in the neck. (b) A 44-year-old male patient with a traumatic fracture of the right corpus of the mandible during a car accident and a lesion of the inferior alveolar nerve. The patient suffers from ongoing pain and aggravation of pain during tactile stimuli in an area corresponding to the innervation territory of the mental nerve, the most peripheral part of the inferior alveolar nerve. (c) A 40-year-old male patient with a brainstem infarct (Wallenberg's syndrome) on the right side. In the right side of

the nociceptive input; care should be taken to disentangle these phenomena (Bennett and Ochoa 1991). A complete transection of the nerve may at first produce vasodilation due to the loss of vasoconstrictor tone, and later cause vasoconstriction due to denervation supersensitivity of blood vessels (Cannon and Rosenbleuth 1949; Fleming and Westfall 1988). In addition, both nociceptive and low-threshold mechanoreceptive input may reflexively evoke vasoconstrictor/sudomotor responses (Ochoa 1993). Not infrequently, such physiological somatosympathetic reflex activity, which is the result of the painful condition, is mistakenly interpreted as its cause, i.e., sympathetically maintained pain.

The outcome of intravenous pharmacological testing should never be used as the sole diagnostic criterion. The outcome of testing (e.g., with lidocaine or morphine) may, however, be used to guide treatment interventions and may be relevant for future discussion of pathophysiological mechanisms.

In summary, the diagnosis of peripheral or central neuropathic pain should be made only when the history and signs are indicative of neuropathy in conjunction with a neuroanatomically correlated pain distribution and sensory abnormalities within the area of pain. The cornerstones of the diagnostic work-up in neuropathic pain, listed in Table III, can also disclose the etiology of the pain.

MECHANISM-BASED CLASSIFICATION:
CRITICISM AND PROPOSAL

Neuropathic pain has been classified according either to the etiological diagnosis (painful diabetic neuropathy, postherpetic neuralgia, and post-traumatic neuralgia), or to the anatomical site of the lesion (central pain or peripheral neuralgia). Unfortunately, chronic painful conditions have often been grouped together based on symptoms, signs, anatomical distribution,

---

the face and in the left thoracic and abdominal regions he reported numbness only. In the left arm he experienced numbness and pricking sensations and in the left leg ongoing pain and numbness, as well as pain aggravation from tactile stimuli. (d) A 78-year-old female with a thalamic infarct reporting pain and pricking sensations in the left side of the head and face and in the lower part of the left arm. (The face and hand/arm areas are represented in close proximity in the ventral posteromedial nucleus and ventral posterolateral nucleus, respectively, of the thalamus.) (e) A 52-year-old female patient who sustained a lesion of the right n. cutaneous femoris lateralis during hysterectomy. After several years of pain distribution (and sensory abnormalities, including dynamic mechanical allodynia) within the innervation territory of the damaged nerve, the pain spread to the medial aspect of the thigh innervated by cutaneous branches of the femoral nerve.

Table III
Cornerstones of the diagnostic work-up

Primary Diagnostic Examination
Medical history
Pain drawing
A comprehensive neurological examination including a focused survey of somatosensory functions
Detailed Work-up
Neurophysiological testing
Electroneurography
Electromyography
Evoked potentials
Quantitative sensory testing
Thermography
Diagnostic nerve block (ischemia/compression cuff block, placebo-controlled local anesthetic nerve block) in selected cases
Central nervous system imaging

and an unproven etiology under inappropriate names such as "failed back surgery syndrome" or misdiagnoses such as "reflex sympathetic dystrophy." Under such circumstances it is impossible to gain reliable information from the published outcomes of therapy, or to plan a rational pharmacological trial of drugs for neuropathic pain. Data from basic research indicate that multiple pathophysiological mechanisms underlie neuropathic pain. Furthermore, different mechanisms may coexist in a single patient and might change over time. Alternatively, etiologically different clinical conditions may harbor similar pathophysiological mechanisms.

In 1998 Woolf and colleagues, reiterating and elaborating concepts introduced by others (Hansson and Kinnman 1996), proposed a classification of pain based on mechanisms in parallel to classical diagnosis by anatomy or cause. According to the authors, a mechanism-based classification would enable us to answer questions such as: "(a) what is the contribution of primary afferent sensitization to the pain, (b) is there evidence for ectopic discharges in the primary afferent neuron, (c) is there an involvement of the sympathetic nervous system, (d) is there evidence for CNS sensitization or CNS disinhibition?" The concept of a mechanism-based classification of pain has been refined in more recent papers (Woolf and Decosterd 1999; Woolf and Mannion 1999).

Due to shortcomings in our ability to determine detailed pathophysiological mechanisms from the clinical examination, we are rarely able to definitively link clinical findings with basic mechanisms. Dynamic mechanical allodynia in widespread areas of the innervation territory of a damaged peripheral nerve is a good example of a phenomenon in which pain mechanisms cannot be determined from the clinical examination. At least three pathophysiological mechanisms could explain the conversion of Aβ-mediated input from tactile to painful sensation: (1) central sensitization, i.e., opening of previously existing but silent synaptic connections between large myelinated afferents and nociceptive-specific neurons in the spinal cord (Cook et al. 1987); (2) central sensitization of wide-dynamic-range neurons (Roberts 1986); and (3) sprouting of mechanoreceptive fibers in the dorsal horn, i.e., central terminals of such fibers making new synaptic connections with nociceptive neurons (Woolf et al. 1992). By currently available clinical testing procedures we cannot determine which of these mechanisms is contributing to a particular patient's pain. We also lack good insights into the biochemical events underlying these phenomena. A detailed mechanism-based classification is currently not feasible, although it is often possible to differentiate likely mechanisms based on signs of somatosensory dysfunction (Hansson and Kinnman 1996; Rowbotham and Fields 1996). Mechanism-based classification of pain is a sound approach and should be pursued to facilitate mechanism-tailored treatment strategies in the future.

Several investigators have attempted to subdivide the effects of drugs on different clinical phenomenologies of neuropathic pain (Attal et al. 1998), including spontaneous and stimulus-evoked pain. Such studies represent an attempt to disclose the mechanisms of different facets of the pain condition, but they do not address detailed pain mechanisms because such details are usually not revealed on a clinical level.

In concert with Woolf et al. (1998), we feel that it is mandatory to retain the traditional organ-based diagnostic work-up, which should precede a further in-depth characterization of specific pain mechanisms (Marchettini and Barbieri 2000). Mechanism-based treatment strategies will depend on extensive preparatory work on how to link certain symptoms and signs to specific mechanisms (Hansson and Kinnman 1996). To develop this area, close collaboration between animal and human researchers is a prerequisite. From a clinical perspective, somatosensory aberrations of different sensory channels may prove important to scrutinize, using quantitative sensory testing techniques, to characterize in detail negative as well as positive sensory phenomena. In peripheral neuropathic pain states the fibers remaining after injury may be subjected to quantitative physiological stimuli of various sensory modalities to further our understanding of clinical neuropathic pain. This approach allows dissociation between somatosensory functions dependent on conduction in myelinated and unmyelinated fibers (Campbell et al.

1988; Ochoa and Yarnitsky 1993). In addition, conduction block by local anesthetic may be used to study the importance of different fiber subpopulations in spontaneous and stimulus-evoked pain (Nurmikko et al. 1991). Associations between spontaneous ongoing pain and stimulus-evoked pain may also be further elucidated (Lindblom 1985; Koltzenburg et al. 1994; Rowbotham and Fields 1996).

TREATMENT OF NEUROPATHIC PAIN

Pharmacological management of neuropathic pain lacks a fully validated rationale. In individual patients we are currently unable to predict the response of spontaneous or stimulus-evoked pain to drug therapy. Recently, however, through systematic reviews, information on the number needed to treat (NNT) has provided insight into the overall effect of drugs in groups of patients in different neuropathic pain states (McQuay et al. 1995, 1996; Sindrup and Jensen 1999). NNT represents the number of patients that must be treated, after correction for placebo responders, to obtain one patient with at least 50% pain relief (Cook and Sackett 1995). The strength of conclusions drawn from such studies regarding the clinical efficacy of a specific treatment critically depends on the quality of the evidence contained in the scientific literature. Further, papers included in systematic reviews, based on ratings of quality, escape adequate scrutiny if the reviewer lacks proper training in the field of the review, which should be taken into account when evaluating such surveys.

Treatment studies in patients with neuropathic pain generally have been designed to monitor the intensity of the spontaneous pain, usually in diagnostic entities such as diabetic neuropathy and postherpetic neuralgia. Judging by the clinical expression of neuropathic pain conditions, similar diagnostic entities may well include multiple mechanisms related to spontaneous and stimulus-evoked pain. For example, one group of patients with postherpetic neuralgia may demonstrate a clinical picture of deafferentation and anesthesia in an area with ongoing pain, whereas another group may report spontaneous pain and severe dynamic mechanical allodynia (Nurmikko and Bowsher 1990; Rowbotham and Fields 1996). In treatment studies of neuropathic pain it seems reasonable to move beyond merely monitoring fluctuations in spontaneous pain. Within a study comprising one diagnostic entity, patients could be subgrouped on the basis of common clinical phenomenology and possible common pathophysiological mechanisms, and various techniques could be used to validate this grouping (Attal et al. 1998). This strategy may aid in demonstrating relief of different aspects of neuropathic pain and in tailoring optimal treatment strategies for individual patients.

The results of scientific treatment studies in humans may not coincide with clinical experience of efficacy, as is the case for mexiletine (Dejgard et al. 1988) and paroxetine (Sindrup et al. 1990). Possible explanations include bias due to patient and physician expectations, which could lead to correct identification of the active treatment versus placebo and hence overinterpretation; too short a follow-up to detect a declining placebo response; a genuine habituation to the active treatment; and imprecise pain ratings (e.g., global pain intensity over a week). Crucial points to consider when evaluating the methodological quality of studies are listed in Table IV.

Several authors have proposed that the outcome of studies using intravenous administration of drugs can be used to predict the long-term effects of oral doses of the same or similar substances (Galer et al. 1996; Canavero and Bonicalzi 1998). The clinical relevance of this approach is questionable and is at odds with our clinical experience. The ability of potentially pain-relieving agents to control chronic pain on an ongoing basis cannot be extrapolated from patients' short-term responses. Furthermore, drugs that may be effective on a long-term basis, such as opioids, may have side effects caused by acute administration that prevent identification of their pain-relieving properties. Such drugs must be tested on an outpatient basis with progressive titration, which may allow patients to adapt to side effects.

ANIMAL MODELS: CRITICISM AND PROPOSAL

Animal models have offered insights into mechanisms of the neurological dysfunction that follows injury to the peripheral or central nervous system (Bennett and Xie 1988; Seltzer et al. 1990; Kim and Chung 1992;

Table IV
Methodological issues to consider when evaluating or conducting treatment trials

Adequate (nonbiased) selection of patients
Description of diagnostic criteria
Assignment of patients to subgroups based on pain characteristics and sensory dysfunctions
Description of criteria for exclusion and inclusion
Blinded randomization (described in detail)
Blinding (described in detail) of patients and research team
Assessment of compliance with treatment
Description of withdrawals and reasons for withdrawals
Description of outcome measures
Independent third-party evaluation
Follow-up period

Yezierski 1996). These seemingly reproducible models have demonstrated striking electrophysiological and behavioral effects of several classes of drugs proposed for the treatment of neuropathic pain (Hunter et al. 1997; Chapman et al. 1998). However, an obvious discrepancy between animal models of peripheral nerve injury and clinical traumatic neuropathy is the extremely high incidence of "pain-like" behavior and facilitated withdrawal reflexes in animals versus the relatively rare painful sequelae of nerve lesions in humans. Indeed, the most common sensory complaints in clinical peripheral neuropathies are tingling paresthesia and numbness, rather than pain. One explanation for this discrepancy is that the highly focal and reproducible injury of the experimental setting differs from the random type of nerve injury in humans. It is also possible that animal models express pathophysiological abnormalities in sensory channels unrelated to pain. "Pain-like" behavior and withdrawal reflexes in animals may not necessarily be equivalent to spontaneous and stimulus-induced pain, respectively, in humans. While avoidance and protective behavior are often interpreted as related to pain, they may be induced by paresthesia or dysesthesia as well as by pain. Zeltser and Seltzer (1994) have attempted to distinguish between hyperesthesia and presumed allodynia in animal models, based on the expression of a complex nocifensive behavior related to allodynia. Also, interpretation of abnormal electrophysiological activity at various levels of the neuraxis is difficult in animal models of neuropathic pain. A relevant example of the problem of symptom interpretation in animals is the widely used chronic constriction injury model, a pain model proposed by Bennett and Xie (1988). The model may to some extent mimic clinical conditions such as median nerve entrapment in the carpal tunnel. However, the most common complaint in patients with median nerve entrapment is numbness with tingling paresthesia; only infrequently do they report neuropathic pain. A more cautious extrapolation from behavioral test outcomes in animal models to clinical conditions is warranted, and future studies using old and new animal "pain models" deserve a better interdisciplinary discussion between pain clinicians or clinical scientists and basic scientists on their clinical relevance. This effort may also reduce the number of less important animal studies.

In our experience, drugs such as mexiletine (Jett et al. 1997) and dextrorphan (Tal and Bennett 1993), effective on a group level in animal models of neuropathic pain, have a limited effect on spontaneous and stimulus-evoked pain in neuropathic pain patients. Even with the few drugs proven effective in animal studies and in patients with neuropathic pain, such as amitriptyline and gabapentin, we are only able to reduce pain in subgroups of patients. These discrepancies may be due to the animal models differing significantly from the clinical conditions. They may also, at least in part, be explained by the limitation of the treatment in humans due to side effects such as cognitive dysfunction and dizziness, which are poorly assessed in animal models.

SUMMARY AND CONCLUSIONS

Lesions of the peripheral or central nervous system may cause neuropathic pain in subgroups of patients. The diagnosis of peripheral or central neuropathic pain should be made only when the history and signs are indicative of neuropathy, in conjunction with a neuroanatomically correlated pain distribution and sensory abnormalities within the area of pain. Although it is mandatory to retain the traditional organ-based diagnostic work-up, future studies of neuropathic pain should aim at developing a mechanism-based classification of such conditions because multiple mechanisms may be involved. A detailed mechanism-based classification is currently not feasible, although it is possible to differentiate likely mechanisms based on signs of somatosensory dysfunction. The development of new treatment strategies based on a pain mechanism classification should be given priority, and clinical trials should monitor treatment effects not only on spontaneous pain but also on stimulus-evoked pain, such as allodynia. Various problems hamper the extrapolation of results from animal studies of neuropathic pain mechanisms and treatment interventions to the clinical situation. The major problem is the often questionable relevance of the experimental model to any given patient. Interdisciplinary discussions among pain clinicians or clinical scientists and basic scientists on matters related to this issue would enhance this area of research.

REFERENCES

Andersen G, Vestergaard K, Ingeman-Nielsen M, Jensen TS. Incidence of central post-stroke pain. *Pain* 1995; 61:187–193.

Arnér S, Meyerson BA. Lack of analgesic effect of opioids on neuropathic and idiopathic forms of pain. *Pain* 1988; 11–23.

Asbury AK. Pain in generalized neuropathies. In: Fields HL (Ed). *Pain Syndromes in Neurology*. London: Butterworths, 1990, pp 131–141.

Attal N, Brasseur L, Parker F, Chauvin M, Bouhassira D. Effects of gabapentin on the different components of peripheral and central neuropathic pain syndromes: a pilot study. *Eur Neurol* 1998; 40:191–200.

Bennett GJ, Ochoa JL. Thermographic observations on rats with experimental neuropathic pain. *Pain* 1991; 45:61–67.

Bennett GJ, Xie YK. A peripheral mononeuropathy in rat that produces disorders of pain sensation like those seen in man. *Pain* 1988; 33:87–107.

Boivie J. Central pain. In: Wall PD, Melzack R (Eds). *Textbook of Pain.* Edinburgh: Churchill Livingstone, 1999, pp 879–914.

Boivie J, Leijon G, Johansson I. Central post-stroke pain: a study of mechanisms through analyses of the sensory abnormalities. *Pain* 1989; 855–860.

Campbell JN, Raja SN, Meyer RA, Mackinnon SE. Myelinated afferents signal the hyperalgesia associated with nerve injury. *Pain* 1988; 32:89–94.

Canavero S, Bonicalzi V. The neurochemistry of central pain: evidence from clinical studies, hypothesis and therapeutic implications. *Pain* 1998; 74:109–114.

Cannon WB, Rosenbleuth A. *The Supersensitivity of Denervated Structures: A Law of Denervation.* New York: Macmillan, 1949.

Chapman V, Suzuki R, Chamarette HL, Rygh LJ, Dickenson AH. Effects of systemic carbamazepine and gabapentin on spinal neuronal responses in spinal nerve ligated rats. *Pain* 1998; 75:261–272.

Cook RJ, Sackett DL. The number needed to treat: a clinically useful measure of treatment effect (published erratum appears in *BMJ* 1995; 310:1056). *BMJ* 1995; 310:452–454.

Cook AJ, Woolf CJ, Wall PD, McMahon SB. Dynamic receptive field plasticity in rat spinal cord dorsal horn following C-primary afferent input. *Nature* 1987; 325:151–153.

Dejgard A, Petersen P, Kastrup J. Mexiletine for treatment of chronic painful diabetic neuropathy. *Lancet* 1988; 1:9–11.

Fleming WB, Westfall DP. Adaptive supersensitivity. In: Trendelenburg U, Weiner N (Eds). *Handbook of Experimental Pharmacology,* Vol. 90/I. New York: Springer 1988, pp 509–559.

Galer BS, Harle J, Rowbotham MC. Response to intravenous lidocaine infusion predicts subsequent response to oral mexiletine: a prospective study. *J Pain Symptom Manage* 1996; 12:161–167.

Hansson P. Possibilities and potential pitfalls of combined bedside and quantitative somatosensory analysis in pain patients. In: Boivie J, Hansson P, Lindblom U (Eds). *Touch, Temperature, and Pain in Health and Disease: Mechanisms and Assessments,* Progress in Pain Research and Management, Vol. 3. Seattle: IASP Press, 1994a, pp 113–132.

Hansson P. Neurogenic pain. *Pain: Clinical Updates* 1994b; II:1–4.

Hansson P, Kinnman E. Unmasking of neuropathic pain mechanisms in a clinical perspective. *Pain Reviews* 1996; 3:272–292.

Hunter JC, Gogas KR, Hedley LR, et al. The effect of novel anti-epileptic drugs in rat experimental models of acute and chronic pain. *Eur J Pharmacol* 1997; 324:153–160.

Jett MF, McGuirk J, Waligora D, Hunter JC. The effects of mexiletine, desipramine and fluoxetine in rat models involving central sensitization. *Pain* 1997; 69:161–169.

Kim SH, Chung JM. An experimental model for peripheral neuropathy produced by segmental spinal nerve ligation in the rat. *Pain* 1992; 50:355–363.

Koltzenburg M, Torebjork HE, Wahren LK. Nociceptor modulated central sensitization causes mechanical hyperalgesia in acute chemogenic and chronic neuropathic pain. *Brain* 1994; 117:579–591.

Kosek E, Ordeberg G. Lack of pressure pain modulation by heterotopic noxious conditioning stimulation in patients with painful osteoarthritis before, but not following, surgical pain relief. *Pain* 2000; 88:69–78.

Kosek E, Ekholm J, Hansson P. Sensory dysfunction in fibromyalgia patients with implications for pathogenic mechanisms. *Pain* 1996; 68:375–383.

Kouyanou K, Pither CE, Rabe-Hesketh S, Wessely S. A comparative study of iatrogenesis, medication abuse, and psychiatric morbidity in chronic pain patients with and without medically explained symptoms. *Pain* 1998; 76:417–426.

Kupers RC, Konings H, Adriaensen H, Gybels JM. Morphine differentially affects the sensory and affective pain ratings in neurogenic and idiopathic forms of pain. *Pain* 1991; 47:5–12.

Lacerenza M, Marchettini P, Formaglio F, et al. Extra-territorial mechanical hyperalgesia in patients with proven nerve damage involves adjacent undamaged nerves. *Abstracts: 8th World Congress on Pain.* Seattle: IASP Press, 1996, p 37.

Lavigne G, Zucconi M, Castronovo C, et al. Sleep arousal response to experimental thermal stimulation during sleep in human subjects free of pain and sleep problems. *Pain* 2000; 84:283–290.

Leijon G, Boivie J, Johansson I. Central post-stroke pain—neurological symptoms and pain characteristics. *Pain* 1989; 36:13–25.

Lindblom U. Assessment of abnormal evoked pain in neurological pain patients and its relation to spontaneous pain: a descriptive and conceptual model with some analytical results. In: Fields HL, Dubner R, Cervero F (Eds). *Advances in Pain Research and Therapy,* Vol. 9. New York: Raven Press, 1985, pp 409–423.

Marchettini P, Barbieri A. Commentary: the peripheral mechanisms of abnormal temporal summation. *Eur J Pain* 2000; 4:15–17.

Marchettini P, Formaglio F, Barbieri A, Tirloni L, Lacerenza M. Pain syndromes that may develop as a result of treatment interventions. In: Devor M, Rowbotham M, Wiesenfeld-Hallin Z (Eds). *Proceedings of the 9th World Congress on Pain,* Progress in Pain Research and Management, Vol. 16. Seattle: IASP Press, 2000, pp 675–688.

Marshall JC, Halligan PW, Fink GR, Wade DT, Frackowiak RS. The functional anatomy of a hysterical paralysis. *Cognition* 1997; 64:B1–8.

McQuay H, Carroll D, Jadad AR, Wiffen P, Moore A. Anticonvulsant drugs for management of pain: a systematic review. *BMJ* 1995; 311:1047–1052.

McQuay HJ, Tramer M, Nye BA, et al. A systematic review of antidepressants in neuropathic pain. *Pain* 1996; 68:217–227.

Merskey H, Bogduk N. *Classification of Chronic Pain: Descriptions of Chronic Pain Syndromes and Definitions of Pain Terms,* 2nd ed. Seattle: IASP Press, 1994, p 222.

Nurmikko T, Bowsher D. Somatosensory findings in postherpetic neuralgia. *J Neurol Neurosurg Psychiatry* 1990; 53:135–141.

Nurmikko T, Wells C, Bowsher D. Pain and allodynia in postherpetic neuralgia: role of somatic and sympathetic nervous systems. *Acta Neurol Scand* 1991; 84:146–152.

Ochoa JL. The human sensory unit and pain: new concepts, syndromes, and tests. *Muscle Nerve* 1993; 16:1009–1016.

Ochoa JL, Yarnitsky D. Mechanical hyperalgesias in neuropathic pain patients: dynamic and static subtypes. *Ann Neurol* 1993; 33:465–472.

Osterberg A, Boivie J, Holmgren H, Thuomas K-Å, Johansson I. The clinical characteristics and sensory abnormalities of patients with central pain caused by multiple sclerosis. In: Gebhart GF, Hammond DL, Jensen TS (Eds). *Proceedings of the 7th World Congress on Pain*, Progress in Pain Research and Management, Vol. 2. Seattle: IASP Press, 1994, pp 789–796.

Petersen KL, Fields HL, Brennum J, Sandroni P, Rowbotham MC. Capsaicin evoked pain and allodynia in post-herpetic neuralgia. *Pain* 2000; 88:125–133.

Roberts WJ. A hypothesis on the physiological basis for causalgia and related pains. *Pain* 1986; 24:297–311.

Ron MA. Somatisation in neurological practice. *J Neurol Neurosurg Psychiatry* 1994; 57:1161–1164.

Rowbotham MC, Fields HL. The relationship of pain, allodynia and thermal sensation in post-herpetic neuralgia. *Brain* 1996; 119:347–354

Rowbotham MC, Reisner-Keller LA, Fields HL. Both intravenous lidocaine and morphine reduce the pain of postherpetic neuralgia. *Neurology* 1991; 41:1024–1028.

Seltzer Z, Dubner R, Shir Y. A novel behavioral model of neuropathic pain disorders produced in rats by partial sciatic nerve injury. *Pain* 1990; 205–218.

Sindrup SH, Jensen TS. Efficacy of pharmacological treatments of neuropathic pain: an update and effect related to mechanism of drug action. *Pain* 1999; 83:389–400.

Sindrup SH, Gram LF, Brösen K, Eshöj O, Mogensen EF. The selective serotonin reuptake inhibitor paroxetine is effective in the treatment of diabetic neuropathy symptoms. *Pain* 1990; 42:135–144.

Sotgiu ML, Biella G. Spinal expansion of saphenous afferents after sciatic nerve constriction. *Neuroreport* 1995; 6:2305–2308.

Sunderland S. *Nerves and Nerve Injuries.* London: Churchill Livingstone, 1993.

Tal M, Bennett GJ. Dextrorphan relieves neuropathic heat-evoked hyperalgesia in the rat. *Neurosci Lett* 1993; 151:107–110.

Tal M, Bennett GJ. Extra-territorial pain in rats with a peripheral mononeuropathy: mechano-hyperalgesia and mechano-allodynia in the territory of an uninjured nerve. *Pain* 1994; 57:375–382.

Tiihonen J, Kuikka J, Viinamaki H, Lehtonen J, Partanen J. Altered cerebral blood flow during hysterical paresthesia. *Biol Psychiatry* 1995; 37:134–135.

Wallace PF, Fitzmorris CS. The S-H-A-F-T syndrome in the upper extremity. *J Hand Surg (Am)* 1978; 3:492–494.

Verdugo R, Ochoa JL. Quantitative somatosensory thermotest. *Brain* 1992; 115:893–913.

Woolf CJ, Decosterd I. Implications of recent advances in the understanding of pain pathophysiology for the assessment of pain in patients. *Pain* 1999; (Suppl 6):S141–147.

Woolf CJ, Mannion RJ. Neuropathic pain: aetiology, symptoms, mechanisms, and management. *Lancet* 1999; 353:1959–1964.

Woolf CJ, Shortland P, Coggeshall RE. Peripheral nerve injury triggers central sprouting of myelinated afferents. *Nature* 1992; 355:75–78.

Woolf CJ, Bennett GJ, Doherty M, et al. Towards a mechanism-based classification of pain? *Pain* 1998; 77:227–229.

Yezierski RP. Pain following spinal cord injury: the clinical problem and experimental studies. *Pain* 1996; 68:185–194.

Zeltser R, Seltser Z. A practical guide for the use of animal models of neuropathic pain. In: Boivie J, Hansson P, Lindblom U (Eds). *Touch, Temperature, and Pain in Health and Disease: Mechanisms and Assessments,* Progress in Pain Research and Management, Vol. 3. Seattle: IASP Press, 1994, pp 295–338.

Correspondence to: Per Hansson, MD, PhD, DDS, Neurogenic Pain Unit, Multidisciplinary Pain Center and Department of Rehabilitation Medicine, Karolinska Hospital/Institute, 17176 Stockholm, Sweden. Tel: 46-8-51775435; Fax: 46-8-51776641; email: per.hansson@kirurgi.ki.se.

Neuropathic Pain: Pathophysiology and Treatment,
Progress in Pain Research and Management, Vol. 21,
edited by Per T. Hansson, Howard L. Fields, Raymond G.
Hill, and Paolo Marchettini, IASP Press, Seattle, © 2001.

2

Sodium Channels as Therapeutic Targets in Neuropathic Pain

Joel A. Black,[a,b] Sulayman Dib-Hajj, [a,b] Theodore R. Cummins,[a,b] Kenji Okuse,[c] Mark Baker,[c] John N. Wood,[c] and Stephen G. Waxman [a,b]

[a]*Department of Neurology and PVA/EPVA Neuroscience Research Center, Yale University School of Medicine, New Haven, Connecticut, USA;* [b]*Rehabilitation Research Center, Veterans Affairs Hospital, West Haven, Connecticut, USA;* [c]*Department of Biology, University College London, London, United Kingdom*

Pain pathways begin with spinal sensory neurons of the dorsal root ganglia (DRG) and trigeminal neurons, which constitute the first relays in the nociceptive system. These primary sensory neurons send their axons peripherally to the body surface, muscles, and viscera, and centrally to enter the ascending pathways that carry information to the brain, and they encode sensory messages in the form of series of action potentials. Healthy DRG and trigeminal neurons are relatively quiescent, unless they are stimulated by sensory inputs; when stimulated they produce highly modulated series of action potentials that convey quantitative information about stimuli in the external world. Voltage-dependent sodium channels produce the inward trans-membrane current that depolarizes the cell membrane, and thus are critically important contributors to action potential electrogenesis. Spinal sensory and trigeminal neurons can become hyperexcitable after nerve injury and can give rise to spontaneous action potential activity or abnormal high-frequency activity that contributes to neuropathic pain (Ochoa and Torebjörk 1980; Wall and Devor 1981; Nordin et al. 1984; Zhang et al. 1997). Considerable attention has thus focused over the past 5 years on sodium channels as players in the pathophysiology of neuropathic pain. This chapter combines the perspectives of two laboratories that work on sodium channels and reviews the available data from our research groups, and from others, that link sodium channels and neuropathic pain.

It is now clear that at least nine distinct voltage-gated sodium channels are encoded by different genes, and that most of these are expressed within the nervous system. The different sodium channels share a common overall structure, but as a result of their different amino acid sequences they are functionally distinct (exhibiting different kinetics and voltage dependences) and pharmacologically distinguishable (with different sensitivities to tetro-dotoxin [TTX], for example). Most types of sodium channels are expressed in regionally and temporally specific patterns within the nervous system.

Molecular and electrophysiological methods have converged in indicat-ing that a complex ensemble of sodium channels is expressed in DRG neu-rons, with some types coexpressing two or more types of sodium channels. Interestingly, three sodium channels (Nav1.7, also termed PN1; Nav1.8, also termed SNS ["sensory-neuron-specific"] or PN3; and Nav1.9, also termed NaN or SNS-2) are preferentially expressed in DRG and trigeminal neurons. It has also become apparent that hyperexcitability of DRG neurons after ax-onal injury results, at least in part, from changes in the expression of the genes that encode sodium channels in these cells. These changes include the downregulation of transcription of several sodium channel genes and the upregulation of transcription of at least one previously silent sodium chan-nel gene.

SPINAL SENSORY NEURONS EXPRESS MULTIPLE SODIUM CHANNELS

It is fortunate for pain research that DRG neurons have been especially well studied in terms of sodium channel expression. Early patch-clamp stud-ies (see, e.g., Kostyuk et al. 1981) demonstrated that DRG neurons have multiple, distinct sodium currents that can be differentiated on the basis of different voltage dependences and kinetics. Pharmacological differences noted in these currents, including varying degrees of sensitivity to TTX, have been used to broadly classify sodium channels as TTX-sensitive or TTX-resistant. Patch-clamp studies have revealed different repertoires of sodium channels within different functional classes of DRG neurons. For example, cutaneous afferents and muscle afferents express physiologically distinct repertoires of sodium channels (Honmou et al. 1994). When studied by patch-clamp methods, some DRG neurons produce multiple distinct so-dium currents, supporting the idea that they coexpress several types of so-dium channels (Caffrey et al. 1992; Elliott and Elliott 1993; Cummins and Waxman 1997; Cummins et al. 1999; Dib-Hajj et al. 1999c).

Consistent with the idea that different channels produce the multiple sodium currents that are generated by DRG neurons, at least seven mRNAs encoding different sodium channels are detectable in these cells (Black et al. 1996; Cummins et al. 2000b; Baker and Wood 2001). Sodium channels Nav1.1 and Nav1.6 (which are also expressed at high levels by other neuronal cell types within the central nervous system) produce TTX-sensitive sodium currents and are expressed at high levels in large and medium-sized DRG neurons and at lower levels in small ones (Black et al. 1996). As noted above, DRG neurons express the mRNAs for three sodium channels that are not present at significant levels in other neuronal cell types, except for trigeminal neurons in the normal nervous system: (1) Nav1.7 or PN1 (Toledo-Aral et al. 1997) is present in virtually all DRG neurons (Black et al. 1996) and encodes a TTX-sensitive channel characterized by slow closed-state inactivation (Cummins et al. 1998). Studies using in vitro model systems suggest that Nav1.7/PN1 channels are preferentially localized near the terminals of DRG neurons (Toledo-Aral et al. 1997), where their slow closed-state inactivation may poise them to amplify sensory generator potentials (Cummins et al. 1998). (2) Nav1.8/SNS/PN3, first cloned by Akopian et al. (1996) and Sangameswaran et al. (1996), is expressed preferentially in small and medium-diameter DRG neurons, and produces a slowly inactivating sodium current that is relatively resistant to TTX (Akopian et al. 1996; Sangameswaran et al. 1996). Nav1.8/SNS channels contribute substantially to the inward current flow during the upstroke of the action potential in cells containing this channel (Renganathan et al. 2001). The gene for Nav1.8/SNS has been localized at chromosome 3p22–24 in humans, adjacent to the other TTX-resistant channels encoding the cardiac channel Nav1.5 and Nav1.9. (3) Nav1.9/NaN, first cloned by Dib-Hajj et al. (1998b) and then by Tate et al. (1998), who call it SNS-2, is expressed preferentially in small DRG neurons, especially in IB4-positive neurons that are responsive to glial-derived neurotrophic factor (GDNF) (Fjell et al. 1999b). The gene for Nav.1.9/NaN has been mapped to locus 3p21–24 on human chromosome 3 (Dib-Hajj et al. 1999a). On the basis of the presence of a serine at a critical position (355) within Nav1.9/NaN, Dib-Hajj et al. (1998b) predicted that this channel is a TTX-resistant sodium channel. Using SNS-knockout mice produced by Akopian et al. (1999), Cummins et al. (1999) demonstrated a persistent TTX-resistant sodium current with a large overlap between activation and steady-state inactivation, which is attributable to Nav1.9/NaN. Because it is nonactivating and is activated close to resting potential, Nav1.9/NaN contributes a depolarizing influence (which can be as large as 10–20 mV; Herzog et al. 2001) to resting potential in cells in which it is present (Cummins et al. 1999).

The presence of two TTX-resistant sodium channels, Nav1.8/SNS and Nav1.9/NaN, within small DRG neurons provides a molecular basis for the observation of TTX-resistant sodium currents in these cells (Kostyuk et al. 1981; Caffrey et al. 1992; Roy and Narahashi 1992; Elliott and Elliott 1993; Rush et al. 1998; Scholz et al. 1998). Consistent with a contribution of one or both of these channels to electrogenesis, electrophysiological results indicate that TTX-resistant sodium channels participate in the generation and/or conduction of action potentials within nociceptive sensory neurons and their axons (Jeftinija 1994; Quasthoff et al. 1995; Brock et al. 1998).

SODIUM CHANNELS AND NEURONAL HYPEREXCITABILITY

Even prior to the demonstration that specific sodium channel subtypes can contribute to hyperexcitability of injured sensory neurons, a number of studies implicated sodium channels in this phenomenon. A role of sodium channels in the hyperexcitability of injured neurons was suggested by early microelectrode studies (Eccles et al. 1958; Kuno and Llinas 1970) that demonstrated long-term alterations in the excitability of motor neurons following axonal transection and indicated that sodium channel density was increased over the cell body and the dendrites. Similar changes in excitability were subsequently observed following axonal injury in sensory neurons (Gurtu and Smith 1988). Immunocytochemical studies with panspecific sodium channel antibodies have demonstrated abnormal accumulations of sodium channels at the distal tips of injured axons (Devor et al. 1989; England et al. 1994, 1996a). Together with results suggesting that increased sodium conductance can lower threshold so that neurons produce inappropriate, repetitive action potential activity (Waxman and Brill 1978; Matzner and Devor 1994), and given reports of partial efficacy of sodium channel-blocking agents in animal models of experimental neuropathic pain and in humans with chronic neuropathic pain (see, e.g., Chabal et al. 1989; Devor et al. 1992; Omana-Zapata et al. 1997; Rizzo 1997), these observations indicate that sodium channels can contribute to sensory neuron hyperexcitability associated with chronic pain. However, the results cited above do not reveal the identities of the sodium channels involved in neuronal hyperexcitability after injury, and do not differentiate between increased membrane incorporation of pre-existing channels from a cytoplasmic pool, upregulation of transcription of an already-active sodium channel gene, or activation of a previously silent sodium channel gene. Answers to these questions have come from application of molecular techniques to injured DRG neurons.

ABNORMAL SODIUM CHANNEL GENE EXPRESSION
IN INJURED DRG NEURONS

In situ hybridization studies by Waxman et al. (1994) provided the first evidence for upregulation of expression of the Nav1.3/type III mRNA in DRG neurons following axonal transection within the sciatic nerve. Polymerase chain reaction (PCR) and in situ hybridization studies by Dib-Hajj et al. (1996) subsequently demonstrated that there is also a downregulation of Nav1.8/SNS (Dib-Hajj et al. 1996) and Nav1.9/NaN expression (Dib-Hajj et al. 1998b) in DRG neurons following axonal transection. Okuse et al. (1997) demonstrated downregulation of Nav1.8/SNS mRNA in several models of neuropathic pain, including streptozotocin-induced diabetes and the tight spinal ligature model. The downregulation of Nav1.8/SNS expression in DRG neurons can persist for 210 days after axonal transection (Dib-Hajj et al. 1996). Fig. 1 illustrates these changes in sodium channel gene expression after transection of the peripheral axons of DRG neurons.

Patch-clamp studies show that Nav1.8/SNS and Nav1.9/NaN encode TTX-resistant sodium channels with characteristic physiological signatures (Cummins et al. 1999), and a reduction in each of these TTX-resistant sodium currents would be expected in DRG neurons following axotomy. As seen in Fig. 2 there is, in fact, a significant loss of both TTX-resistant sodium currents in DRG neurons following axonal transection within the sciatic nerve (Sleeper et al. 2000); this downregulation persists for at least 60 days (Cummins and Waxman 1997), consistent with the long-lasting changes in sodium channel gene expression that have been described in these cells after peripheral axotomy.

Cummins and Waxman (1997) also showed that axonal injury is accompanied by a discrete switch in the properties of the TTX-sensitive sodium currents in DRG neurons (Fig. 3), the most notable change being the emergence of a current that recovers (reprimes) rapidly from inactivation (Cummins and Waxman 1997).

The time constant for recovery of TTX-sensitive sodium currents from inactivation is accelerated about fourfold following axotomy (Cummins and Waxman 1997). The proposal (Cummins and Waxman 1997) that newly formed Nav1.3/type III sodium channels are responsible, at least in part, for the rapidly repriming sodium current is supported by several observations: (1) rapidly repriming TTX-sensitive current and Nav1.3/type III sodium channel protein display parallel patterns of upregulation after transection of the peripherally directed (sciatic nerve) axons of DRG neurons but not following transection of the centrally directed (dorsal root) axons of these cells

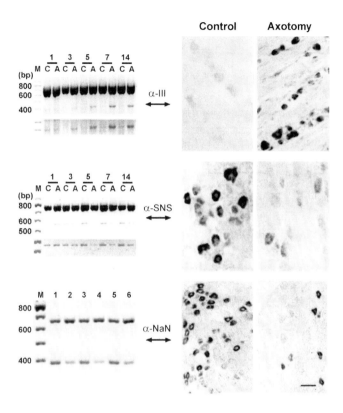

Fig. 1. Expression of sodium channel Nav1.3 mRNA (top) is upregulated, and Nav1.8/SNS mRNA (middle) and Nav1.9/NaN mRNA (bottom) are downregulated, in dorsal root ganglion (DRG) neurons following axonal transection within the sciatic nerve. In situ hybridizations in control DRG neurons and 5–7 days post-axotomy are shown on the right. Reverse transcription polymerase chain reaction (left side) shows products of co-amplification of Nav1.3 (top) and Nav1.8/SNS (middle) together with β-actin transcripts in control and axotomized DRG (days post-axotomy are indicated above gels), with computer-enhanced images of amplification products shown below gels. Co-amplification of Nav1.9/NaN (392 base pairs) and GAPDH (606 bp) (bottom) shows decreased expression of Nav1.9/NaN mRNA 7 days post-axotomy (lanes 2,4,6) compared to controls (lanes 1,3,5). Top and middle panels are modified with permission from Dib-Hajj et al. (1996); bottom panels are modified with permission from Dib-Hajj et al. (1998b).

(Black et al. 1999). (2) Nav1.3/type III sodium channels display rapid repriming when expressed in a mammalian expression system (HEK 293 cells) and in DRG neurons (Cummins et al. 2001). (3) Nav1.3/type III sodium channel protein accumulates close to the tips of injured axons within experimental neuromas (Black et al. 1999), a site where hyperexcitability has been demonstrated (Scadding 1981; Burchiel 1988; Matzner and Devor 1994).

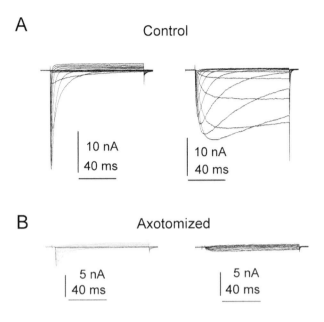

Fig. 2. In parallel with downregulation of Nav1.8/SNS and Nav1.9/NaN channels, TTX-resistant sodium currents in small DRG neurons are attenuated following axonal transection within the sciatic nerve. Left side (A,B): patch-clamp recordings from typical control (A) and axotomized (B, 6 days post-axotomy) DRG neurons showing the reduction in slowly inactivating TTX-resistant sodium current following axotomy within the sciatic nerve. Right side (A,B): Reduction of TTX-resistant persistent sodium currents in axotomized DRG neurons. Reprinted with permission from Cummins et al. (2000a).

In addition to the accumulation of Nav1.3/type III channels, immunocytochemistry with subtype-specific antibodies has demonstrated the accumulation of Nav1.8/SNS channels in these experimental neuromas (Novakovic et al. 1998). As noted below, several studies implicate Nav1.8/SNS channels as potential contributors to neuropathic pain.

There are several reasons why changes in sodium channel expression might predispose DRG neurons to fire spontaneously, or at inappropriately high frequencies, following injury to their axons. Matzner and Devor (1994) suggested that increased sodium conductance, due to increased numbers of channels per se, should lower the threshold for action potential generation. Rizzo et al. (1986) provided evidence suggesting that, as a result of overlap between steady-state activation and inactivation and the relatively weak voltage dependence of TTX-resistant sodium channels, coexpression of abnormal repertoires of channels might permit subthreshold potential oscillations, supported by TTX-resistant channels, to cross-activate TTX-sensitive

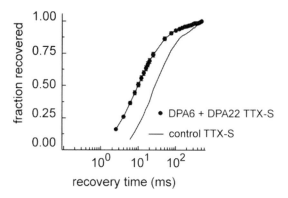

Fig. 3. A rapidly repriming TTX-sensitive sodium current emerges in DRG neurons following axonal transection. The graph shows recovery of the TTX-sensitive sodium current from inactivation (repriming) in DRG neurons following axonal transection within the sciatic nerve (6 and 22 days post-axotomy [DPA], results pooled). The leftward shift in the recovery curve, compared to controls, indicates that recovery from inactivation is accelerated post-axotomy. Modified with permission from Cummins and Waxman (1997).

sodium channels, thus producing abnormal action potential activity. Cummins and Waxman (1997) suggested that, because of the rapid repriming of the TTX-sensitive sodium current that is expressed in DRG neurons following axotomy, the refractory period would be reduced, a change that would sustain higher firing frequencies. Finally, if Nav1.9/NaN persistent sodium channels contribute to resting potential in DRG neurons or their axons as suggested by Cummins et al. (1999) and as demonstrated by Stys et al. (1993) in axons within the optic nerve, downregulation of Nav1.9/NaN following axotomy could lead to a hyperpolarizing shift in resting potential in DRG neurons. Because TTX-sensitive sodium current in DRG neurons has relatively hyperpolarized steady-state inactivation (Kostyuk et al. 1981; Cummins and Waxman 1997), this shift in membrane potential could increase the availability of TTX-sensitive sodium channels by relieving resting inactivation, thereby increasing cell excitability (Cummins and Waxman 1997).

Downregulation of transcription of Nav1.8/SNS and Nav1.9/NaN and upregulation of Nav1.3/type III sodium channels also occur in the chronic constriction injury (CCI) model of neuropathic pain (Dib-Hajj et al. 1999b). In parallel with these changes in gene transcription, TTX-resistant sodium currents are reduced and repriming of TTX-sensitive currents is accelerated in DRG neurons in this model of neuropathic pain. The changes in the CCI model are similar to those seen after sciatic nerve ligation, but are smaller, possibly because only some axons are transected (80% loss of myelinated fibers and 60–80% loss of unmyelinated fibers; Carlton et al. 1991), in the CCI model.

NEUROTROPHINS AND SODIUM CHANNEL EXPRESSION IN DRG NEURONS

Early in vitro experiments suggested that nerve growth factor (NGF) can affect sodium channel expression in DRG neurons (Aguayo and White 1992; Zur et al. 1995) and raised the possibility that peripheral nerve injury might affect sodium channel expression in DRG neurons by interrupting access to a peripheral supply of NGF. Studying an in vitro model of axotomy, Black et al. (1997) demonstrated that NGF, delivered to the cell bodies of small DRG neurons, downregulates expression of Nav1.3/type III sodium channel mRNA and upregulates expression of Nav1.8/SNS mRNA. Dib-Hajj et al. (1998a) subsequently showed that delivery of exogenous NGF to the axotomized nerve stump in vivo results in a partial rescue of Nav1.8/SNS mRNA levels and TTX-resistant sodium current in small DRG neurons. NGF also appears to be required for Nav1.8/SNS expression in uninjured DRG neurons of adult rats, suggesting that NGF participates in maintaining Nav1.8/SNS levels in the adult nervous system in vivo (Fjell et al. 1999a). Changes in Nav1.3/type III and Nav1.8/SNS expression in DRG neurons following nerve injury may thus, at least in part, reflect loss of access to peripheral pools of NGF.

In an effort to determine whether GDNF modulates TTX-resistant channel expression in DRG neurons, Fjell et al. (1999) exposed cultured DRG neurons to GDNF. They observed an increase in both Nav1.8/SNS and Nav1.9/NaN mRNA levels, together with an increase in total TTX-resistant sodium current after 7 days in vitro. In a subsequent study, Cummins et al. (2000a) used patch-clamp methods to isolate the currents attributable to Nav1.8/SNS and Nav1.9/NaN channels, and observed that exposure to GDNF can significantly increase both of these currents, with parallel increases in Nav1.8/SNS and Nav1.9/NaN mRNA and protein levels in axotomized DRG neurons in vitro. Cummins et al. (2001) also showed that intrathecal administration of GDNF increases the levels of both currents as well as the Nav1.8/SNS and Nav1.9/NaN channel protein levels.

Boucher et al. (2000) conducted several studies that showed that exposure of axotomized DRG neurons in vivo to GDNF prevents the abnormal expression of the Nav1.3/type III sodium channel, restores Nav1.8/SNS and Nav1.9/NaN transcript levels, reduces ectopic discharges within DRG neurons, and, importantly, prevents and reverses sensory abnormalities that develop in neuropathic pain models, without affecting pain-related behavior in normal animals. Consistent with a role of GDNF in modulating sodium channel expression in axotomized DRG neurons in vivo, Bennett et al. (1998) found that intrathecal GDNF ameliorates the reduction in conduction velocity that is seen in C fibers following axotomy. Taken together, these observations

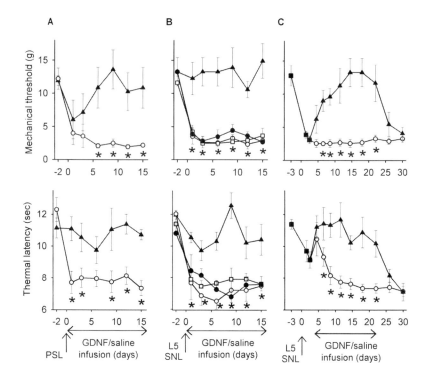

Fig. 4. Mechanical and thermal thresholds in treated (▲) versus untreated (○) animals following either partial sciatic ligation (PSL) or L5 spinal nerve ligation (SNL). GDNF prevents the development of hyperalgesia, and also reverses an established neuropathy. (A) PSL results in mechanical and thermal hyperalgesia in vehicle-treated animals. Concurrent infusion of GDNF over the 2-week testing period prevents the development of this neuropathy. (B) SNL establishes hyperalgesia that can be prevented by GDNF, but not by NGF (□) or NT-3 (●). (C) The delayed infusion of GDNF reverses manifestations of neuropathy induced by SNL. The cessation of GDNF infusion results in the re-emergence of hyperalgesia. Filled squares (■) denote pretreatment thresholds. Asterisks (✱) denote significant difference between vehicle- and GDNF-treated animals on each testing day; error bars denote standard error. Reprinted with permission from Boucher et al. (2000).

indicate that GDNF can play a significant modulatory role in axotomized DRG neurons, maintaining expression of at least some sodium channels at near-normal levels so as to reduce hyperexcitability and neuropathic pain.

SODIUM CHANNEL EXPRESSION IS ALTERED IN INFLAMMATORY PAIN

Although inflammatory pain may occur alone, neuropathic pain is often associated with tissue damage that contributes an inflammatory component to the development of chronic pain. Sodium channels are known to play a critical role in setting pain thresholds in inflammatory hyperalgesia. Inflammatory molecules such as prostaglandins and serotonin can modulate TTX-resistant sodium currents in DRG neurons (Gold et al. 1996), possibly via a cyclic adenosine monophosphate–protein kinase A cascade (England et al. 1996b). The rapid time course of these changes suggest that they involve the modulation of pre-existing channels, for example by phosphorylation. These events can be replicated in heterologous expression systems, where the Nav1.8 channel, in response to phosphorylation on serine residues, shows increased peak current amplitude of sodium channels (Fitzgerald et al. 1999). In addition, changes in sodium channel gene expression occur in inflammatory pain models. Tanaka et al. (1998) studied sodium channel expression in DRG neurons 4 days following injection of the inflammatory agent carrageenan into the hindpaw of rats. SNS mRNA expression was significantly increased in DRG neurons projecting to the inflamed limb, compared with DRG neurons from the contralateral side or from naive (uninjected) controls. Accompanying the upregulation of SNS mRNA expression was a significant increase in TTX-resistant sodium current amplitude in DRG neurons projecting to the inflamed limb, suggesting the insertion of an increased number of functional channels in the cell membrane (Tanaka et al. 1998).

Other studies have demonstrated increased levels of Nav1.9/NaN mRNA 7 days after injection of complete Freund's adjuvant (CFA; Tate et al. 1998), and have shown increased sodium channel immunoreactivity in DRG neurons for at least 2 months after injection of CFA into their peripheral projection field (Gould et al. 1998). Altered neurotrophin levels may contribute to these changes in sodium channel gene expression in inflammatory pain. Fibroblasts, Schwann cells, and keratinocytes normally produce NGF within peripheral target tissues; inflammation stimulates NGF production in immune cells, and increased NGF concentrations have been observed within tissues exposed to inflammatory agents (Weskamp and Otten 1978; Woolf et al. 1994).

CAN WE IDENTIFY SPECIFIC SODIUM CHANNELS AS MOLECULAR TARGETS IN NEUROPATHIC PAIN?

In view of the preferential expression of Nav1.7/PN1, Nav1.8/SNS, and Nav1.9/NaN in DRG and trigeminal neurons (particularly the expression of Nav1.8/SNS and Nav1.9/NaN in small/medium and small DRG neurons, respectively), and given the upregulation of the Nav1.3/type III sodium channel in axotomized DRG neurons and in DRG neurons in models of neuropathic pain, each of these channels might be considered as a candidate molecular target in the search for more effective drugs to treat neuropathic pain. An important step in evaluating these potential targets will be to determine whether neuropathic pain can be attenuated or abolished via the selective blockade or selective activation of one of these channels. Unfortunately, ligands that specifically block or activate these channel subtypes are not yet available. The application of molecular genetics has generated some information about the role of specific subtypes, however. The twin approaches of antisense downregulation and conventional knockout technology have been applied to several sodium channel genes.

Porreca et al. (1999) used antisense oligodeoxynucleotide knockdown of Nav1.8/SNS and Nav1.9/NaN in an attempt to produce selective, reversible block of channel protein expression. They reported that selective knockdown of Nav1.8/SNS prevented and reversed tactile allodynia and thermal hyperalgesia in a sciatic nerve ligation model of neuropathic pain. These results are surprising, given the TTX sensitivity of ectopic action potential propagation in neuropathic pain models. Although the antisense oligonucleotides were directed against the Nav1.8 channel, the possible effects on expression on other channels were not investigated, allowing the possibility that other channels, perhaps Nav1.3, may also have been affected. Nevertheless, the authors concluded that knockdown of Nav1.9/NaN protein has little or no effect on nerve-injury-induced behavioral responses. They interpreted their results as suggesting that relief from neuropathic pain might be achieved via selective inhibition or blockade of Nav1.8/SNS sodium channels. It should be noted in this context that Nav1.9/NaN mRNA levels fall in DRG neurons following axotomy (Dib-Hajj et al. 1998b) and that this decline is accompanied by a reduction in the persistent TTX-resistant current attributable to Nav1.9/NaN in these cells (Sleeper et al. 2000). Cummins and Waxman (1997) proposed that attenuation of the persistent current would lead to a hyperpolarizing shift in resting potential that could reduce resting inactivation of TTX-sensitive channels; this proposal implies that increases in Nav1.9/NaN, rather than knockdown, may reduce neuropathic pain.

Akopian et al. (1999) used transgenic techniques to generate a null-mutant mouse for the Nav1.8/SNS channel. The null mutants were viable, fertile, and apparently normal. However, they displayed lower threshold for electrical activation of C fibers and increased current densities of TTX-sensitive sodium channels, suggesting compensatory upregulation of TTX-sensitive currents in spinal sensory neurons. Behavioral studies (Akopian et al. 1999) demonstrated pronounced analgesia to noxious mechanical stimuli, small deficits in noxious thermoreception, and delayed development of inflammatory hyperalgesia. Interestingly, NGF-induced hyperalgesia is significantly attenuated in the Nav1.8 null mutants (Kerr et al. 2001). These results demonstrate that Nav1.8/SNS is involved in information transfer along nociceptive pathways, and suggest that blockade of Nav1.8/SNS expression and/or function may produce analgesia, particularly in inflammation, without side effects. In contrast, there were no deficits in the development of mechanical or thermal allodynia in the null mutants (Kerr et al. 2001), arguing against a role for Nav1.8 in the development of neuropathic pain.

SODIUM CHANNELS AND NEUROPATHIC PAIN

The question of whether a specific, single sodium channel generates neuropathic pain remains unanswered. No singular candidate has been identified to date, although Nav1.3 is an attractive possibility. It may be significant that not only are functional α-subunits dysregulated in neuropathic pain conditions, but accessory subunits are also affected. Beta subunits play a critical role in regulating channel expression and their subcellular localization. The upregulation of the newly discovered β_3 subunit in a chronic constriction model of neuropathic pain (Shah et al. 2000) may result in increased densities of sodium channel expression, leading to hyperexcitability.

Compelling evidence indicates that sodium channels participate substantially to the hyperexcitability of sensory neurons that contributes to neuropathic pain. The identification of three sodium channels (Nav1.7, Nav1.8, and Nav1.9) that are preferentially expressed within DRG and trigeminal neurons and the abnormal upregulation of a fourth channel (Nav1.3), which is expressed at only low levels in the normal nervous system, suggest that it may be possible to target hyperexcitable sensory neurons along the nociceptive pathway without producing significant side effects. Several converging lines of evidence implicate Nav1.8/SNS as a potentially attractive molecular target in this respect, whilst the Nav1.3 channel (also expressed within the human central nervous system) may also present an important target if it can be downregulated peripherally. The available evidence also suggests that Nav1.9/NaN exerts a significant effect on membrane potential, making it an interesting target.

To date, research on sodium channels as they relate to pain has concentrated on primary sensory neurons, i.e., DRG and trigeminal neurons. Waxman et al. (2000) have suggested that secondary sensory neurons along nociceptive pathways, located postsynaptic to primary sensory cells, may display dysregulation of sodium channel gene expression in chronic pain states. Dynamic changes in sodium channel expression within normal neurons as they pass between quiescent and bursting states (Tanaka et al. 1999) suggest that this hypothesis is not unreasonable. A single study has demonstrated that noxious versus innocuous input can be distinguished by sodium channel blockers within the dorsal horn (Blackburn-Munro and Fleetwood-Walker 1997), providing some support for the hypothesis that specific types of sodium channels within secondary or higher-order neurons can contribute to pain-related signaling. If this conjecture is correct, other therapeutic targets may appear on the horizon.

ACKNOWLEDGMENTS

Work in the authors' laboratories has been supported in part by grants from the National Multiple Sclerosis Society, and the Rehabilitation Research Service and Medical Research Service, Department of Veterans Affairs, and the Paralyzed Veterans of America/Eastern Paralyzed Veterans Association (S.G. Waxman); and from the Wellcome Trust and Medical Research Council (J.N. Wood). We are grateful to our coworkers, especially S. McMahon, for permission to summarize results from previously published papers. T.R. Cummins, S. Dib-Hajj, and S.G. Waxman are consultants to TransMolecular, Inc.

REFERENCES

Aguayo LG, White G. Effects of nerve growth factor on TTX- and capsaicin-sensitivity in adult rat sensory neurons. *Brain Res* 1992; 570:61–67.

Akopian AN, Sivilotti L, Wood JN. A tetrodotoxin-resistant voltage-gated sodium channel expressed by sensory neurons. *Nature* 1996; 379:257–262.

Akopian AN, Souslova V, England S, et al. The tetrodotoxin-resistant sodium channel SNS has a specialized function in pain pathways. *Nat Neurosci* 1999; 2:541–548.

Baker MD, Wood JN. Involvement of Na channels in pain pathways. *Trends Pharmacol Sci* 2001; 22:27–31.

Bennett DL, Michael GJ, Ramachandran N, et al. A distinct subgroup of small DRG cells express GDNF receptor components and GDNF is protective for these neurons after nerve injury. *J Neurosci* 1998; 18:3059–3072.

Black JA, Dib-Hajj S, McNabola K, et al. Spinal sensory neurons express multiple sodium channel α-subunit mRNAs. *Mol Brain Res* 1996; 43:117–132.

Black JA, Langworthy K, Hinson AW, Dib-Hajj SD, Waxman SG. NGF has opposing effects on Na+ channel III and SNS gene expression in spinal sensory neurons. *Neuroreport* 1997; 8:2331–2335.

Black JA, Fjell J, Dib-Hajj S, et al. Abnormal expression of SNS/PN3 sodium channel in cerebellar Purkinje cells following loss of myelin in the taiep rat. *Neuroreport* 1999a; 10:913–918.

Black JA, Cummins TR, Plumpton C, et al. Upregulation of a previously silent sodium channel in axotomized DRG neurons. *J Neurophysiol* 1999b; 82:2776–2785.

Black JA, Dib-Hajj S, Baker D, et al. Sensory neuron specific sodium channel SNS is abnormally expressed in the brains of mice with experimental allergic encephalomyelitis and humans with multiple sclerosis. *Proc Natl Acad Sci USA* 2000; 97:11598–11602.

Blackburn-Munro G, Fleetwood-Walker SM. The effects of Na$^+$ channel blockers on somatosensory processing by rat dorsal horn neurones. *Neuroreport* 1997; 8:1549–1554.

Boucher TJ, Okuse K, Bennett DLH, et al. Potent analgesic effects of GDNF on neuropathic pain states. *Science* 2000; 290:124–127.

Brock JA, McLachlan EM, Belmonte C. Tetrodotoxin-resistant impulses in single nociceptor nerve terminals in guinea-pig cornea. *J Physiol* 1998; 512:211–217.

Burchiel KJ. Carbamazepine inhibits spontaneous activity in experimental neuromas. *Exp Neurol* 1988; 102:249–253.

Caffrey JM, Eng DL, Black JA, Waxman SG, Kocsis JD. Three types of sodium channels in adult rat dorsal root ganglion neurons. *Brain Res* 1992; 592:283–297.

Carlton SM, Dougherty PM, Pover CM, Coggeshall RE. Neuroma formation and numbers of axons in a rat model of experimental peripheral neuropathy. *Neurosci Lett* 1991; 131:88–92.

Chabal C, Russell LC, Burchiel KJ. The effect of intravenous lidocaine, tocainide, and mexiletine on spontaneously active fibers originating in rat sciatic neuromas. *Pain* 1989; 38:333–338.

Cummins TR, Waxman SG. Downregulation of tetrodotoxin-resistant sodium currents and up-regulation of a rapidly repriming tetrodotoxin-sensitive sodium current in small spinal sensory neurons after nerve injury. *J Neurosci* 1997; 17:3503–3514.

Cummins TR, Howe JR, Waxman SG. Slow closed-state inactivation: a novel mechanism underlying ramp currents in cells expressing the hNE/PN1 sodium channel. *J Neurosci* 1998; 18:9607–9619.

Cummins TR, Dib-Hajj SD, Black JA, et al. A novel persistent tetrodotoxin-resistant sodium current in small primary sensory neurons. *J Neurosci* 1999; 19:RC43.

Cummins TR, Black JA, Dib-Hajj SD, Waxman SG. Glial-derived neurotrophic factor upregulates expression of functional SNS and NaN sodium channels and their currents in axotomized dorsal root ganglion neurons. *J Neurosci* 2000a; 20:8754–8761.

Cummins TR, Dib-Hajj SD, Black JA, Waxman SG. Sodium channels and the molecular pathophysiology of pain. *Prog Brain Res* 2000b; 129:3–19.

Cummins TR, Aglieco F, Renganathan M, et al. Na$_v$1.3 sodium channels: rapid repriming and slow closed-state inactivation display quantitative differences following expression in a mammalian cell line and in spinal sensory neurons. *J Neurosci* 2001, in press.

Devor M, Keller CH, Deerinck TJ, Ellisman MH. Na channel accumulation on axolemma of afferents in nerve end neuromas in *Apteronotus. Neurosci Lett* 1989;102:149–154.

Devor M, Wall PD, Catalan N. Systemic lidocaine silences ectopic neuroma and DRG discharge without blocking nerve conduction. *Pain* 1992; 48:261–268.

Dib-Hajj S, Black JA, Felts P, Waxman SG. Down-regulation of transcripts for Na channel alpha-SNS in spinal sensory neurons following axotomy. *Proc Natl Acad Sci USA* 1996; 93:14950–14954.

Dib-Hajj SD, Black JA, Cummins TR, et al. Rescue of alpha-SNS sodium channel expression in small dorsal root ganglion neurons after axotomy by nerve growth factor in vivo. *J Neurophysiol* 1998a; 9:2668–2678.

Dib-Hajj SD, Tyrrell L, Black JA, Waxman SG. NaN, a novel voltage-gated Na channel, is expressed preferentially in peripheral sensory neurons and down-regulated after axotomy. *Proc Natl Acad Sci USA* 1998b; 95:8963–8969.

Dib-Hajj SD, Tyrrell L, Escayg A, et al. Coding sequence, genomic organization, and conserved chromosomal localization of the mouse gene Scn11a encoding the sodium channel NaN. *Genomics* 1999a; 59:309–318.

Dib-Hajj SD, Fjell J, Cummins TR, et al. Plasticity of sodium channel expression in DRG neurons in the chronic constriction injury model of neuropathic pain. *Pain* 1999b; 83:591–600.

Dib-Hajj SD, Tyrell L, Cummins TR, et al. Two tetrodotoxin-resistant sodium channels in human dorsal root ganglion neurons. *FEBS Lett* 1999c; 462:117–120.

Eccles JC, Libet B, Young RR. The behavior of chromatolysed motoneurons studied by intracellular recording. *J Physiol Lond* 1958; 143:11–40.

Elliott AA, Elliott JR. Characterization of TTX-sensitive and TTX-resistant sodium currents in small cells from adult rat dorsal root ganglia. *J Physiol Lond* 1993; 463:39–56.

England JD, Gamboni F, Ferguson MA, Levinson SR. Sodium channels accumulate at the tips of injured axons. *Muscle Nerve* 1994; 17:593–598.

England JD, Happel LT, Kline DG, et al. Sodium channel accumulation in humans with painful neuromas. *Neurology* 1996a; 47:272–276.

England S, Bevan S, Docherty RJ. PGE2 modulates the tetrodotoxin-resistant sodium current in neonatal rat dorsal root ganglion neurones via the cyclic AMP-protein kinase A cascade. *J Physiol Lond* 1996b; 495:429–440.

Fitzgerald EM, Okuse K, Wood JN, Dolphin AC, Moss SJ. cAMP-dependent phosphorylation of the tetrodotoxin-resistant voltage-dependent sodium channel SNS. *J Physiol* 1999; 516(Pt 2):433–436.

Fjell J, Cummins TR, Fried K, Black JA, Waxman SG. In vivo NGF deprivation reduces SNS/ PN3 expression and TTX-R sodium currents in IB4-negative DRG neurons. *J Neurophysiol* 1999a; 81:803–810.

Fjell J, Cummins TR, Dib-Hajj SD, et al. Differential role of GDNF and NGF in the maintenance of two TTX-resistant sodium channels in adult DRG neurons. *Mol Brain Res* 1999b; 67:267–282.

Gold MS, Reichling DB, Shuster MJ, Levine JD. Hyperalgesic agents increase a tetrodotoxin-resistant Na⁺ current in nociceptors. *Proc Natl Acad Sci USA* 1996; 93:1108–1112.

Gould HJ III, England JD, Liu ZP, Levinson SR. Rapid sodium channel augmentation in response to inflammation induced by complete Freund's adjuvant. *Brain Res* 1998; 802:69–74.

Gurtu S, Smith PA. Electrophysiological characteristics of hamster dorsal root ganglion cells and their response to axotomy. *J Neurophysiol* 1988; 59:408–423.

Herzog RI, Cummins TR, Waxman SG. Persistent TTX-resistant Na⁺ current affects resting potential and response to depolarization in simulated spinal sensory neurons. *J Neurophysiol* 2001, in press.

Honmou O, Utzschneider DA, Rizzo MA, et al. Delayed depolarization and slow sodium currents in cutaneous afferents. *J Neurophysiol* 1994; 71:1627–1641.

Jeftinija S. The role of tetrodotoxin-resistant sodium channels of small primary afferent fibers. *Brain Res* 1994; 639:125–134.

Jung H-Y, Mickus T, Spruston N. Prolonged sodium channel inactivation contributes to dendritic action potential attenuation in hippocampal pyramidal neurons. *J Neurosci* 1997; 17:6639–6646.

Kerr B, Souslova V, McMahon S, Wood JN. A role for the TTX-resistant sodium channel Nav 1.8 in NGF-induced hyperalgesia, but not neuropathic pain. *Neuroreport* 2001, in press.

Kostyuk PG, Veselovsky NS, Tsyandryenko AY. Ionic currents in the somatic membrane of rat dorsal root ganglion neurons. I. Sodium currents. *Neuroscience* 1981; 6:2423–2430.

Kuno M, Llinas R. Enhancement of synaptic transmission by dendritic potentials in chromatolysed motoneurons of the cat. *J Physiol Lond* 1970; 210:807–821.

Matzner O, Devor M. Na conductance and the threshold for repetitive neuronal firing. *Brain Res* 1992; 597:92–98.

Matzner O, Devor M. Hyperexcitability at sites of nerve injury depends on voltage-sensitive Na⁺ channels. *J Neurophysiol* 1994; 72:349–359.

Nordin M, Nyström B, Wallin U, Hagbarth K-E. Ectopic sensory discharges and paresthesiae in patients with disorders of peripheral nerves, dorsal roots and dorsal columns. *Pain* 1984; 20:231–245.

Novakovic SD, Tzoumaka E, McGivern JG, et al. Distribution of the tetrodotoxin-resistant sodium channel PN3 in rat sensory neurons in normal and neuropathic conditions. *J Neurosci* 1998; 18:2174–2187.

Ochoa J, Torebjörk HE. Paresthesiae from ectopic impulse generation in human sensory nerves. *Brain* 1980; 103:835–854.

Okuse K, Chaplan SR, McMahon SB, et al. Regulation of expression of the sensory neuron-specific sodium channel SNS in inflammatory and neuropathic pain. *Mol Cell Neurosci* 1997; 10:196–207.

Omana-Zapata I, Khabbaz MA, Hunter JC, Bley KR. QX-314 inhibits ectopic nerve activity associated with neuropathic pain. *Brain Res* 1997; 771:228–237.

Porreca F, Lai J, DiBian, Wegert S, et al. A comparison of the potential role of the tetrodotoxin-insensitive sodium channels, PN3/SNS and NaN/SNS2, in rat models of chronic pain. *Proc Natl Acad Sci USA* 1999; 96:7640–7644.

Quasthoff S, Grosskreutz J, Schroder JM, Schneider U, Grafe P. Calcium potentials and tetrodotoxin-resistant sodium potentials in unmyelinated C fibres of biopsied human sural nerve. *Neuroscience* 1995; 69:955–965.

Renganathan M, Cummins TR, Waxman SG. The contribution of Nav1.8 sodium channels to action potential electrogenesis in DRG neurons. *J Neurophysiol* 2001, in press.

Rizzo MA. Successful treatment of painful traumatic mononeuropathy with carbamazepine: insights into a possible molecular pain mechanism. *J Neurol Sci* 1997; 152:103–106.

Rizzo MA, Kocsis JD, Waxman SG. Mechanisms of paresthesiae, dysesthesiae, and hyperesthesiae: role of Na+ channel heterogeneity. *Eur Neurol* 1986; 36:3–12.

Rizzo MA, Kocsis JD, Waxman SG. Selective loss of slow and enhancement of fast Na+ currents in cutaneous afferent dorsal root ganglion neurones following axotomy. *Neurobiol Dis* 1995; 2:87–96.

Roy ML, Narahashi T. Differential properties of tetrodotoxin-sensitive and tetrodotoxin-resistant sodium channels in rat dorsal root ganglion neurons. *J Neurosci* 1992; 12:2104–2111.

Rush AM, Brau ME, Elliott AA, Elliott JR. Electrophysiological properties of sodium current subtypes in small cells from adult rat dorsal root ganglia. *J Physiol* 1998; 511(Pt 3):771–789.

Sangameswaran L, Delgado SG, Fish LM, et al. Structure and function of a novel voltage-gated tetrodotoxin-resistant sodium channel specific to sensory neurons. *J Biol Chem* 1996; 271:5953–5956.

Scadding JW. Development of ongoing activity, mechanosensitivity, and adrenalin sensitivity in severed peripheral nerve axons. *Exper Neurol* 1981; 73:345–364.

Scholz A, Appel N, Vogel W. Two types of TTX-resistant and one TTX-sensitive Na+ channel in rat dorsal root ganglion neurons and their blockade by halothane. *Eur J Neurosci* 1998; 10:2547–2556.

Shah BS, Stevens EB, Gonzalez MI, et al. Beta 3, a novel auxiliary subunit for the voltage-gated sodium channel, is expressed preferentially in sensory neurons and is upregulated in the chronic constriction injury model of neuropathic pain. *Eur J Neurosci* 2000; 12:3985–3990.

Sleeper AA, Cummins TR, Hormuzdiar W, et al. Changes in expression of two tetrodotoxin-resistant sodium channels and their currents in dorsal root ganglion neurons following sciatic nerve injury, but not rhizotomy. *J Neurosci* 2000; 20:7279–7289.

Stys PK, Sontheimer H, Ransom BR, Waxman SG. Noninactivating, tetrodotoxin-sensitive Na+ conductance in rat optic nerve axons. *Proc Natl Acad Sci USA* 1993; 90(15):6976–6980.

Tanaka M, Cummins TR, Ishikawa K, et al. SNS Na channel expression increases in dorsal root ganglion neurons in the carrageenan inflammatory pain model. *Neuroreport* 1998; 9:967–972.

Tanaka M, Cummins TR, Ishikawa K, et al. Molecular and functional remodeling of electrogenic membrane of hypothalamic neurons in response to changes in their input. *Proc Natl Acad Sci USA* 1999; 96:1088–1093.

Tate S, Benn S, Hick C, et al. Two sodium channels contribute to the TTX-resistant sodium current in primary sensory neurons. *Nat Neurosci* 1998; 1:653–655.

Titmus MJ, Faber DS. Altered excitability of goldfish mauthner cell following axotomy. II. Localization and ionic basis. *J Neurophysiol* 1986; 55:1440–1454.

Toledo-Aral JJ, Moss BL, He Z-J, et al. Identification of PN1, a predominant voltage-dependent sodium channel expressed principally in peripheral neurons. *Proc Natl Acad Sci USA* 1997; 94:1527–1532.

Wall PD, Devor M. The effect of peripheral nerve injury on dorsal root potentials and on transmission of afferent signals into the spinal cord. *Brain Res* 1981; 209:95–111.

Waxman SG, Brill MH. Conduction through demyelinated plaques in multiple sclerosis: computer simulations of facilitation by short internodes. *J Neurol Neurosurg Psychiatry* 1978; 41:408–417.

Waxman SG, Kocsis JK, Black JA. Type III sodium channel mRNA is expressed in embryonic but not adult spinal sensory neurons, and is reexpressed following axotomy. *J Neurophysiol* 1994; 72:466–471.

Waxman SG, Cummins TR, Dib-Hajj SD, Black JA. Voltage-gated sodium channels and the molecular pathogenesis of pain. *J Rehab Res* 2000; 3:517–529.

Weskamp G, Otten U. An enzyme-linked immunoassay for nerve growth factor (NGF): a tool for studying regulatory mechanisms involved in NGF production in brain and in peripheral tissues. *J Neurochem* 1978; 48:1779–1786.

Woolf CJ, Safieh-Garabedian B, Ma Q-P, Crilly P, Winters J. Nerve growth factor contributes to the generation of inflammatory sensory hypersensitivity. *Neuroscience* 1994; 62:327–331.

Zhang J-M, Donnelly DF, Song X-J, LaMotte RH. Axotomy increases the excitability of dorsal root ganglion cells with unmyelinated axons. *J Neurophysiol* 1997; 78:2790–2794.

Zur KB, Oh Y, Waxman SG, Black JA. Different up-regulation of sodium channel alpha- and beta 1-subunit mRNAs in cultured embryonic DRG neurons following exposure to NGF. *Molec Brain Res* 1995; 30:97–103.

Correspondence to: Stephen G. Waxman, MD, PhD, Department of Neurology, LCI 707, Yale Medical School, 333 Cedar Street, New Haven, CT 06510, USA. Tel: 203-785-6351; Fax: 203-785-7826; email: stephen.waxman@yale.edu.

Neuropathic Pain: Pathophysiology and Treatment,
Progress in Pain Research and Management, Vol. 21,
edited by Per T. Hansson, Howard L. Fields, Raymond G.
Hill, and Paolo Marchettini, IASP Press, Seattle, © 2001.

3

Cytokines and Neuropathic Pain

Claudia Sommer

Department of Neurology, University of Würzburg,
Würzburg, Germany

Cytokines are a heterogeneous group of polypeptides that activate the immune system and mediate inflammatory responses, acting on a variety of tissues, including the peripheral and central nervous system (Hopkins and Rothwell 1995). Cytokines are extracellular signaling proteins that form part of a bidirectional circuit between the immune system and the nervous system (Bianchi et al. 1998). Cytokines act at hormonal concentrations through high-affinity receptors and produce endocrine, paracrine, and autocrine effects. In contrast to circulating endocrine hormones, they exert their effects on nearby cells over short extracellular distances at low concentrations, and thus serum levels may not reliably reflect local activation (Kelley 1990). Because of their broad range of action, cytokines are said to be *pleiotropic.* Cytokine activation or dysregulation is implied in various disease states including sepsis, rheumatoid arthritis, Crohn's disease, multiple sclerosis, and skin diseases. Some cytokines are labeled *pro-inflammatory* and others *anti-inflammatory,* depending on their effects on immune cells.

Interest in the modulation of pain by cytokines arose through observations on the "illness response," the organism's response to infection, which is associated with fever, fatigue, loss of appetite, and hyperalgesia (Watkins et al. 1995a). In this context hyperalgesia is regarded as part of the larger set of cytokine-mediated adaptive changes that occur during illness or injury. These adaptive changes are proposed to promote recuperation in part by decreasing energy use. The pathway from the peripheral cytokines to the brain may involve vagal afferents terminating in the nucleus tractus solitarius and circumventricular sites that lack a blood-brain barrier (Watkins et al. 1994, 1995).

This chapter reviews the distribution and regulation of interleukins IL-1, IL-6, and IL-10 and tumor necrosis factor α in the intact nervous system and in the lesioned peripheral nervous system. Influences of cytokines upon the central nervous system (CNS) are well established, but the vast literature on cytokines in lesions and diseases of the CNS is beyond the scope of this chapter. To facilitate understanding of the role of cytokines in neuropathic pain, I will summarize data on cytokines and non-neuropathic pain. Finally, I will discuss possible mechanisms of the algesic and analgesic actions of cytokines in peripheral nerve disease.

CYTOKINES IN THE INTACT NERVOUS SYSTEM

Cytokines were initially described as products of peripheral immune cells, but cells in the brain also produce cytokines. However, the strong stimulus-dependent dissociation between transcription and translation of certain cytokines often results in discrepant results between studies measuring mRNA and those measuring protein (Roux-Lombard 1998).

Interleukin-1 (IL-1) occurs as two products of different genes, IL-1α and IL-1β, which act on the same receptors, IL-1RI and IL-1RII. IL-RI is considered the active receptor, while IL-1RII lacks a transduction molecule and is a functional antagonist. IL-1 has another naturally occurring antagonist, the IL-1 receptor antagonist (IL-1Ra) (for review see Dinarello 1991; Martin and Falk 1997). IL-1β mRNA has been detected in the normal brain of mice and rats as well as humans, although not all investigators could replicate this finding (for review see Vitkovic et al. 2000). After lipopolysaccharide injection, IL-1 was found in microglia of the thalamus, the dorsal hypothalamus, and the parietal and frontal cortex, as well as in monocytes in the circumventricular organs and the pituitary gland (Eriksson et al. 2000). IL-1 follows a diurnal rhythm (Taishi et al. 1997). IL-1 immunoreactivity is also detectable in several regions of the normal brain, and has been found in brain neurons (Breder et al. 1988; Bandtlow et al. 1990; Lechan et al. 1990; Molenaar et al. 1993).

Interleukin-6 (IL-6) is a member of the IL-6 cytokine family, which also includes leukemia inhibitory factor (LIF) and ciliary neurotrophic factor (CNTF). IL-6 requires IL-6 receptor-α (IL-6R) and the gp130 subunit to exert its action. IL-6 is expressed at low levels in astrocytes and possibly in neurons of the normal brain; it is upregulated in disease (Van Wagoner and Benveniste 1999; Gao et al. 2000). IL-6 protein exists in the cortex of normal mice (Tha et al. 2000), and mRNA of IL-6 and its receptor are present in rat midbrain and hypothalamus (Miyahara et al. 2000).

Tumor necrosis factor alpha (TNF or TNFα) is produced by a wide variety of cells. The structurally related peptide lymphotoxin (LTα, formerly

TNFβ) is primarily expressed by lymphocytes and has not received major attention in the context of pain. Both the transmembrane and the secreted form of TNF are biologically active (Aggarwal and Natarajan 1996). Several other structurally related proteins belong to the "TNF superfamily." There are two TNF receptors: TNF receptor 1 (TNFR1, also called p55 or p60), and TNF receptor 2 (TNFR2, or p75, p80) that belong to the TNF receptor superfamily, which also includes the receptor for p75 nerve growth factor (NGF) (Aggarwal and Natarajan 1996). TNF is regulated at various levels; the second messenger pathways are reasonably well known (Darnay and Aggarwal 1999). TNF mRNA has been detected in the normal mouse, rat, and human CNS (Vitkovic et al. 2000).

TNF has been localized to the hypothalamus, hippocampus, cortex, cerebellum, and brainstem, although data are conflicting (Gatti and Bartfai 1993; Bredow et al. 1997). In the CNS of normal mice, TNF was found using immunohistochemistry and Western blot analysis in neurons of the hypothalamus, in the bed nucleus of the stria terminalis, in the caudal raphe nuclei, and on the ventral pontine and medullary surface (Breder et al. 1993; Ignatowski et al. 1997). A bioassay detected a diurnal variation of brain TNF with about 10-fold greater levels at light onset than at night-time in the hypothalamus and hippocampus (Floyd and Krueger 1997). As with IL-1, not all researchers agree that TNF is constitutively present in normal brain (Vitkovic et al. 2000).

IL-10 was originally described as *cytokine synthesis inhibitory factor* because it inhibits production of cytokines by activated T cells and macrophages. It is synthesized in neuroendocrine and neural tissues (Smith et al. 1999).

CYTOKINES IN PERIPHERAL NERVE INJURY

Studies on cytokines in the nervous system after peripheral nerve injury are summarized in Table I. Injury to an axon upregulates production of a series of inflammatory mediators, including cytokines, in the peripheral nerve (Stoll and Müller 1999). IL-1α is synthesized in the mouse sciatic nerve after axotomy (Rotshenker et al. 1992). Plasma levels of IL-1 and TNF rise on days 1–2 and days 10–14 after a unilateral crush injury of the rat sciatic nerve (Wells et al. 1992). In a model of nerve transection and regeneration, concentrations of IL-1β, IL-6, and TNF mRNA peaked on day 2 after transection, the earliest time point studied (Bizette et al. 1996). In nerve transection without regeneration, IL-6 mRNA peaked 12 hours after transection, with a greater increase in the proximal than in the distal stump (Bourde et al. 1996).

Table I

Cytokines in the nervous system after peripheral nerve injury

Cytokine(s)	Location/Cell Type	Type of Nerve Injury	Method(s)	Reference
IL-1α	mouse sciatic nerve	↑, axotomy	bioassay	Rotshenker et al. 1992
IL-1β	rat sciatic nerve	↑, crush	RT-PCR	Gillen et al. 1998
IL-1β	rat and mouse sciatic nerve	↑, CCI	IHC	George et al. 2000; Sommer and Schäfers 1998
IL-1β	rat L4 and L5 DRG	↑, sciatic nerve transection	RT-PCR	Murphy et al. 1995
IL-1β	rat sciatic nerve	↑, transection and regeneration	RT-PCR	Bizette et al. 1996
IL-1β	lumbar spinal cord	↑, SCN, CCI	IHC	DeLeo et al. 1997
IL-1β	rat sciatic nerve	↑, EAN	ISH	Zhu et al. 1997
IL-6	rat sciatic nerve	↑, crush	RT-PCR	Bolin et al. 1995
IL-6	rat sciatic nerve	↑, transection	RT-PCR	Bourde et al. 1996
IL-6	rat sciatic nerve	↑, EAN	ISH	Zhu et al. 1997
IL-6	spinal cord	↑, SCN, SNL	ISH	Arruda et al. 1998
IL-6	rat L4 and L5 DRG	↑, sciatic nerve transection	RT-PCR, ISH, bioassay	Murphy et al. 1995
IL-6	rat sciatic nerve	↑, transection and regeneration	RT-PCR	Bizette et al. 1996
IL-10	rat sciatic nerve, Schwann cells	↓, transection	ISH	Jander et al. 1996
IL-10	rat sciatic nerve	↑, crush	RT-PCR	Gillen et al. 1998
IL-10	rat sciatic nerve	↑, transection	RT-PCR	Taskinen et al. 2000
IL-10	rat sciatic nerve, Schwann cells and macrophages	↓, CCI	IHC, ELISA	George et al. 2000; A. George et al., unpublished manuscript

IL-10	rat L5 DRG	↑, crush, CCI	IHC	George and Sommer 2000; A. George and C. Sommer, unpublished manuscript
TNF	rat sciatic nerve macrophages	↑, axotomy	ISH	Griffin et al. 1993
TNF	rat sciatic nerve, macrophages	↑, EAN	IHC	Stoll et al. 1993
TNF	rat L4 and L5 DRG	↑, sciatic nerve transection	RT-PCR	Murphy et al. 1995
TNF	mouse sciatic nerve	↑, crush	RT-PCR	La Fleur et al. 1996
TNF	rat sciatic nerve	↑, transection and regeneration	RT-PCR	Bizette et al. 1996
TNF	rat sciatic nerve	↑, EAN	ISH	Zhu et al. 1997
TNF	lumbar spinal cord	↑, SCN, CCI	IHC	DeLeo et al. 1997
TNF	rat sciatic nerve Schwann cells and endothelial cells	↑, CCI	IHC, ISH	Wagner and Myers 1996
TNF	rat sciatic nerve Schwann cells, fibroblasts	↑, CCI	ELISA, IHC	George et al. 1999
TNF	rat sciatic nerve	↑, transection	RT-PCR	Taskinen et al. 2000
TNF	rat sciatic nerve	↑, CCI	Western blot	Shubayev and Myers 2000
TNF	rat hippocampus, LC, spinal cord DH	↑, CCI	bioassay	Covey et al. 2000; Ignatowski et al. 1999

↑: cytokine upregulated; ↓: cytokine downregulated.

Abbreviations: Animal models and cell type: CCI = chronic constrictive injury of the sciatic nerve; DH = dorsal horn; DRG = dorsal root ganglion; EAN = experimental autoimmune neuritis; LC = locus ceruleus; SCN = sciatic nerve cryoneurolysis; SNL = spinal nerve ligation. Methods: ELISA = enzyme-linked immunospecific assay; IHC = immunohistochemistry; ISH: in situ hybridization; RT-PCR = reverse transcription polymerase chain reaction.

After a crush injury, IL-6 mRNA peaked at 3 and 6 hours, increasing more in the distal than in the proximal portion of the nerve (Bolin et al. 1995). TNF mRNA increased on days 1 and 4 after a crush injury (La Fleur et al. 1996). IL-1β and IL-10 mRNA were upregulated in the distal stump after nerve crush on day 1 (the first time point investigated) and slowly declined until day 14. In experimental autoimmune neuritis (EAN), IL-1β and IL-10 peaked at the onset of clinical disease (Gillen et al. 1998). Taskinen et al. (2000) found three peaks of TNF mRNA after sciatic nerve transection, at 14 hours, 5 days, and 2 weeks after the lesion, and noted a continuous upregulation of IL-10 mRNA during this period.

Cytokines in peripheral nerve tissue have been mostly localized to Schwann cells or macrophages, and occasionally to fibroblasts. Rat Schwann cells in culture produce IL-1 and release it into the microenvironment after appropriate stimulation (Bergsteinsdottir et al. 1991). TNF is constitutively expressed in the sciatic nerve and increases in macrophages after injury, as demonstrated by in situ hybridization (Griffin et al. 1993). In Wallerian degeneration, only prephagocytotic macrophages had TNF immunoreactivity, whereas TNF was consistently seen in macrophages in experimental autoimmune neuritis (EAN) (Stoll et al. 1993). After nerve crush, TNF mRNA was localized to infiltrating macrophages and Schwann cells (La Fleur et al. 1996). In Wallerian degeneration only Schwann cells expressed IL-10, but in EAN macrophages also did so (Jander et al. 1996).

In a model of painful nerve injury, chronic constrictive injury (CCI) to the sciatic nerve (Bennett and Xie 1988), TNF was expressed in Schwann cells from injured and non-injured nerves and in endothelial cells on day 7 (Wagner and Myers 1996b). TNF protein, as determined by enzyme-linked immunospecific assay (ELISA), peaked 12 hours after CCI (George et al. 1999) (Fig. 1). Mice with delayed Wallerian degeneration (C57BL/6Wld) had a delayed increase in endoneurial TNF (Sommer and Schäfers 1998). Using double-staining immunofluorescence, we found TNF in Schwann cells and fibroblasts. TNF was rare in endoneurial macrophages after CCI, whereas epineurial macrophages were more often TNF positive. Shubayev and Myers (2000) found two peaks in TNF protein after CCI, at 6 hours and at 5 days after injury, and proposed an interaction with metalloproteinases. IL-10 protein was downregulated immediately after CCI in the peripheral nerve and slowly recovered during the following weeks (George et al. 2000). This postoperative reduction of IL-10 could be attenuated by administration of the TNF-synthesis inhibitor thalidomide.

In dorsal root ganglion (DRG) neurons from axotomized sciatic nerves, IL-6 mRNA increased after 2 and 4 days, being localized within large and medium-sized neurons. IL-1 and TNF mRNA was also expressed in the DRG

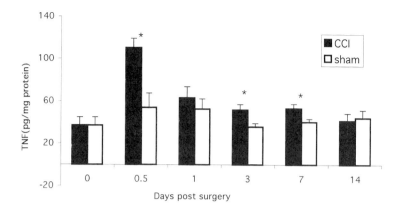

Fig. 1. Levels of endogenous tumor necrosis factor (TNF) in rat sciatic nerve homogenates as determined by ELISA of controls (day 0), after ipsilateral constrictive injury (CCI, black bars), and in sham-operated nerves (open bars), on days 0.5, 1, 3, 7, and 14. $N = 12$ animals per time point. Note the rapid increase at 12 hours after surgery. Asterisks (*) denote $P < 0.05$. Data are from George et al. (1999).

in this model, although the cellular sources of these cytokines could not be defined (Murphy et al. 1995a). Endogenous IL-6 contributes to the survival of axotomized neurons, and the upregulation of IL-6 in the DRG depends on axonal transport (Murphy et al. 1999). We found that TNF is expressed in small to medium-sized DRG cells after nerve injury (Fig. 2a). IL-10 was present in some DRG cells after injury, but we rarely found it in normal tissue (Fig. 2b).

Expression of pro-inflammatory cytokines changes in other parts of the CNS after nerve injury. Increases in lumbar spinal IL-1β-, TNF-, and TGFβ-like immunoreactivity were found in both sciatic cryoneurolysis (SCN) and CCI models (DeLeo et al. 1997). IL-6 mRNA in neurons was significantly elevated at 3 and 7 days after SCN and 7 days after a spinal nerve ligation (SNL) in both dorsal and ventral horns (Arruda et al. 1998). A bioassay showed increased TNF in the rat hippocampus, locus ceruleus, and spinal cord dorsal horn after CCI (Ignatowski et al. 1999; Covey et al. 2000).

Cytokine expression increases in human neuropathies such as chronic inflammatory demyelinating polyneuropathy (Mathey et al. 1999) and Guillain-Barré syndrome (Putzu et al. 2000). In nerve biopsies of patients with various peripheral disorders, TNF was mainly associated with phagocytosing macrophages in acute axonal injury, most frequently in patients with vasculitis (Oka et al. 1998). We found increased cytokine content, particularly of IL-6, in sural nerve biopsies from patients with acute painful vasculitic neuropathies (Fig. 3).

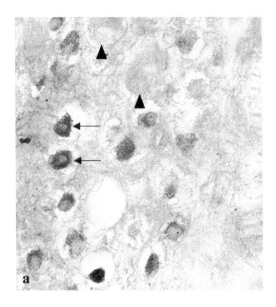

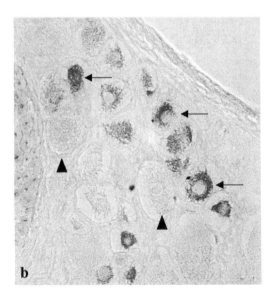

Fig. 2. Cryosection of L5 dorsal root ganglion (DRG) from a mouse 6 hours after ipsilateral constrictive injury (CCI) of the sciatic nerve, immunostained for (a) TNF (polyclonal antibody from Serotec) and (b) IL-10 (monoclonal antibody from Pharmingen). Specificity of immunostaining was verified by preabsorption of the respective antigens. Note cytokine immunoreactivity in small DRG cells (arrows), but not in large DRG cells (arrows). Bar = 20 μm. From C. Sommer and A. George (unpublished manuscript).

Although cytokine receptors are thought to exist on all cell types (Aggerwal and Natarajan 1996), evidence of their presence on neurons is scarce. For example, although mRNA for IL-1 receptors has been demonstrated in the brain, no double-labeling studies have been done for neurons. Functional studies, however, strongly suggest the presence of IL-1 receptors on neurons (Vitkovic et al. 2000). TNF receptors have been found in cultured oligodendrocytes and on neurons in some regions of the brain (Tchelingerian et al. 1996). We found TNF-receptor immunoreactivity on sciatic nerve Schwann cells (as previously shown by Wagner et al. 1998b) and on freshly dissociated DRG cells (Sommer 2000; C. Sommer, unpublished manuscript). After CCI, ELISA showed a rapid increase in TNFR2 in the mouse sciatic nerve (George and Sommer 1999).

CYTOKINES AND PAIN

MODELS USING CYTOKINE INJECTION

In animal models, pro-inflammatory cytokines influence pain. Evidence for pain modulation by cytokines in non-neuropathic models will be presented briefly to clarify the role of cytokines in neuropathic pain.

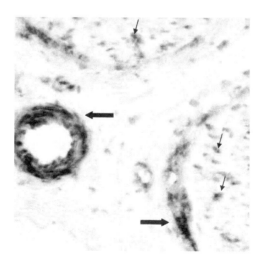

Fig. 3. Cryosection of a human sural nerve biopsy in a case of acute painful vasculitic neuropathy, immunostained for IL-6 (monoclonal antibody from R&D). Note dense IL-6 staining around an epineurial vessel and in the perineurium (large arrows), and also in endoneurial cells (small arrows). From C. Sommer and T. Lindenlaub (unpublished manuscript).

IL-1 is by far the most extensively studied cytokine in the context of pain and hyperalgesia. Applied by intraplantar (i.pl.) injection in rats, IL-1β reduced mechanical nociceptive thresholds (Ferreira et al. 1988). This effect was blocked by a local cyclooxygenase inhibitor and thus was judged to be prostaglandin dependent. Further studies have confirmed that IL-1 induces mechanical hyperalgesia, and possibly thermal hyperalgesia (Schweizer et al. 1988; Follenfant et al. 1989; Perkins and Kelly 1994; Poole et al. 1995). Perkins and colleagues (1995) found IL-1 hyperalgesia to be dependent on bradykinin B1 receptors. In the hands of Fukuoka et al. (1994), intraplantar IL-1β (100 pg–1 μg) increased the number of discharges in response to thermal and mechanical stimuli and induced spontaneous activity in afferent fibers within 1 minute. The authors concluded that IL-1β has a direct action on nerve endings.

IL-1β given intraperitoneally (i.p., 10 μg/kg) reduced tail-flick latency to noxious heat between 10 and 55 minutes after injection (Maier et al. 1993; Watkins et al. 1994b). IL-1Ra blocked lipopolysaccharide- and lithium-induced hyperalgesia (Maier et al. 1993). The action of i.p. IL-1 may be partially mediated by vagal afferents (Watkins et al. 1994).

Large doses of IL-1α administered into the cerebral ventricles (i.c.v.) had analgesic effects in the writhing test in mice (48 ng/kg; Nakamura et al. 1988) and in the hot-plate test in rats (2.5–15 ng/kg; Bianchi et al. 1992b). This analgesic action was not naloxone sensitive and was not mediated by prostaglandins (Bianchi et al. 1992). In contrast, corticotropin-releasing hormone and the noradrenergic system seemed to be involved in IL-1 mediated analgesia (Bianchi and Panerai 1995). A lower dose of 10 pg to 1 ng/kg of IL-1β reduced paw-licking latency in the hot-plate test, indicating hyperalgesia (Oka et al. 1993). This dose also enhanced the response of wide-dynamic-range (WDR) neurons in the trigeminal nucleus caudalis to noxious pinch (Oka et al. 1994). Injection of IL-1β at doses of 40 and 400 pg/kg i.c.v. caused mechanical hyperalgesia, whereas higher doses of 4 and 40 ng/kg induced analgesia (Yabuuchi et al. 1996). These findings indicate a biphasic effect of IL-1β on nociceptive thresholds, with lower doses inducing hyperalgesia and higher doses, analgesia. IL-1β injected into the preoptic area of the hypothalamus induced hyperalgesia in the hot-plate test, the dose being five times lower than that needed in i.c.v. application (Oka et al. 1995b). Injection into the ventromedial hypothalamus produced analgesia in the same test (Oka et al. 1995b). Hori et al. (1998) suggest that at lower doses IL-1β induces hyperalgesia through prostaglandin EP3 receptors in the preoptic area and that at higher doses it produces analgesia through EP1 receptors in the ventromedial hypothalamus. Watkins et al. (1994b) found that IL-1β induces pain when delivered i.c.v. (0.5–50 ng) and i.p. (10 μg/kg), but not intrathecally (i.t.).

IL-6 had a hyperalgesic effect in the hot-plate test when given i.c.v. (6 pg–300 ng, (Oka et al. 1995a). IL-8 given i.pl. produced mechanical hyperalgesia, which could be blocked by a β-blocker and by guanethidine (Cunha et al. 1991).

When given in i.pl. doses of 0.0025–2.5 pg/100 μL, TNF produced dose-dependent mechanical hyperalgesia both ipsi- and contralaterally between 1 and 6 hours after injection (Cunha et al. 1992). TNF given i.pl. at a dose of 100 U had an ipsilateral hyperalgesic effect, maximal at 1 and 6 hours (Perkins et al. 1995). TNF applied topically at low concentrations (0.001–0.01 ng/mL) along a restricted portion of the sciatic nerve elicited a dose-dependent, rapid-onset (1–3-minute) increase in discharge in C fibers and to a lesser extent in Aδ fibers; higher concentrations led to reduced firing rates (Sorkin et al. 1997). Mechanical thresholds were unchanged by this method of application. Subcutaneous (s.c.) injection within the distribution of the sural nerve (50 pg) led to ectopic discharge and a decrease in mechanical thresholds. TNF injected s.c. sensitized C nociceptors in rats. The optimal dose (5 ng) lowered thresholds in two-thirds of the single fibers tested. Sensitization occurred within 30 minutes and could last for over 2 hours. Injected TNF had no effect on Aβ mechanoreceptive fibers. In addition, TNF evoked ongoing activity in 14% of C nociceptors and increased vascular permeability in glabrous skin (Junger and Sorkin 2000). Epineurial administration of TNF led to mechanical allodynia to von Frey hairs at doses of 0.9 and 7.7 ng, but not at doses of 90 ng, with little effect on thermal thresholds (Sorkin and Doom 2000).

Intraperitoneal injection of TNF induced thermal hyperalgesia that could be blocked by IL-1Ra and by subdiaphragmatic vagotomy, indicating that in this paradigm TNF hyperalgesia is mediated by release of endogenous IL-1β acting through vagal afferents (Watkins et al. 1995a). Injections of TNF at doses of 10 pg, 100 pg, and 1 ng i.c.v. reduced paw-withdrawal latency in the hot-plate test, with a maximal response at a dose of 10 pg, peaking 60 minutes after injection (Oka et al. 1996). When administered i.c.v. by a continuous osmotic pump at doses of 1000 ng/24 hours, TNF induced thermal hyperalgesia in rats in a 58° hot-plate test, while doses of 30 ng/24 hours were ineffective (Ignatowski et al. 1999).

IL-10 pretreatment reduced the hyperalgesic responses to i.pl. carrageenan and IL-1β, IL-6, and TNF (Poole et al. 1995). Intraperitoneal injection of IL-10 downregulated local levels of IL-1β, TNF, and NGF after endotoxin injection into the hindpaw and reduced thermal and mechanical hyperalgesia (Kanaan et al. 1998).

In humans, IL-1β and TNF have been used for adjuvant chemotherapy; many patients develop pain and tenderness at the injection site (Kemeny et al. 1990; Del Mastro et al. 1995; Elkordy et al. 1997).

In models of inflammatory pain, pain is generally enhanced by pro-inflammatory cytokines and reduced by cytokine blockade (for review see Watkins et al. 1995b). However, analgesia is briefly induced by injection of IL-1β, IL-6, or TNF into an inflamed rat hindpaw, an effect probably mediated by the liberation of endorphins from inflammatory cells (Czlonkowski et al. 1993; Schäfer et al. 1994).

EVIDENCE FROM KNOCKOUT STUDIES

Studies with knockout animals often lead to different conclusions than pharmacological studies due to compensatory mechanisms in knockout animals that can complicate interpretation of results. Several investigators have studied IL-6 knockout mice, with varying results. Mice deficient for IL-6 had normal thermal thresholds but reduced opioid responses in one study (Bianchi et al. 1999). In another study, IL-6 knockout mice had reduced temperature sensitivity in the absence of nerve injury and impaired sensory regeneration after nerve crush (Zhong et al. 1999). In a study using the CCI model, IL-6 knockout mice did not develop thermal hyperalgesia or mechanical allodynia and had reduced substance P in sensory neurons (Murphy et al. 1999b). Other investigators found a significantly lower response threshold to both mechanical and thermal stimulation in IL-6 knockout mice, and found reduced hyperalgesia and plasma extravasation after carrageenan injection (Xu et al. 1997). The results must be interpreted with care because IL-6 knockout mice have a markedly increased production of TNF (Fattori et al. 1994).

Mice overexpressing TNF in thalamic neurons had increased heat thresholds to a 50°C hot-plate test at postnatal day 90, but not at a younger age (Fiore et al. 1996). Mice overexpressing TNF in astrocytes had increased mechanical allodynia after L5 spinal nerve transection (DeLeo et al. 2000). We studied mice deficient for TNFR1, TNFR2, or both. The most consistent finding was the absence of thermal hyperalgesia in TNFR1 knockout mice after CCI compared to wild-type mice (Vogel et al. 2000). The i.pl. injection of 100 pg of TNF induced mechanical allodynia in wild-type mice and in TNFR2-deficient mice, but not in TNFR1 knockouts (C. Vogel and C. Sommer, unpublished manuscript). IL-10 knockout mice increase their production of TNF and IL-1β after stimulation, so that we would expect increased hyperalgesia in pain models, but behavioral data are unavailable (Agnello et al. 2000).

CYTOKINES IN NEUROPATHIC PAIN

Models of painful nerve injury reveal changes in cytokine expression in the injured nerve itself, in the DRG, in the spinal cord dorsal horn, and in the CNS. In the CCI model, TNF and IL-1β increase in the nerve, the spinal cord dorsal horn, the hippocampus, and the locus ceruleus, as described in detail above. Lumbar spinal IL-1β-, TNF-, and TGFβ-like immunoreactivity increases in both sciatic cryoneurolysis (SCN) and sciatic nerve CCI(DeLeo et al. 1997). IL-6 mRNA in neurons was significantly elevated at 3 and 7 days after SCN and 7 days after SNL in both dorsal and ventral horns (Arruda et al. 1998).

Much information is available on IL-1 in models of inflammatory pain, but we lack data on its role in neuropathic pain. It is unclear what happens on direct injection of IL-1α or IL-1β into a nerve. IL-1β increases in the nerve, the spinal cord, and the serum after nerve injury. Neutralizing antibodies to IL-1RI reduced thermal hyperalgesia and mechanical allodynia in mice with CCI and attenuated the endoneurial increase of TNF immunoreactivity (Sommer et al. 1999a).

IL-6 directly injected into rat sciatic nerve induces inflammatory infiltrates and may cause demyelination between days 4 and 7 after injection (Deretzi et al. 1999); it also increases the percentage of neuronal profiles in L4 and L5 DRG with galanin immunoreactivity (Thompson et al. 1998). Examining the role of IL-6 in neuropathic pain, Arruda et al. (1998) used in situ hybridization and a digoxigenin-labeled oligonucleotide to demonstrate significant elevation of IL-6 mRNA in neurons 3 and 7 days after SCN and 7 days after SNL in both dorsal and ventral horns. Serial staining confirmed that the cellular localization of the IL-6 mRNA expression was predominantly neuronal. Intrathecal IL-6 produced touch-evoked allodynia in normal rats and thermal hyperalgesia in rats with SCN (DeLeo et al. 1996). Anti-IL-6 antibodies and IgG i.t. in doses of 0.01–0.001 μg decreased tactile allodynia in the SNL model (Arruda et al. 2000). Epineurial injection of antibodies to the IL-6 receptor attenuated thermal hyperalgesia and mechanical allodynia in CCI (Sommer 1999a).

Mice deficient in the IL-6 gene are less susceptible to spinal nerve lesion-induced mechanoallodynia and adrenergic sprouting in sensory ganglia (Ramer et al. 1998). In IL-6 knockout mice, CCI does not cause thermal or mechanical hyperalgesia; loss of substance P in sensory neurons is excessive in these knockouts, and induction of galanin in central sensory projections is reduced (Murphy et al. 1999b). Other investigators found reduced temperature sensitivity in naive IL-6 knockout mice and noted impaired sensory regeneration after nerve crush (Zhong et al. 1999). Female IL-6 knockout mice had increased autotomy after section of the sciatic nerve (Xu et al. 1997).

Injection of TNF into the sciatic nerves induces vascular changes, demyelination, and axonal degeneration (Said and Hontebeyrie-Joskowicz 1992; Redford et al. 1995). Doses of 100 and 1000 U caused inflammation but no axonal or myelin damage (Uncini et al. 1999). Intraneurally injected TNF produced thermal hyperalgesia and mechanical allodynia for 3 days (Wagner and Myers 1996a), but these effects were attenuated with prosaptide (Wagner et al. 1998b). In an invertebrate model using *Aplysia,* hyperexcitability after nerve injury was mediated by the release of IL-1β and TNF from amebocytes; additional exposure of the nerve stumps to TNF increased the hyperexcitability (Walters 1994).

Spengler's laboratory has investigated intracerebral TNF levels under nerve injury conditions. After CCI, TNF bioactivity increased in the hippocampus, locus ceruleus, and spinal cord dorsal horn, whereas stimulated norepinephrine release decreased (Ignatowski et al. 1999). Intracerebroventricular administration of anti-TNF antibodies on day 4 after CCI reduced thermal hyperalgesia. Administration of TNF (1 μg in 24 hours) increased thermal hyperalgesia in naive rats and in rats with CCI. Alpha-2-receptor- and TNF-induced inhibition of norepinephrine release increased and stimulated norepinephrine release decreased on day 8 after CCI (Covey et al. 2000). Spengler's team concluded that TNF antagonizes the endogenous pain-suppressing system and thus could block the action of tricyclic antidepressants.

Pain-related behavior after CCI was reduced by substances blocking the production of TNF, its release from the cell membrane, or its function (Sommer et al. 1997, 1998a; Wagner et al. 1998a; Lindenlaub et al. 2000). The CCI model combines nerve lesion with epineurial inflammation (Sommer et al. 1993), so anti-TNF antibodies might reduce the inflammatory reaction without influencing neuropathic events directly. This explanation is unlikely, however, because anti-TNF antibodies worked equally well in the model of partial sciatic nerve transection (PST), where epineurial inflammation is minimal (Sommer et al. 1999b; Lindenlaub and Sommer 2000). Furthermore, thalidomide, a blocker of TNF production, reduced hyperalgesia in nerve injury models, but not in a model of nerve inflammation (Sommer et al. 1998a; Bennett 2000). The TNF synthesis inhibitors, thalidomide and pentoxifylline, had to be administered before induction of nerve injury. Delayed administration did not reduce hyperalgesia in CCI, perhaps due to the early peak in TNF increase after nerve injury (George et al. 1999). However, compounds directly inhibiting TNF-like neutralizing antibodies or the recently developed TNF-receptor fusion protein etanercept reversed pre-existing hyperalgesia in mice with CCI (Sommer et al. 1999b, 2000; Fig. 4). The hyperalgesic action of TNF seems to be mediated by TNFR1 because neutralizing antibodies

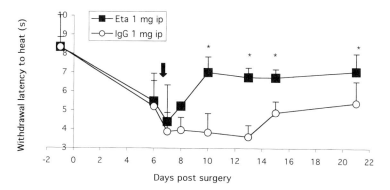

Fig. 4. Withdrawal latencies to heat of the CCI-operated hindpaws of mice treated with etanercept (Eta, 1 mg) or human IgG (1 mg) i.p. daily from day 6 after surgery. Latencies are elevated starting on day 10 in etanercept-treated mice compared to IgG-treated mice, indicating a reduction in thermal hyperalgesia. The arrow shows the start of treatment. Asterisks (*) denote $P < 0.05$. Data are from Sommer et al. (2001).

to TNFR1, but not to TNFR2, can reduce hyperalgesia (Sommer et al. 1998b).

Studies on the mechanism of TNF hyperalgesia suggested retrograde transport of TNF (Watkins et al. 1995b). We used the double ligature model to study transport of endogenous TNF and used rat recombinant ^{125}I-TNF to study transport of exogenously applied TNF in the rat sciatic nerve (Tonra et al. 1998). Calcitonin gene-related peptide (CGRP) served as a positive control for anterograde transport, and NGF as a control for retrograde transport. Both methods demonstrated that TNF is anterogradely transported in peripheral nerve and that it accumulates in muscle after intraneural injection (Schäfers et al. 2000) (Fig. 5). Thus, muscular pain may contribute to nerve injury pain, as ectopic activity occurs in muscle afferents after nerve injury (Michaelis et al. 2000). Retrograde transport of TNF was not present in our model, although we confirmed retrograde transport of ^{125}I-NGF. However, retrograde transport of TNF in rat sciatic nerve recently was demonstrated using biotinylated TNF (Shubayev and Myers 2001).

Mice overexpressing TNF in astrocytes have increased mechanical allodynia after L5 spinal nerve transection (DeLeo et al. 2000). Mice deficient in TNFR1 do not develop thermal hyperalgesia after CCI (Vogel et al. 2000). They also have diminished upregulation of cyclooxygenase (COX)-2, nitric oxide synthase (NOS), and intracellular adhesion molecule (ICAM)-1 in the peripheral nerve (Schäfers and Sommer 1999; Marziniak and Sommer 2000). The consequences for the electrophysiological properties of C fibers in these animals remain to be investigated.

Intraneural injection of the anti-inflammatory cytokine IL-10 reduced thermal hyperalgesia in rats with CCI (Wagner et al. 1998a). Anti-IL-10 antibodies

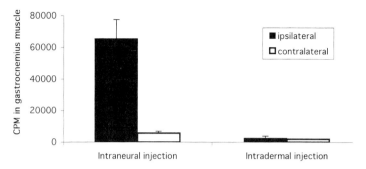

Fig. 5. Radioactive count in gastrocnemius muscle 6 hours after intraneural injection of ^{125}I-TNF. TNF is anterogradely transported in the peripheral nerve and accumulates in the muscle after intraneural injection. No accumulation occurred contralaterally or after intradermal injection, indicating specific axonal transport. CPM = counts per minute. Data are from M. Schäfers and C. Sommer (unpublished manuscript).

(100 µg daily) administered epineurially to mice with CCI did not alter the time course of hyperalgesia (A. George and C. Sommer, unpublished manuscript).

RELEVANCE OF CYTOKINES TO NEUROPATHIC PAIN IN HUMANS

Serum levels of TNF and IL-1 are elevated in a subgroup of leprosy patients (Sarno et al. 1991). Treatment of the painful neuropathic condition of erythema nodosum leprosum with thalidomide, 100–200 mg/day, reduces TNF secretion in peripheral blood mononuclear cells by >90% and greatly reduces pain (Barnes et al. 1992). Anti-TNF strategies have been used in various non-neuropathic painful conditions such as AIDS-associated proctitis (Georghiou and Alworth 1992), rheumatoid arthritis (Elliott et al. 1994; Moreland et al. 1999), and HIV-associated aphthous ulcers (Jacobson et al. 1997; for review see Sommer 1999b). The potential of drugs that inhibit TNF-α bioactivity, such as etanercept and infliximab, now available for human use, remains to be explored in neuropathic pain.

In patients, post-diskectomy pain correlates with high serum IL-6 levels (Geiss et al. 1997), and IL-1β in the synovial fluid is associated with hyperalgesia and spontaneous pain in temporomandibular joint pain (Kopp 1998). In Schwann cells from different individuals, the cytokines IL-8, IL-6, and IL-1β are produced at very different levels, which might be one factor determining differences in regeneration and pain after nerve injury (Rutkowski et al. 1999). In human neuropathies, preliminary data point to a correlation between acuteness of the axonal degeneration, cytokine expression, and pain. In vasculitic neuropathy, patients whose nerve biopsy revealed a higher content of IL-6 and whose neuropathy was of short duration had more pain (Empl et al. 2000).

Intravenous immunoglobulin (IVIG, 0.4 g/kg) reduces IL-1α and IL-1β levels in the plasma of patients with previously elevated levels, and markedly increases levels of IL-1Ra and neutralizing antibodies to IL-1 (Aukrust et al. 1999). Given that IVIG reduced pain in a subgroup of patients with chronic pain (Goebel et al. 1999), the reduction of IL-1-activity might be one mechanism of the analgesic property of IVIG.

TNF genes show strong linkage disequilibrium with genes in the major histocompatibility complex, such that polymorphisms in these genes may contribute not only to autoimmune diseases (Probert and Selmaj 1997; Makhatadze 1998), but also to the susceptibility to develop neuropathic pain.

HOW DO CYTOKINES INDUCE PAIN IN NEUROPATHIC CONDITIONS?

IL-1β and TNF may directly activate or sensitize afferent neurons. This process may be receptor dependent, although a low pH, trimeric TNF inserts itself into biological membranes in a receptor-independent fashion and has ion channel activity (Kagan et al. 1992; Baldwin et al. 1996). However, this process has not yet been shown in whole cells or in vivo. If true in vivo, this insertion of the TNF trimer into previously depolarized membranes of damaged neurons might enhance spontaneous activity and sensitization (Sorkin et al. 1997). Furthermore, TNF has a lectin-like activity, which is also independent from both receptors (Lucas et al. 1994).

IL-1β and TNF can stimulate afferent fibers to release CGRP in the rat trachea after systemic lipopolysaccharide injection (Hua et al. 1996), and can increase heat-evoked CGRP release in rat skin within 5 minutes, suggesting a direct action on afferent fibers (Opree and Kress 2000). Intraplantar IL-1β increased evoked and spontaneous activity in afferent fibers within 1 minute, providing further evidence of a direct action of the cytokine on nerve fibers (Fukuoka et al. 1994). The increase in CGRP release is receptor dependent for IL-6 (Opree and Kress 2000) and most likely for IL-1β and TNF, which have same temporal characteristics. The authors suggest a sensitization of heat-activated ion channels by phosphorylation (Cesare and McNaughton 1996; Opree and Kress 2000). These effects were dose dependent, with maximal results at doses of 20 or 50 ng.

Indirect actions of the cytokines, mediated by other algogenic compounds, are likely in many paradigms. Nerve growth factor is one candidate mediator of cytokine-induced hyperalgesia. IL-1 acts on sciatic nerve Schwann cells to induce transcription of NGF (Lindholm et al. 1987). TNF-treated fibroblasts also produce NGF (Hattori et al. 1996). IL-1β induced hyperalgesia can be prevented by anti-NGF antibodies (Safieh-Garabedian et al. 1995), indicating that IL-1β hyperalgesia is mediated via the increase in NGF in inflamed nerve. A similar mechanism was proposed for TNF (Woolf et al. 1997).

Prostaglandins, bradykinin, and neuropeptides may mediate cytokine hyperalgesia. TNF enhances capsaicin sensitivity in rat sensory neurons (Nicol et al. 1997), probably via the neuronal production of prostaglandins. Perkins' team found IL-1 hyperalgesia to be dependent on bradykinin B1 receptors (Davis and Perkins 1994). Long-time exposure of primary afferent neurons to IL-1β induced substance P release via the COX-2 system (Inoue et al. 1999). TNF induced substance P in sympathetic ganglia via induction of IL-1 and leukemia inhibitory factor (LIF) (Ding et al. 1995). IL-6 and LIF promoted the production of galanin in sensory neurons in vivo (Thompson et al. 1998). These changes in neurotransmitter expression might alter pain processing after nerve injury.

Our own studies show that the hyperalgesic effect of endogenous TNF after CCI is mediated by TNFR1 (Sommer et al. 1998b; Vogel et al. 2000). COX-2 may play a role in this model, because both COX-2 upregulation and thermal hyperalgesia were absent in TNFR1 knockout mice. Our studies on axonal transport of TNF do not support the hypothesis that TNF is transported retrogradely to the DRG, where it could induce long-term changes in gene transcription that might further enhance pain messages (Schäfers et al. 2000). However, other investigators used different methods to show retrograde transport of TNF to the DRG (Shubayev and Myers 2001). Furthermore, TNF expression in the DRG itself may be upregulated by nerve injury, therefore several sources of TNF are candidates for acting on the DRG. We could, however, unequivocally demonstrate anterograde transport of TNF in the sciatic nerve to the gastrocnemius muscle. Given recent work implicating muscle afferents in chronic pain (Michaelis et al. 2000), our finding may be relevant to the mechanisms of cytokine hyperalgesia. Cytokine actions on the brain are, at least in part, mediated by the vagus nerve (Goehler et al. 1999), which may also be true for hyperalgesic actions, particularly in intestinal pain (Watkins et al. 1994b, 1995a).

Many studies have shown a biphasic action of cytokines on nociceptive thresholds or on surrogate markers (Yabuuchi et al. 1996; Sorkin et al. 1997; Hori et al. 1998; Junger and Sorkin 2000; Laughlin et al. 2000), with lower doses inducing hyperalgesia and higher doses having no effect. When injected into the cerebral ventricles (but not when injected into one hindpaw), lower doses of IL-1β induced hyperalgesia and higher doses created analgesia (Bianchi et al. 1998). A possible explanation might be that at higher concentrations, the cytokines induce release of their own inhibitors or other molecules attenuating the inflammatory and proalgesic response.

SUMMARY

Ample evidence from experimental studies indicates that proinflammatory cytokines induce or increase both neuropathic and inflammatory pain. Research has demonstrated direct actions of cytokines on afferent nerve fibers as well as actions involving further mediators. Inhibition of proinflammatory cytokines by synthesis inhibitors, by inhibitors of the conversion into the active molecule, by direct antagonists, or by anti-inflammatory antibodies reduces pain and hyperalgesia in most models studied. Cytokine knockout models are now being studied in the context of neuropathic pain. Encouraging preliminary data from human studies indicate that cytokine inhibition may be added to the panel of treatment modalities for neuropathic pain.

ACKNOWLEDGMENTS

Supported by the Deutsche Forschungsgemeinschaft, SFB 353, and by Volkswagen-Stiftung (I/73 833).

REFERENCES

Aggarwal BB, Natarajan K. Tumor necrosis factors: developments during the last decade. *Eur Cytokine Netw* 1996; 7:93–124.

Agnello D, Villa P, Ghezzi P. Increased tumor necrosis factor and interleukin-6 production in the central nervous system of interleukin-10-deficient mice. *Brain Res* 2000; 869:241–243.

Aloe L, Moroni R, Angelucci F, Fiore M. Role of TNF-alpha but not NGF in murine hyperalgesia induced by parasitic infection. *Psychopharmacology (Berl)* 1997; 134:287–292.

Arruda JL, Colburn RW, Rickman AJ, Rutkowski MD, DeLeo JA. Increase of interleukin-6 mRNA in the spinal cord following peripheral nerve injury in the rat: potential role of IL-6 in neuropathic pain. *Brain Res Mol Brain Res* 1998; 62:228–325.

Arruda JL, Sweitzer S, Rutkowski MD, DeLeo JA. Intrathecal anti-IL-6 antibody and IgG attenuates peripheral nerve injury-induced mechanical allodynia in the rat: possible immune modulation in neuropathic pain (1). *Brain Res* 2000; 879:216–225.

Aukrust P, Muller F, Svenson M, et al. Administration of intravenous immunoglobulin (IVIG) in vivo—down-regulatory effects on the IL-1 system. *Clin Exp Immunol* 1999; 115:136–143.

Baldwin RL, Stolowitz ML, Hood L, Wisnieski BJ. Structural changes of tumor necrosis factor alpha associated with membrane insertion and channel formation. *Proc Natl Acad Sci USA* 1996; 93:1021–1026.

Bandtlow CE, Meyer M, Lindholm D, et al. Regional and cellular codistribution of interleukin 1 beta and nerve growth factor mRNA in the adult rat brain: possible relationship to the regulation of nerve growth factor synthesis. *J Cell Biol* 1990; 111:1701–1711.

Barnes PF, Chatterjee D, Brennan PJ, Rea TH, Modlin RL. Tumor necrosis factor production in patients with leprosy. *Infect Immun* 1992; 60:1441–1446.

Bennett GJ. A neuroimmune interaction in painful peripheral neuropathy. *Clin J Pain* 2000; 16:S139–S143.

Bennett GJ, Xie YK. A peripheral mononeuropathy in rat that produces disorders of pain sensation like those seen in man. *Pain* 1988; 33:87–107.

Bergsteinsdottir K, Kingston A, Mirsky R, Jessen KR. Rat Schwann cells produce interleukin-1. *J Neuroimmunol* 1991; 34:15–23.

Bianchi M, Sacerdote P, Ricciardi-Castagnoli P, Mantegazza P, Panerai A. Central effects of tumor necrosis factor and interleukine-1alpha on nociceptive thresholds and spontaneous locomotor activity. *Neurosci Lett* 1992; 148:76–80.

Bianchi M, Panerai AE. CRH and the noradrenergic system mediate the antinociceptive effect of central interleukin-1 alpha in the rat. *Brain Res Bull* 1995; 36:113–117.

Bianchi M, Dib B, Panerai AE. Interleukin-1 and nociception in the rat. *J Neurosci Res* 1998; 53:645–650.

Bianchi M, Maggi R, Pimpinelli F, et al. Presence of a reduced opioid response in interleukin-6 knock out mice. *Eur J Neurosci* 1999; 11:1501–1507.

Bizette C, Chan-Chi-Song P, Fontaine M, Tadie M. Expression des ARNm de l'interleukine 1 beta, de l'interleukine 6 et du Tumor Necrosis Factor alpha au cours de la regeneration du nerf sciatique de rat apres perte de substance. *Chirurgie* 1996; 121:474–481.

Bolin LM, Verity AN, Silver JE, Shooter EM, Abrams JS. Interleukin-6 production by Schwann cells and induction in sciatic nerve injury. *J Neurochem* 1995; 64:850–858.

Bourde O, Kiefer R, Toyka KV, Hartung HP. Quantification of interleukin-6 mRNA in Wallerian degeneration by competitive reverse transcription polymerase chain reaction. *J Neuroimmunol* 1996; 69:135–410.

Breder CD, Dinarello CA, Saper CB. Interleukin-1 immunoreactive innervation of the human hypothalamus. *Science* 1988; 240:321–324.

Breder CD, Tsujimotot M, Terano Y, Scott DW, Saper CB. Distribution and characterization of tumor necrosis factor-alpha-like immunoreactivity in the murine central nervous system. *J Comp Neurol* 1993; 337:543–567.

Bredow S, Guha-Thakurta N, Taishi P, Obal F Jr, Krueger JM. Diurnal variations of tumor necrosis factor alpha mRNA and alpha-tubulin mRNA in rat brain. *Neuroimmunomodulation* 1997; 4:84–90.

Cesare P, McNaughton P. A novel heat-activated current in nociceptive neurons and its sensitization by bradykinin. *Proc Natl Acad Sci USA* 1996; 93:15435–15439.

Covey WC, Ignatowski TA, Knight PR, Spengler RN. Brain-derived TNFalpha: involvement in neuroplastic changes implicated in the conscious perception of persistent pain. *Brain Res* 2000; 859:113–122.

Cunha FQ, Lorenzetti BB, Poole S, Ferreira SH. Interleukin-8 as a mediator of sympathetic pain. *Br J Pharmacol* 1991; 165–167.

Cunha F, Poole S, Lorenzetti B, Ferreira S. The pivotal role of tumor necrosis factor alpha in the development of inflammatory hyperalgesia. *Br J Pharmacol* 1992; 107:660–664.

Czlonkowski A, Stein C, Herz A. Peripheral mechanisms of opioid antinociception in inflammation: involvement of cytokines. *Eur J Pharmacol* 1993; 242:229–235.

Darnay BG, Aggarwal BB. Signal transduction by tumour necrosis factor and tumour necrosis factor related ligands and their receptors. *Ann Rheum Dis* 1999; 58(Suppl 1):I2–I13.

Davis AJ, Perkins MN. The involvement of bradykinin B1 and B2 receptor mechanisms in cytokine-induced mechanical hyperalgesia in the rat. *Br J Pharmacol* 1994; 113:63–68.

Del Mastro L, Venturini M, Giannessi PG, et al. Intraperitoneal infusion of recombinant human tumor necrosis factor and mitoxantrone in neoplastic ascites: a feasibility study. *Anticancer Res* 1995; 15:2207–2212.

DeLeo JA, Colburn RW, Nichols M, Malhotra A. Interleukin-6-mediated hyperalgesia/allodynia and increased spinal IL-6 expression in a rat mononeuropathy model. *J Interferon Cytokine Res* 1996; 16:695–700.

DeLeo JA, Colburn RW, Rickman AJ. Cytokine and growth factor immunohistochemical spinal profiles in two animal models of mononeuropathy. *Brain Res* 1997; 759:50–57.

DeLeo JA, Rutkowski MD, Stalder AK, Campbell IL. Transgenic expression of TNF by astrocytes increases mechanical allodynia in a mouse neuropathy model. *Neuroreport* 2000; 11:599–602.

Deretzi G, Pelidou SH, Zou LP, Quiding C, Zhu J. Local effects of recombinant rat interleukin-6 on the peripheral nervous system. *Immunology* 1999; 97:582–587.

Dinarello C. Interleukin-1 and interleukin-1 antagonism. *Blood* 1991; 77:1627–1652.

Ding M, Hart RP, Jonakait GM. Tumor necrosis factor-alpha induces substance P in sympathetic ganglia through sequential induction of interleukin-1 and leukemia inhibitory factor. *J Neurobiol* 1995; 28:445–454.

Elkordy M, Crump M, Vredenburgh JJ, et al. A phase I trial of recombinant human interleukin-1 beta (OCT-43) following high-dose chemotherapy and autologous bone marrow transplantation. *Bone Marrow Transplant* 1997; 19:315–322.

Elliott MJ, Maini RN, Feldmann M, et al. Randomised double-blind comparison of chimeric monoclonal antibody to tumour necrosis factor alpha (cA2) versus placebo in rheumatoid arthritis. *Lancet* 1994; 344:1105–1110.

Empl M, Renaud S, Erne B, et al. TNF-alpha Expression in schmerzhaften und nicht-schmerzhaften Neuropathien. *Schmerz* 2000; 14(Suppl 1):S70.

Eriksson C, Nobel S, Winblad B, Schultzberg M. Expression of interleukin 1 alpha and beta, and interleukin 1 receptor antagonist mRNA in the rat central nervous system after peripheral administration of lipopolysaccharides. *Cytokine* 2000; 12:423–431.

Fattori E, Cappelletti M, Costa P, et al. Defective inflammatory response in interleukin 6-deficient mice. *J Exp Med* 1994; 180:1243–1250.

Ferreira S, Lorenzetti B, Poole S. Bradykinin initiates cytokine-mediated inflammatory hyperalgesia. *Br J Pharmacol* 1993; 110:1227–1231.

Ferreira S, Lorenzetti B, Bristow A, Poole S. Interleukin-1β as a potent hyperalgesic agent antagonized by a tripeptide analogue. *Nature* 1988; 334:698–700.

Fiore M, Probert L, Kollias G, et al. Neurobehavioral alterations in developing transgenic mice expressing TNF-alpha in the brain. *Brain Behav Immun* 1996; 10:126–138.

Floyd RA, Krueger JM. Diurnal variation of TNF alpha in the rat brain. *Neuroreport* 1997; 8:915–918.

Follenfant RL, Nakamura-Craig M, Henderson B, Higgs GA. Inhibition by neuropeptides of interleukin-1 beta-induced, prostaglandin-independent hyperalgesia. *Br J Pharmacol* 1989; 98:41–43.

Fukuoka H, Kawatani M, Hisamitsu T, Takeshige C. Cutaneous hyperalgesia induced by peripheral injection of interleukin-1β in the rat. *Brain Res* 1994; 657:133–140.

Gao Y, Ng YK, Lin JY, Ling EA. Expression of immunoregulatory cytokines in neurons of the lateral hypothalamic area and amygdaloid nuclear complex of rats immunized against human IgG. *Brain Res* 2000; 859:364–368.

Gatti S, Bartfai T. Induction of tumor necrosis factor-alpha mRNA in the brain after peripheral endotoxin treatment: comparison with interleukin-1 family and interleukin-6. *Brain Res* 1993; 624:291–294.

Geiss A, Varadi E, Steinbach K, Bauer HW, Anton F. Psychoneuroimmunological correlates of persisting sciatic pain in patients who underwent discectomy. *Neurosci Lett* 1997; 237:65–68.

George A, Sommer C. Upregulation of the tumor necrosis factor receptor 1 and 2 in mouse sciatic nerve after chronic constrictive injury. *J Neurol* 1999; 246(Suppl 1):115.

George A, Schmidt C, Weishaupt A, Toyka KV, Sommer C. Serial determination of tumor necrosis factor-alpha content in rat sciatic nerve after chronic constriction injury. *Exp Neurol* 1999; 160:124–132.

George A, Marziniak M, Schäfers M, Toyka KV, Sommer C. Thalidomide treatment in chronic constrictive neuropathy decreases endoneurial tumor necrosis factor-alpha, increases interleukin-10 and has long-term effects on spinal cord dorsal horn met-enkephalin. *Pain* 2000; 88:267–275.

Georghiou PR, Alworth AM. Thalidomide in painful AIDS-associated proctitis. *J Infect Dis* 1992; 166:939–940.

Gillen C, Jander S, Stoll G. Sequential expression of mRNA for proinflammatory cytokines and interleukin-10 in the rat peripheral nervous system: comparison between immune-mediated demyelination and Wallerian degeneration. *J Neurosci Res* 1998; 51:489–496.

Goebel A, Netal S, Schedel R, Sprotte G. Wirkung von gepoolten humanen Immunglobulinen auf das Schmerzniveau bei Fibromyalgiepatienten. *Schmerz* 1999; 13:S73–S74.

Goehler LE, Gaykema RP, Nguyen KT, et al. Interleukin-1beta in immune cells of the abdominal vagus nerve: a link between the immune and nervous systems? *J Neurosci* 1999; 19:2799–2806.

Griffin JW, George R, Ho T. Macrophage systems in peripheral nerves: a review. *J Neuropathol Exp Neurol* 1993; 52:553–560.

Hattori A, Hayashi K, Kohno M. Tumor necrosis factor (TNF) stimulates the production of nerve growth factor in fibroblasts via the 55-kDa type 1 TNF receptor. *FEBS Lett* 1996; 379:157–160.

Hopkins SJ, Rothwell NJ. Cytokines and the nervous system. I: Expression and recognition. *Trends Neurosci* 1995; 18:83–88.

Hori T, Oka T, Hosoi M, Aou S. Pain modulatory actions of cytokines and prostaglandin E2 in the brain. *Ann NY Acad Sci* 1998; 840:269–281.

Hua X-Y, Chen P, Fox A, Myers RR. Involvement of cytokines in lipopolysaccharide-induced facilitation of CGRP release from capsaicin-sensitive nerves in the trachea: studies with interleukin-1β and tumor necrosis factor-α. *J Neurosci* 1996; 16:4742–4748.

Ignatowski TA, Noble BK, Wright JR, et al. Neuronal-associated tumor necrosis factor (TNF alpha): its role in noradrenergic functioning and modification of its expression following antidepressant drug administration. *J Neuroimmunol* 1997; 79:84–90.

Ignatowski TA, Covey WC, Knight PR, et al. Brain-derived TNFalpha mediates neuropathic pain. *Brain Res* 1999; 841:70–77.

Inoue A, Ikoma K, Morioka N, et al. Interleukin-1beta induces substance P release from primary afferent neurons through the cyclooxygenase-2 system. *J Neurochem* 1999; 73:2206–2213.

Jacobson JM, Greenspan JS, Spritzler J, et al. Thalidomide for the treatment of oral aphthous ulcers in patients with human immunodeficiency virus infection. National Institute of Allergy and Infectious Diseases AIDS Clinical Trials Group. *N Engl J Med* 1997; 336:1487–1493.

Jander S, Pohl J, Gillen C, Stoll G. Differential expression of interleukin-10 mRNA in Wallerian degeneration and immune-mediated inflammation of the rat peripheral nervous system. *J Neurosci Res* 1996; 43:254–259.

Junger H, Sorkin LS. Nociceptive and inflammatory effects of subcutaneous TNF-alpha. *Pain* 2000; 85:145–151.

Kagan BL, Baldwin RL, Munoz D, Wisnieski BJ. Formation of ion-permeable channels by tumor necrosis factor-alpha. *Science* 1992; 255:1427–1430.

Kanaan SA, Poole S, Saade NE, Jabbur S, Safieh-Garabedian B. Interleukin-10 reduces the endotoxin-induced hyperalgesia in mice. *J Neuroimmunol* 1998; 86:142–150.

Kelley J. Cytokines of the lung. *Am Rev Respir Dis* 1990; 141:765–788.

Kemeny N, Childs B, Larchian W, Rosado K, Kelsen D. A phase II trial of recombinant tumor necrosis factor in patients with advanced colorectal carcinoma. *Cancer* 1990; 66:659–663.

Kopp S. The influence of neuropeptides, serotonin, and interleukin 1-beta on temporomandibular joint pain and inflammation. *J Oral Maxillofac Surg* 1998; 56:189–191.

La Fleur M, Underwood JL, Rappolee DA, Werb Z. Basement membrane and repair of injury to peripheral nerve: defining a potential role for macrophages, matrix metalloproteinases, and tissue inhibitor of metalloproteinases 1. *J Exp Med* 1996; 184:2311–2326.

Laughlin TM, Bethea JR, Yezierski RP, Wilcox GL. Cytokine involvement in dynorphin-induced allodynia. *Pain* 2000; 84:159–167.

Lechan RM, Toni R, Clark BD, et al. Immunoreactive interleukin-1 beta localization in the rat forebrain. *Brain Res* 1990; 514:135–410.

Lindenlaub T, Sommer C. Partial sciatic nerve transection as a model of neuropathic pain: a qualitative and quantitative neuropathological study. *Pain* 2000; 89:97–106.

Lindenlaub T, Teuteberg P, Hartung T, Sommer C. Effects of neutralizing antibodies to TNF-alpha on pain-related behavior and nerve regeneration in mice with chronic constriction injury. *Brain Res* 2000; 866:15–22.

Lindholm D, Heumann R, Meyer M, Thoenen H. Interleukin-1 regulates synthesis of nerve growth factor in non-neuronal cells of rat sciatic nerve. *Nature* 1987; 330:658–659.

Lucas R, Magez S, De Leys R, et al. Mapping the lectin-like activity of tumor necrosis factor. *Science* 1994; 263:814–817.

Maier SF, Wiertelak EP, Martin D, Watkins LR. Interleukin-1 mediates the behavioral hyperalgesia produced by lithium chloride and endotoxin. *Brain Res* 1993; 623:321–324.

Makhatadze NJ. Tumor necrosis factor locus: genetic organisation and biological implications. *Hum Immunol* 1998; 59:571–579.

Martin MU, Falk W. The interleukin-1 receptor complex and interleukin-1 signal transduction. *Eur Cytokine Netw* 1997; 8:5–17.

Marziniak M, Sommer C. Upregulation of cyclooxygenase 2 is dependent on tumor necrosis factor receptor 1 and 2 after chronic constriction injury. *J Neurol* 2000; 247(III):125.

Mathey EK, Pollard JD, Armati PJ. TNF alpha, IFN gamma and IL-2 mRNA expression in CIDP sural nerve biopsies. *J Neurol Sci* 1999; 163:47–52.

Michaelis M, Liu X, Jänig W. Axotomized and intact muscle afferents but no skin afferents develop ongoing discharges of dorsal root ganglion origin after peripheral nerve lesion. *J Neurosci* 2000; 20:2742–2748.

Miyahara S, Komori T, Fujiwara R, et al. Effects of repeated stress on expression of interleukin-6 (IL-6) and IL-6 receptor mRNAs in rat hypothalamus and midbrain. *Life Sci* 2000; 66:L93–L98.

Molenaar GJ, Berkenbosch F, van Dam AM, Lugard CM. Distribution of interleukin 1 beta immunoreactivity within the porcine hypothalamus. *Brain Res* 1993; 608:169–174.

Moreland LW, Schiff MH, Baumgartner SW, et al. Etanercept therapy in rheumatoid arthritis: a randomized, controlled trial. *Ann Intern Med* 1999; 130:478–486.

Murphy PG, Grondin J, Altares M, Richardson PM. Induction of interleukin-6 in axotomized sensory neurons. *J Neurosci* 1995; 15:5130–5138.

Murphy PG, Borthwick LS, Johnston RS, Kuchel G, Richardson PM. Nature of the retrograde signal from injured nerves that induces interleukin-6 mRNA in neurons. *J Neurosci* 1999a; 19:3791–3800.

Murphy PG, Ramer MS, Borthwick L, et al. Endogenous interleukin-6 contributes to hypersensitivity to cutaneous stimuli and changes in neuropeptides associated with chronic nerve constriction in mice. *Eur J Neurosci* 1999b; 11:2243–2253.

Nakamura H, Nakanishi K, Kita A, Kadokawa T. Interleukin-1 induces analgesia in mice by a central action. *Eur J Pharmacol* 1988; 149:49–54.

Nicol GD, Lopshire JC, Pafford CM. Tumor necrosis factor enhances the capsaicin sensitivity of rat sensory neurons. *J Neurosci* 1997; 17:975–982.

Oka N, Akiguchi I, Kawasaki T, et al. Tumor necrosis factor-alpha in peripheral nerve lesions. *Acta Neuropathol (Berl)* 1998; 95:57–62.

Oka T, Aou S, Hori T. Intracerebroventricular injection of interleukin-1β induces hyperalgesia in rats. *Brain Res* 1993; 624:61–68.

Oka T, Aou S, Hori T. Intracerebroventricular injection of interleukin-1 beta enhances nociceptive neuronal responses of the trigeminal nucleus caudalis in rats. *Brain Res* 1994; 656:236–244.

Oka T, Oka K, Hosoi M, Hori T. Intracerebroventricular injection of interleukin-6 induces thermal hyperalgesia in rats. *Brain Res* 1995a; 692:123–128.

Oka T, Oka K, Hosoi M, Aou S, Hori T. The opposing effects of interleukin-1 beta microinjected into the preoptic hypothalamus and the ventromedial hypothalamus on nociceptive behavior in rats. *Brain Res* 1995b; 700:271–278.

Oka T, Wakugawa Y, Hosoi M, Oka K, Hori T. Intracerebroventricular injection of tumor necrosis factor-alpha induces thermal hyperalgesia in rats. *Neuroimmunomodulation* 1996; 3:135–140.

Opree A, Kress M. Involvement of the proinflammatory cytokines tumor necrosis factor-alpha, IL-1beta, and IL-6 but not IL-8 in the development of heat hyperalgesia: effects on heat-evoked calcitonin gene-related peptide release from rat skin. *J Neurosci* 2000; 20:6289–6293.

Perkins MN, Kelly D. Interleukin-1β induced desArg[9] bradykinin-mediated thermal hyperalgesisa in the rat. *Neuropharmacology* 1994; 33:657–660.

Perkins MN, Kelly D, Davis AJ. Bradykinin B1 and B2 receptor mechanisms and cytokine-induced hyperalgesia in the rat. *Can J Physiol Pharmacol* 1995; 73:832–836.

Poole S, Cunha FQ, Selkirk S, Lorenzetti BB, Ferreira SH. Cytokine-mediated inflammatory hyperalgesia limited by interleukin-10. *Br J Pharmacol* 1995; 115:684–688.

Probert L, Selmaj K. TNF and related molecules: trends in neuroscience and clinical applications. *J Neuroimmunol* 1997; 72:113–117.

Putzu GA, Figarella-Branger D, Bouvier-Labit C, et al. Immunohistochemical localization of cytokines, C5b-9 and ICAM-1 in peripheral nerve of Guillain-Barre syndrome. *J Neurol Sci* 2000; 174:16–21.

Ramer MS, Murphy PG, Richardson PM, Bisby MA. Spinal nerve lesion-induced mechano-allodynia and adrenergic sprouting in sensory ganglia are attenuated in interleukin-6 knockout mice. *Pain* 1998; 78:115–121.

Redford EJ, Hall SM, Smith KJ. Vascular changes and demyelination induced by the intraneural injection of tumour necrosis factor. *Brain* 1995; 118:869–878.

Rotshenker S, Aamar S, Barak V. Interleukin-1 activity in lesioned peripheral nerve. *J Neuroimmunol* 1992; 39:75–80.

Roux-Lombard P. The interleukin-1 family. *Eur Cytokine Netw* 1998; 9:565–576.

Rutkowski JL, Tuite GF, Lincoln PM, et al. Signals for proinflammatory cytokine secretion by human Schwann cells. *J Neuroimmunol* 1999; 101:47–60.

Safieh-Garabedian B, Poole S, Allchorne A, Winter J, Woolf CJ. Contribution of interleukin-1 beta to the inflammation-induced increase in nerve growth factor levels and inflammatory hyperalgesia. *Br J Pharmacol* 1995; 115:1265–1675.

Safieh-Garabedian B, Kanaan SA, Jalakhian RH, Jabbur SJ, Saade NE. Involvement of interleukin-1 beta, nerve growth factor, and prostaglandin-E2 in the hyperalgesia induced by intraplantar injections of low doses of thymulin. *Brain Behav Immun* 1997; 11:185–200.

Said G, Hontebeyrie-Joskowicz M. Nerve lesions induced by macrophage activation. *Res Immunol* 1992; 143:589–599.

Sarno EN, Grau GE, Vieira LM, Nery JA. Serum levels of tumour necrosis factor-alpha and interleukin-1 beta during leprosy reactional states. *Clin Exp Immunol* 1991; 84:103–108.

Schäfer M, Carter L, Stein C. Interleukin 1 beta and corticotropin-releasing factor inhibit pain by releasing opioids from immune cells in inflamed tissue. *Proc Natl Acad Sci USA* 1994; 91:4219–4223.

Schäfers M, Sommer C. ICAM and TNF: ICAM regulation in mice with painful mononeuropathy. *J Peripher Nerv Syst* 1999; 4:150.

Schäfers M, Toyka KV, Sommer C. Retrograde transport of tumor necrosis factor-alpha is unlikely to cause neuropathic pain. *Soc Neurosci Abstracts* 2000; 26:1956.

Schweizer A, Feige U, Fontana A, Muller K, Dinarello CA. Interleukin-1 enhances pain reflexes: mediation through increased prostaglandin E2 levels. *Agents Actions* 1988; 25:246–251.

Shubayev VI, Myers RR. Upregulation and interaction of TNFalpha and gelatinases A and B in painful peripheral nerve injury. *Brain Res* 2000; 855:83–89.

Shubayev VI, Myers RR. Axonal transport of TNF-alpha in painful neuropathy: altered distribution of ligand and receptors. *Neuroimmunology* 2001; 114:48–56.

Smith EM, Cadet P, Stefano GB, Opp MR, Hughes TK, Jr. IL-10 as a mediator in the HPA axis and brain. *J Neuroimmunol* 1999; 100:140–148.

Sommer C. Tierexperimentelle Untersuchungen bei neuropathischem Schmerz: die pathogene und therapeutische Bedeutung von Zytokinen und Zytokinrezeptoren. *Schmerz* 1999a; 13:315–323.

Sommer C. Thalidomide as a blocker of TNF production. *Drugs Future* 1999b; 24:67–75.

Sommer C, Schäfers M. Painful mononeuropathy in C57BL/Wld mice with delayed Wallerian degeneration: differential effects of cytokine production and nerve regeneration on thermal and mechanical hypersensitivity. *Brain Res* 1998; 784:154–162.

Sommer C, Galbraith JA, Heckman HM, Myers RR. Pathology of experimental compression neuropathy producing hyperesthesia. *J Neuropathol Exp Neurol* 1993; 52:223–233.

Sommer C, Schmidt C, George A, Toyka KV. A metalloprotease-inhibitor reduces pain associated behavior in mice with experimental neuropathy. *Neurosci Lett* 1997; 237:45–48.

Sommer C, Marziniak M, Myers RR. The effect of thalidomide treatment on vascular pathology and hyperalgesia caused by chronic constriction injury of rat nerve. *Pain* 1998a; 74:83–91.

Sommer C, Schmidt C, George A. Hyperalgesia in experimental neuropathy is dependent on the TNF receptor 1. *Exp Neurol* 1998b; 151:138–142.

Sommer C, Petrausch S, Lindenlaub T, Toyka KV. Neutralizing antibodies to interleukin 1-receptor reduce pain associated behavior in mice with experimental neuropathy. *Neurosci Lett* 1999a; 270:25–28.

Sommer C, Lindenlaub T, Teuteberg P, Hartung T, Toyka K. Anti-TNF neutralizing antibodies reduce pain-related behavior in two models of painful mononeuropathy. *J Peripher Nerv Syst* 1999b; 4:151.

Sommer C, Schäfers M, Marziniak M, Toyka KV. Etanercept reduces hyperalgesia in experimental painful neuropathy. *J Peripher Nerv Syst* 2001; in press.

Sorkin LS, Doom CM. Epineurial application of TNF elicits an acute mechanical hyperalgesia in the awake rat. *J Peripher Nerv Syst* 2000; 5:96–100.

Sorkin LS, Xiao WH, Wagner R, Myers RR. Tumour necrosis factor-alpha induces ectopic activity in nociceptive primary afferent fibres. *Neuroscience* 1997; 81:255–262.

Stoll G, Müller HW. Nerve injury, axonal degeneration and neural regeneration: basic insights. *Brain Pathol* 1999; 9:313–325.

Stoll G, Jung S, Jander S, Meide PVD, Hartung H-P. Tumor necrosis factor-alpha in immune-mediated demyelination and Wallerian degeneration of the rat peripheral nervous system. *J Neuroimmunol* 1993; 45:175–182.

Taishi P, Bredow S, Guha-Thakurta N, Obal F Jr, Krueger JM. Diurnal variations of interleukin-1 beta mRNA and beta-actin mRNA in rat brain. *J Neuroimmunol* 1997; 75:69–74.

Taskinen HS, Olsson T, Bucht A, et al. Peripheral nerve injury induces endoneurial expression of IFN-gamma, IL-10 and TNF-alpha mRNA. *J Neuroimmunol* 2000; 102:17–25.

Tchelingerian JL, Le Saux F, Jacque C. Identification and topography of neuronal cell populations expressing TNF alpha and IL-1 alpha in response to hippocampal lesion. *J Neurosci Res* 1996; 43:99–106.

Tha KK, Okuma Y, Miyazaki H, et al. Changes in expressions of proinflammatory cytokines IL-1beta, TNF-alpha and IL-6 in the brain of senescence accelerated mouse (SAM) P8. *Brain Res* 2000; 885:25–31.

Thompson SW, Priestley JV, Southall A. gp130 cytokines, leukemia inhibitory factor and interleukin-6, induce neuropeptide expression in intact adult rat sensory neurons in vivo: time-course, specificity and comparison with sciatic nerve axotomy. *Neuroscience* 1998; 84:1247–1255.

Tonra JR, Curtis R, Wong V, et al. Axotomy upregulates the anterograde transport and expression of brain-derived neurotrophic factor by sensory neurons. *J Neurosci* 1998; 18:4374–4383.

Uncini A, Di Muzio A, Di Guglielmo G, et al. Effect of rhTNF-alpha injection into rat sciatic nerve. *J Neuroimmunol* 1999; 94:88–94.

Van Wagoner NJ, Benveniste EN. Interleukin-6 expression and regulation in astrocytes. *J Neuroimmunol* 1999; 100:124–139.

Vitkovic L, Bockaert J, Jacque C. "Inflammatory" cytokines: neuromodulators in normal brain? *J Neurochem* 2000; 74:457–471.

Vogel C, Lindenlaub T, Tiegs G, Toyka KV, Sommer C. Pain-related behavior in TNF-receptor-deficient mice. In: Devor M, Rowbotham MC, Wiesenfeld-Hallin Z (Eds). *Proceedings of the 9th World Congress on Pain,* Progress in Pain Research and Management, Vol. 16. Seattle: IASP Press, 2000, pp 249–257.

Wagner R, Myers RR. Endoneurial injection of TNF-alpha produces neuropathic pain behaviors. *Neuroreport* 1996a; 7:2897–2901.

Wagner R, Myers RR. Schwann cells produce tumor necrosis factor alpha: expression in injured and non-injured nerves. *Neuroscience* 1996b; 73:625–629.

Wagner R, Janjigian M, Myers RR. Anti-inflammatory interleukin-10 therapy in CCI neuropathy decreases thermal hyperalgesia, macrophage recruitment, and endoneurial TNF-alpha expression. *Pain* 1998a; 74:35–42.

Wagner R, Myers RR, O'Brien JS. Prosaptide prevents hyperalgesia and reduces peripheral TNFR1 expression following TNF-alpha nerve injection. *Neuroreport* 1998b; 9:2827–2831.

Walters ET. Injury-related behavior and neuronal plasticity: an evolutionary perspective on sensitization, hyperalgesia, and analgesia. *Int Rev Neurobiol* 1994; 36:325–427.

Watkins LR, Wiertelak EP, Goehler LE, et al. Neurocircuitry of illness-induced hyperalgesia. *Brain Res* 1994a; 639:283–299.

Watkins LR, Wiertelak EP, Goehler LE, et al. Characterization of cytokine-induced hyperalgesia. *Brain Res* 1994b; 654:15–26.

Watkins L, Goehler L, Rekton J, Brewer M, Maier S. Mechanisms of tumor necrosis factor α (TNF-α) hyperalgesia. *Brain Res* 1995a; 692:244–250.

Watkins LR, Maier SF, Goehler LE. Immune activation: the role of pro-inflammatory cytokines in inflammation, illness responses and pathological pain states. *Pain* 1995b; 63:289–302.

Wells MR, Racis SP Jr, Vaidya U. Changes in plasma cytokines associated with peripheral nerve injury. *J Neuroimmunol* 1992; 39:261–268.

Woolf CJ, Allchorne A, Safieh-Garabedian B, Poole S. Cytokines, nerve growth factor and inflammatory hyperalgesia: the contribution of tumour necrosis factor alpha. *Br J Pharmacol* 1997; 121:417–424.

Xu XJ, Hao JX, Andell-Jonsson S, et al. Nociceptive responses in interleukin-6-deficient mice to peripheral inflammation and peripheral nerve section. *Cytokine* 1997; 9:1028–1033.

Yabuuchi K, Nishiyori A, Minami M, Satoh M. Biphasic effects of intracerebroventricular interleukin-1 beta on mechanical nociception in the rat. *Eur J Pharmacol* 1996; 300:59–65.

Zhong J, Dietzel ID, Wahle P, Kopf M, Heumann R. Sensory impairments and delayed regeneration of sensory axons in interleukin-6-deficient mice. *J Neurosci* 1999; 19:4305–4313.

Zhu J, Bai XF, Mix E, Link H. Cytokine dichotomy in peripheral nervous system influences the outcome of experimental allergic neuritis: dynamics of mRNA expression for IL-1 beta, IL-6, IL-12, TNF-alpha, TNF-beta, and cytolysin. *Clin Immunol Immunopathol* 1997; 84:85–94.

Correspondence to: Claudia Sommer, MD, Neurologische Universitätsklinik, Josef-Schneider-Str. 11, 97080 Würzburg, Germany. Tel: 49 931 201 2621; Fax: 49 931 201 2697; email: sommer@mail.uni-wuerzburg.de.

Neuropathic Pain: Pathophysiology and Treatment,
Progress in Pain Research and Management, Vol. 21,
edited by Per T. Hansson, Howard L. Fields, Raymond G.
Hill, and Paolo Marchettini, IASP Press, Seattle, © 2001.

4

Human Studies of Primary Nociceptors in Neuropathic Pain

Jordi Serra,[a] José Ochoa,[b,c] and Mario Campero[d]

[a]*Neuropathic Pain Unit, Sagrada Familia Clinic, Barcelona, Spain;*
[b]*Neuromuscular Unit, Good Samaritan Hospital and Medical Center,
Portland, Oregon, USA;* [c]*Oregon Health Sciences University, Portland,
Oregon, USA;* [d]*Department of Neurology, University of Chile,
Santiago, Chile*

According to the specificity theory, distinct somatic sensations are normally experienced when afferent impulses generated in the receptors of specific tactile, thermal, or nociceptor sensory units are transmitted to conscious levels (Sinclair 1967). Pain, as a normal sensory experience, reflects activation of particular centers of the sensing brain, including the somatosensory cortex and the prefrontal and limbic affective areas (Talbot et al. 1991; Derbyshire et al. 1994; Wall and Melzack 1994; Iadarola et al. 1998; Treede et al. 1999). Pain as an elementary sensation is naturally evoked by C or Aδ nociceptors without necessary contribution from low-threshold Aβ units (Ochoa and Torebjörk 1983, 1989; Macefield et al. 1990; Marchettini et al. 1996). C nociceptors receive noxious stimuli, transmit impulses decoded in the brain as pain sensation, and mediate neurogenic inflammation.

Recent scientific medical advances shed light on nociceptor function and disease and provide new methods for their investigation in man. These include: (a) identification of dedicated voltage- and heat-sensitive ion channels, and their blockers, in the excitable membranes of C nociceptor neurons (in animals), (b) biophysical differentiation of subtypes of human C units, (c) discovery of an "insensitive nociceptor" in humans, (d) characterization of receptor properties of C nociceptors from human muscle, (e) objective measurement through skin microdialysis or thermography of vascular responses to excitation of antidromic C nociceptors, (f) recognition of abnormal catecholamine sensitivity of surviving nociceptor axons in (animal) neuropathy, and (g) experimental endorsement of secondary central neuronal "wind-up" and sensitization (in animals).

NEUROPATHIC PAIN SYMPTOMS

Damage or dysfunction may affect the normal functioning of the nervous system in several different ways. According to Jackson (1932), nervous system dysfunction may cause both negative and positive phenomena (Table I). Negative symptoms and signs depend on the functional system affected, and include paralysis (motor system), hypoesthesias (somatosensory system), and hypohidrosis (autonomic system). Positive phenomena will also depend on the affected system, and may include fasciculations (motor system), paresthesias, pain (sensory system), or "goose bumps" (autonomic system). It is useful to use this approach when assessing patients suffering from neurological dysfunction, including patients with neuropathic pain. It is important to understand that neuropathic pain is not a disease itself, but only a symptom of neurological dysfunction. Therefore, it is mandatory that neuropathic pain patients be examined by physicians with a neurological background; a neurological examination must always be performed.

Neuropathic pain patients characteristically express a variety of positive and negative sensory and motor symptoms, as well as autonomic symptoms. Therefore, clinical evaluation must address all symptoms and not just the pain component. Some of these symptoms escape conventional medical examination, particularly the mapping and quantification of positive and negative sensory dysfunction. Sensory examination is time consuming, and requires special training and facilities that are not universally available to clinicians. Also, the use of sensory terms must be standardized, as many cultural and medical traditions give different meanings to similar words. According to the Taxonomy Task Force of the International Association for

Table I

Negative Phenomena	Positive Phenomena
Motor	
Paresia, paralysis	Myokymia, fasciculations, dystonia
Sensory	
Hypoesthesia, hypoalgesia, anosmia, blindness, deafness	Paresthesia, dysesthesia, pain, photopsia, tinnitus
Autonomic	
Vasodilation, hypo/anhidrosis	Vasoconstriction, hyperhidrosis, piloerection

the Study of Pain (Merskey and Bogduk 1994), the term *dysesthesia* is preferred to indicate an unpleasant, abnormal sensation, whether spontaneous or evoked. The term *paresthesia* is used to denote an abnormal sensation, whether spontaneous or evoked. Additionally, *hyperalgesia* refers to an increased response to a stimulus that is normally painful, and *allodynia* to pain due to a stimulus that does not normally provoke pain. These last two terms, *hyperalgesia* and *allodynia,* are used frequently, and most neuropathic pain patients present variable combinations of both symptoms, usually overlapping the same skin area. We believe that the term *allodynia* has led to confusion among clinicians and basic scientists because it is difficult to agree upon the definition of a "normally painful stimulus."

TYPES OF NEUROPATHIC PAIN SYMPTOMS

It is easy to envisage that when ectopic impulses are generated along a damaged large myelinated axon that maintains its connection to the sensing brain, the subject will predictably experience a tactile sensation in the absence of an actual skin stimulus; this is known as a tactile paresthesia. Following the same reasoning, ectopic impulse generation along nociceptor axons predictably results in the experience of pain. However, this apparent simplicity becomes blurred when dealing with patients, as they have difficulty in defining the sensory experience in terms of touch, pain, a combination of both, or unpleasantness. This difficulty in describing symptoms makes the study of neuropathic pain patients particularly complicated. When a patient describes a positive sensory symptom as painless, we may assume that ectopic impulses are being generated along non-nociceptor afferent axons (sensations of touch, warmth, cold, etc.). However, the opposite—that painful symptoms only stem from ectopic impulse generation along nociceptor axons—is not always true. Several experimental studies (nerve blocks, reaction times, etc.) seem to confirm that pain is sometimes experienced when large myelinated Aβ fibers are activated.

Different (and conflicting) pathophysiological mechanisms are proposed to explain this departure from the law of specificity. One theory is that central changes at the dorsal horn level cause sensitized wide-dynamic-range neurons to become activated by normally non-noxious Aβ impulses, resulting in pain (LaMotte et al. 1991; Simone et al. 1991; Torebjörk et al. 1992). These abnormal primary central mechanisms have been well rationalized but remain hypothetical for human disease (Boivie et al. 1989; Beric 1993). The other theory attempts to explain most positive sensory symptoms through the changes in excitability of the damaged axon (Ochoa 1985;

Campero et al. 1998). Proven primary peripheral sources of hyperalgesia and allodynia, accessible to testing in humans, include sensitization of nociceptor end organs (Ochoa 1986) and defective primary afferent modulation of coactivated nociceptor-thermoreceptor input causing central release of the nociceptor component (Craig and Bushnell 1994; Ochoa and Yarnitsky 1994) and abnormal afterdischarges in hyperexcitable peripheral axons (Campero et al. 1998).

SECONDARY SENSITIZATION OF CENTRAL NEURONS

Some investigators hypothesize that primary injury to peripheral nociceptors may cause chronic pain as a consequence of secondary central dysfunction of pain-signaling neurons in the dorsal horns and higher up (Hardy et al. 1952; Lindblom and Verrillo 1979; Wall 1984; Meyer et al. 1987; Torebjörk et al. 1992; Coderre and Katz 1997). This concept was entertained intuitively in the 1940s by clinicians who could not explain through the laws of nerve anatomy and physiology certain atypical and expansive neuropathic sensorimotor painful profiles (Evans 1946; Livingston 1947). During the past decade the concept has become revitalized through animal experiments demonstrating unquestionable temporary hyperexcitability of central sensory neurons following nerve irritation (Dickenson and Sullivan 1987; Dubner 1991; Woolf and Thompson 1991). While the experiments on central neuronal "wind-up" induced by primary nociceptor input are impeccable, it remains true that all of the typical sensorimotor dysfunction and pain caused by organic nerve injury, and the recovery course, can be explained by primary mechanisms (Head 1905). For that reason, secondary "centralization" as a hypothetical determinant of clinical dysfunction in neuropathic pain patients remains the favored explanation for nonanatomical and expansive sensorimotor profiles. Those painful profiles are preferentially displayed by patients who harbor little clinical or physiological evidence of dysfunction in their primary sensory or lower motor neurons, or in spinal reflex loops (Campero et al. 1992).

The concept that the larger area of "secondary hyperalgesia" induced experimentally by skin irritants is necessarily due to central neuronal changes is also in question because primary peripheral mechanisms may explain both the vascular flare and the sensory hyperalgesic phenomena within that area in human volunteers (Serra et al. 1998). The objective area of peripherally mediated flare coincides with the broad area of "secondary hyperalgesia," thus challenging the prevalent hypothesis. Preliminary studies in human subjects, applying nociceptor irritants while recording with microneurography, suggest that the psychophysical, presumed-to-be-secondary pains and hyperalgesias may be explained through sensitization of a subtype of nociceptor, the mechanically "insensitive" afferents (Serra et al. 1995; but see Schmelz et al. 1997). The issue remains unresolved.

CONCEPTUALIZING A NEUROPATHIC SYNDROME CAUSED BY CENTRAL RELEASE OF COLD PAIN

Application of a painless low-temperature stimulus to the skin activates cold-specific channels subserved by small-caliber myelinated fibers (MacKenzie et al. 1975; Adriaensen et al. 1983). For low-temperature stimuli of noxious intensity, simultaneous coactivation of nociceptor channels subserved by unmyelinated C polymodal nociceptors is believed to mediate the characteristic painful cold sensation (Torebjörk 1974; LaMotte and Thalhammer 1982; Saumet et al. 1985; Campero et al. 1996). For high-temperature stimuli of noxious intensity, activation of unmyelinated C polymodal nociceptors mediates the familiar burning pain sensation (Van Hees and Gybels 1981; Ochoa and Torebjörk 1989; Torebjörk and Ochoa 1990; Yarnitsky et al. 1992). In turn, noxious mechanical stimuli to skin normally evoke a sharp or dull burning pain devoid of any thermal quality. However, noxious mechanical stimulation of skin during differential nerve block that selectively spares C-fiber input in normal volunteers evokes delayed burning pain without a mechanical sharp or dull component (Hallin and Torebjörk 1976; Ochoa and Torebjörk 1989). Correspondingly, intraneural microstimulation of identified C nociceptors typically evokes burning pain after a relatively long reaction time; such pain is resistant to selective unmyelinated fiber block (Ochoa and Torebjörk 1989). Nevertheless, during noxious low-temperature stimulation of human skin, the normal subjective experience is cold pain rather than burning pain (Yarnitsky and Ochoa 1990).

Selective experimental blockade of cold-specific cutaneous input releases the magnitude of pain induced by noxious low temperature and changes its subjective quality into "a burn" (Yarnitsky and Ochoa 1990). This paradoxical phenomenon, like the thermal grill illusion of Thunberg (Craig and Bushnell 1994), is interpreted as due to central disinhibition or unmasking. The modulation normally exerted by cold-specific Aδ neural input upon the quality and magnitude of C-fiber-mediated pain (induced by low temperature) was found to be defective in certain patients with small-caliber fiber neuropathy. The abnormal condition is not related to etiology, but to pathophysiology. These patients typically express a combination of cold hyperalgesia (featuring a paradoxical burning quality), cold hypoesthesia, and cold skin (Ochoa and Yarnitsky 1994). The cutaneous hypothermia prevailing in symptomatic areas in these patients is due to vasospasm caused by partial sympathetic denervation supersensitivity secondary to unmyelinated fiber loss. The minimal requirement for spatial summation of painful input from polymodal nociceptors explains the prominence of nociceptor-mediated cold hyperalgesia, even with substantial loss of small-caliber fibers. The failing neural function follows a dynamic gradient along the limbs, in keeping with the "dying back" process. Indeed, proximally in the symptomatic limb, these patients display normal thresholds for cold pain and cold sensation, whereas in the symptomatic area there is cold hypoesthesia associated with cold hyperalgesia. Occasionally, distal to the hyperalgesic region there is global hypoesthesia and hypoalgesia. Descriptively this syndrome is the mirror image of erythralgia (erythromelalgia) or ABC syndrome (described below). Both syndromes emerge as independent clinical entities with definable ab-normal mechanisms that should be retrieved out of the all-embracing and purely descriptive diagnostic category of complex regional pain syndrome types I and II (CRPS-I, formerly called reflex sympathetic dystrophy, and CRPS-II, formerly causalgia).

MEMBRANE HYPEREXCITABILITY AS THE CAUSE
OF POSITIVE SENSORY SYMPTOMS

The basic function of axons is nerve conduction (Waxman 1986). For the system to be reliable, conduction must be accomplished both without loss and without gain. Impulse conduction without loss means that if a single action potential is generated at the receptor level, a single action potential must reach the spinal cord. If the impulse is lost during transmission, then a sensory deficit will occur. Impulse conduction without gain means that if a single action potential is generated at the receptor level, not more than one action potential reaches the spinal cord. Generation of extra impulses during transmission would distort the sensory message.

Axonal membrane hyperexcitability may lead to the generation of ec-topic impulses (Bostock et al. 1994) at the mid-axon level where the injury took place. Generation of ectopic impulses was also observed in the neu-ronal bodies of dorsal root ganglion cells whose peripheral axons had been damaged (Liu et al. 2000). Although several authors provide direct evidence that ectopic impulse generation does occur both in the experimental (Wall and Devor 1983; Baker and Bostock 1992; Tal et al. 1999) and the human setting (Ochoa and Torebjörk 1980; Nyström and Hagbarth 1981; Nordin et al. 1984; Campero et al. 1998), research has not traditionally focused on its basic underlying mechanisms. Additionally, until recently the pharmaceutical industry has shown little interest in generating new membrane-stabilizing agents.

The only available method to study ectopic impulse generation in human axons is microneurography. This method consists of the introduction of microelectrodes into the nerve of an awake, conscious person (Vallbo and Hagbarth 1973), allowing selective recordings from individual axons. In patients experiencing positive sensory symptoms, it is possible to record abnormal activity, similar to that reported in animals by Adrian (1930) in his article "The effects of injury on mammalian nerve fibers." It is clear that this spontaneous activity can account for spontaneous pain and paresthesias or dysesthesias, depending on the modality of the activated axon.

Another aspect of this increased excitability of nerve fibers in response to injury is that the nerve fibers generate ectopic impulses not only spontaneously, but also in response to mechanical deformation or to changes in the chemical environment surrounding the damaged axon (Devor 1994). Moreover, trains of impulses may be generated by a preceding impulse traveling along the damaged segment of axon. This phenomenon, called "afterdischarge" or "multiplication of impulses," has recently been well documented in animals (Burchiel 1980) and in human Aβ axons (Campero et al. 1998).

As previously mentioned, ectopic impulse activity arising in Aβ fibers will lead to the experience of tactile sensations, but under certain circumstances it will also evoke a sensory experience of pain. As stated above, this phenomenon poses an important question regarding somatosensory physiology because there appears to be an exception to the law of specificity. A clue is provided when we take into consideration the difficulty patients have in verbalizing the type of sensations they experience. Some of these patients have tactile allodynia—that is, very gentle touch stimuli are able to evoke what their examiners interpret as pain. However, when the symptom is investigated in more detail, interesting insight may emerge. For example, when mechanical stimuli above the touch threshold but below the known nociceptor receptor threshold are applied, the sensation described by patients is similar to that described in the postischemic paresthesia period after cuff deflation during nerve block experiments (J. Serra et al., unpublished observations). During the postischemic period, increased axonal membrane hyperexcitability results in chaotic spontaneous discharges and afterdischarges evoked by the passage of impulses through hyperexcitable segments of the axon (Ochoa and Torebjörk 1980). If the skin is touched at that moment, a strange, unpleasant sensation occurs as the consequence of the severe distortion of the natural spatiotemporal sequence of impulses reaching consciousness. Due to the fact that the resulting sensation is highly unpleasant, patients tend to describe it as pain. Therefore, it *is* pain, because it evokes suffering. However, this sensation of pain is not dependent on the activation of nociceptor pathways. This finding suggests that patients with nerve lesions in continuity have hyperexcitable axons that behave similarly to hyperexcitable axons of the postischemic period. This mechanism is what most likely occurs in patients with overt nerve injury, causalgia, and symptoms restricted to the distribution territory of the damaged nerve. Of course, the situation may be different in patients without nerve injury suffering from CRPS type I (reflex sympathetic dystrophy).

PRIMARY NOCICEPTORS AND NEUROPATHIC PAINS

The observations to be described below apply to common C polymodal nociceptors and, in our experience, also to "mechanically insensitive" or "silent" C nociceptors. Data on hyperexcitability of Aδ human nociceptors are apparently unavailable in published form. Microneurography combined with psychophysical and thermographic studies has provided evidence that sensitization of primary nociceptors may explain a spectrum of positive sensory and antidromic vasomotor symptoms (Cline and Ochoa 1986; Cline et al. 1989). The criteria for sensitization under these circumstances include abnormal reduction of the receptor threshold and/or abnormal spontaneous or stimulus-induced afferent discharge.

Clinical and experimental observations on polymodal hyperalgesia and cross-modality threshold modulation in patients and volunteers allowed our group to conceptualize a clinical condition caused by sensitization of primary peripheral nociceptors: the ABC syndrome (Cline et al. 1989). This syndrome is seen in a subgroup of patients with neuropathy, but not commonly. Its prevalence remains to be established. One key clinical feature of sensitization of C polymodal nociceptors is the rubor or erythema of the symptomatic parts, which led Lewis (1936) to term this condition *erythralgia*. The underlying vasodilatation is active, rather than an expression of sympathetic vasoparalysis. Sensitization of primary nociceptors has been recorded as the cause of a combined neurosensory and neurovascular painful syndrome in diabetic neuropathy, in which afferent nerve impulses multiply in response to finite receptor stimulation. This feature partially fits not only the concept of hyperalgesia but also that of "hyperpathia" (Merskey and Bogduk 1994). Such receptor-response anomaly is not necessarily associated with reduced receptor threshold of the C nociceptor.

In the case of the patient reported in detail by Cline et al. (1989), spontaneous discharge of C nociceptors was not a feature. In that patient the

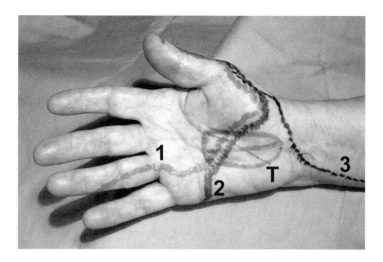

Fig. 1. Mapping of the sensory dysfunction in the hand of a 62-year-old patient with a lesion of the right median and ulnar nerves. The median nerve was injured at the palm level during local surgery for a Dupuytren's contracture. Ulnar nerve entrapment at the elbow level had been present for several months prior to surgery. There is a combination of negative and positive sensory symptoms in the distribution territory of both nerves. 1 = static mechanical hyperalgesia in the median nerve territory, but not in that of the ulnar nerve; 2 = dynamic mechanical hyperalgesia in the median nerve territory and part of the ulnar nerve territory; 3 = touch *hypo*esthesia in the ulnar territory, and touch *an*esthesia in the median territory; T (crossed circle) = Tinel's sign projecting a dysesthetic sensation to fingers 2 and 3, where spontaneous pain was experienced with more intensity, as reported by the patient.

striking abnormalities were reduction of receptor threshold to normally non-noxious levels and prolonged afterdischarges evoked by brief mechanical stimuli. More interestingly, in a recent reported case of erythralgia (Ochoa et al. 2001), microneurography documented ectopic impulse generation in the most distal parts of cutaneous C nociceptors. Microneurography with latency tracking of identified single C nociceptors supplying symptomatic skin (see Serra et al. 1999) revealed evidence of their spontaneous firing and abnormal afterdischarges. Preliminary immunological testing showed cross-reactivity when Western blots containing extracts from VR1-expressing fibroblasts were probed with the patient's serum.

Hyperexcitability of primary C nociceptors carries predictable clinical cognitive correlates. The pathologically prolonged aftersensation of pain is obviously determined by the abnormally prolonged nociceptor afterdischarge. Duration of the afterdischarges matches duration of the hyperalgesic pain, as delineated through the use of a manual analogue device. Another obvious clinical correlate of C nociceptor hyperexcitability obtains for mechanical hyperalgesia: gentle natural mechanical stimuli can activate nociceptors and evoke pain at abnormally low thresholds. The mechanical hyperalgesia determined by sensitized C nociceptors is of the "static" subtype (Ochoa and Yarnitsky 1993). This kind of hyperalgesia has a typical dull or burning painful quality and resists selective A-fiber blockade. The clinical-pathophysiological profile of this kind of hyperalgesia is quite distinct from the "dynamic," "allodynic" subtype of mechanical hyperalgesia.

It is logically anticipated that sensitization of polymodal nociceptors should determine not only static mechanical hyperalgesia but also hyperalgesia to heat and to low temperature. Heat hyperalgesia is indeed a key feature of the human syndrome determined by sensitization of C nociceptors. It is for that reason that this hyperalgesic state was termed *polymodal hyperalgesia* (Culp et al. 1989). Cold hyperalgesia does not emerge as an issue in the context of sensitized C nociceptors for the simple reason that application of low temperature to symptomatic body parts soothes the painful symptoms. This phenomenon has been called *cross-modality receptor threshold modulation*. This term describes relief of both pain and mechanical hyperalgesia by passive cooling of the symptomatic parts (during differential block of tactile and cold-specific input). Increasing the temperature of those parts worsens pain and mechanical hyperalgesia. This striking influence of temperature has been construed as a clinical sign of nociceptor sensitization (Cline et al. 1989) and is taken to reflect modulation of biophysical properties of the excitable membrane of polymodal nociceptors (Culp et al. 1989). We have also observed that, through a cooling effect, sympathetically mediated vasoconstriction also relieves polymodal hyperalgesia. However, by virtue of the theoretical principle of cross-modality threshold modulation, there would exist a critical level below which low temperature no longer soothes but evokes pain in patients with sensitized C-polymodal nociceptors. Lewis (1936) wrote: "cooling abolishes the pain unless a low temperature is reached ... ice gives pain, indistinguishable from that induced by heat."

CLASSIFICATION OF NOCICEPTORS

To date, the only accepted method for classifying human afferent C fibers has been by studying the receptor properties of axons. Conduction velocity distinguishes between myelinated and unmyelinated axons and among different classes of myelinated axons, but has provided no useful subdivision of unmyelinated axons (Lynn 1994), although "itch" fibers have recently been reported to conduct more slowly than other C fibers (Schmelz et al. 1997). During electrophysiological studies both in vitro and in vivo, it is desirable to be able to distinguish between different classes of C fibers without having to study the properties of their receptors. This is particularly true for insensitive units, which represent a significant percentage in both animals and in humans (Meyer et al. 1991; Davis et al. 1993; Schmidt et al. 1995), because they may be either normal unresponsive afferent C units or sympathetic efferent axons.

Repetitive firing in axons can lead to subexcitability and reduced conduction velocity due to prolonged hyperpolarization (Gasser 1935; Bergmans 1970; Bostock and Grafe 1985). Such activity-dependent changes in membrane potential and conduction velocity are much more pronounced in unmyelinated fibers than in myelinated ones (Ritchie and Straub 1957; Grafe et al. 1997), and have been used in microneurographic recordings from humans as a "marking" technique for C fibers activated by natural stimuli (Hallin and Torebjörk 1974; Torebjörk 1974; Schmelz et al. 1995). Most of these studies have implicitly assumed that all C fibers slow to a similar degree when challenged with repetitive stimulation. However, recent evidence from animal studies shows that C fibers segregate into discrete groups when stimulated repetitively, and that these differences may be used to classify the submodality of fiber. Thalhammer and colleagues (1994), in a study of A and C fibers in the rat sciatic nerve, demonstrated that C nociceptors show a greater degree of activity-dependent slowing than do cold-specific C fibers. Gee and colleagues (1996) have confirmed these results, and shown that this differential behavior in response to repetitive stimulation may be used to separate afferent and nonafferent populations of unexcitable C fibers. Human C fibers can be segregated into at least three different classes based on their response to repetitive stimulation, and it is possible unambiguously to differentiate nociceptive from cold-specific C fibers innervating human skin. Therefore, activity-dependent slowing on electrical stimulation, both at 2 Hz (Serra et al. 1999) and at low frequencies (Weidner et al. 1999), can provide a means of classifying C fibers that relate to function (Fig. 2). Application of this method to disease states promises new discoveries about pathophysiological mechanisms.

VASCULAR REACTIONS INDUCED BY ANTIDROMIC EXCITATION OF C NOCICEPTORS, AND THEIR INTERACTIONS WITH SYMPATHETIC VASOMOTOR RESPONSES

Antidromically triggered vasodilatation is a well known event (see, for example, Stricker 1876; Bayliss 1901; Langley 1923; Hinsey and Gasser 1930; Lewis 1937; Chapman et al. 1961). Not surprisingly, electrical stimulation of

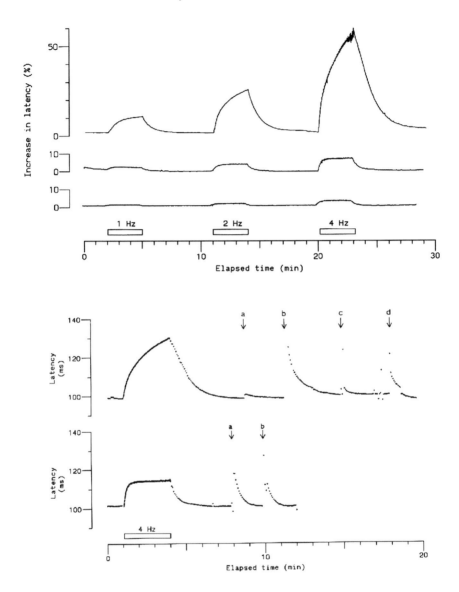

Fig. 2. *Upper panel:* Examples of three types of response to a standard repetitive stimulation protocol. Latencies were tracked during 3-minute periods of stimulation at 1, 2, and 4 Hz, separated by 6-minute periods at 0.25 Hz. From top to bottom: Type 1 units progressively increase in latency and often block, Type 2 units soon reach a plateau, while Type 3 units change little in latency (<2% at 2 Hz). *Lower panel:* "Marking" of units by natural stimulation, compared with responses to repetitive stimulation at 4 Hz. *Top:* A Type 1 unit is stimulated at *a* by a metal rod (at 25°C), at *b* by ice, at *c* by a von Frey hair (6.65 VF), and at *d* by heating to 48°C for 5 s. *Bottom:* A Type 2 unit is excited at *a* and *b* by a metal rod (at 25°C), confirming that it is a "cold" fiber. Rates of recovery after natural stimulation resemble those after repetitive electrical stimulation. From Serra et al. (1999).

the peripheral end of freshly divided nerve roots in humans elicits rubor in dermatomal distribution (Foerster 1933). This chemically based vasodilator reaction, eventually attributed to neurosecretion of substance P, is believed today to be largely mediated by CGRP (Brain and Escott 1994). Prolonged repetitive electrical microstimulation at painful intensities of nerve fascicles projecting to the hand consistently elicits warming of coherent districts of the skin. This is precisely and sensitively detected by thermography (Ochoa et al. 1987).

This regional warming is most likely antidromic because it is not abolished after postganglionic sympathetic denervation of human skin, which rules out the possibility that it might be due to temporary use-dependent blockade of sympathetic efferent vasoconstrictor fibers (Ochoa et al. 1987). The cutaneous receptive field for the nerve fascicle being stimulated matches the discrete territory of skin that displays the antidromic vasodilator phenomenon. This good match provides neuroanatomical evidence that C-nociceptor units contained in individual nerve fascicles are distributed into well-defined partial somatotopic domains within the total nerve territory.

Striking and possibly clinically relevant interactions occur between orthodromic sympathetic vasoconstrictor and antidromic vasodilator effects of C-fiber stimulation. During high-intensity intraneural stimulation, when both sympathetic and somatic systems are coactivated, skin temperature becomes decreased diffusely in the tested limb. This response occurs because reflex sympathetic vasoconstriction overrides the coactivated antidromic vasodilator effect induced by stimulation of C nociceptors. After termination of the stimulus the skin temperature increases regionally, within the territory of the stimulated fascicle. Upon renewed stimulation, the regional warming induced by antidromic neurosecretion from C nociceptors is again rapidly erased (Ochoa et al. 1993). The fact that both sympathetic vasomotor and antidromic sensory mechanisms may determine changes in color and temperature of the skin is clinically relevant. There exist interesting medical conditions of neuropathic origin that feature prominent deviations of skin temperature, such as erythralgia (Lewis 1936), the ABC syndrome (Ochoa 1986), the triple cold syndrome (Ochoa and Yarnitsky 1994), and the heterogeneous "reflex sympathetic dystrophy" (Bonica 1979). Thus it is useful from the diagnostic point of view to remain aware that "neuropathic" painful syndromes associated with vascular phenomena need not necessarily imply sympathetic pathophysiology.

It has been assumed that the neurovascular apparatus and the operant mechanism responsible for antidromically induced vasodilatation of human skin are identical to those responsible for local vasodilatation in response to substances that cause neurogenic inflammation and sensitization of nociceptors. Recent evidence supports the concept that flare and antidromic vasodilatation may have different mechanisms (Serra et al. 1994a, 1998). Langley (1921) suggested that the neural system responsible for the flare response that follows noxious stimulation of the skin is the same system responsible for the antidromic vasodilatation. However, Lewis (1937) cautioned: "When both posterior root vasodilatation and flare were thought to depend on sensory nerves, one system for the two reactions was a natural conception; but the identity of the nerves underlying these two reactions has not been proved." It is known that the skin flush that follows antidromic stimulation is due to capillary dilatation with no intervention of deeper arterioles, as it persists after the aorta is clamped (Langley 1923). Recent histophysiological experiments also suggest that antidromic vasodilatation is a vascular effect primarily at the "minute" vessel level (Kenins 1984; Bharali and Lisney 1992). On the other hand, the flare response is entirely an arteriolar phenomenon (Lewis 1927; Serra et al. 1994b). Antidromic stimulation would activate unmyelinated nociceptor axons and would trigger antidromic release of substances capable of inducing plasma extravasation and visible capillary flushing. In contrast, activation of the neural system mediating the flare response would trigger arteriolar vasodilatation and secondary flushing in a wide area surrounding the injury site. In the clinical context, antidromic vasodilatation is defective or absent in patients who have lost peripheral unmyelinated axons. This is the likely reason why the flare response becomes sluggish with age (Helme et al. 1985).

VASCULAR AND SENSORY REACTIONS OF THE SKIN INDUCED BY LOCAL ADMINISTRATION OF SUBSTANCES THAT EXCITE OR SENSITIZE NOCICEPTORS

Following intradermal injection of the irritant capsaicin, flare and hyperalgesia may develop in a broad surrounding area. The neurogenic flare mechanism is resolved locally in the skin (Lewis 1927) and may spread through local axon reflexes involving C-polymodal nociceptors (Szolcsányi 1992). However, the hypothetical existence of a distinct subset of "nocifensor" nerve fibers specifically arranged for the flare reaction (Lewis 1937) remains viable. In addition to the flare, cutaneous hyperalgesia develops surrounding the injection site (Simone et al. 1989, LaMotte et al. 1991; Torebjörk et al. 1992). A distinction has been made between the hyperalgesia that appears at the site of cutaneous injury, "erythralgia" (Lewis 1942) or primary hyperalgesia (Hardy et al. 1952), and the hyperalgesia beyond it, "nocifensor tenderness" (Lewis 1942) or secondary hyperalgesia (Hardy et al. 1952). Secondary hyperalgesia has been characterized as occurring only in response to mechanical stimuli, without associated heat hyperalgesia (Raja et al. 1984; LaMotte et al. 1991; Ali et al. 1996). There is general agreement that primary hyperalgesia is due to sensitization of cutaneous nociceptor terminals (LaMotte et al. 1982, 1992; Campbell and Meyer 1983; LaMotte et al. 1983; Torebjörk et al. 1984).

Failure to detect sensitization in common C-polymodal nociceptors in the area of secondary hyperalgesia during capsaicin experiments in animals or humans (Baumann et al. 1991; LaMotte 1992; Schmelz et al. 1996) has led to the proposition that secondary hyperalgesia might be mediated by dorsal horn neurons previously sensitized by a C-nociceptor afferent barrage (LaMotte et al. 1991; Simone et al. 1991; Torebjörk et al. 1992). However, recent experiments (Serra et al. 1998) using dynamic telethermography prove that following capsaicin injection, the flare response occurs over an area much larger than usually detected by visual inspection or by laser Doppler blood flow measurement (Fig. 3). Such flare reflects underlying arteriolar dilatation and extends into the area commonly considered to be that in which "secondary" hyperalgesia occurs (Serra et al. 1993). In this

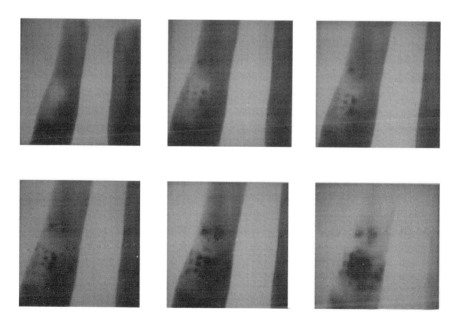

Fig. 3. Typical spatiotemporal development of a flare following capsaicin injection in the anterior forearm (100 μg in 10 μL), as recorded with infrared telethermography. Discrete multifocal areas of increased skin temperature, reflecting dilatation of cutaneous arterioles, appeared in a wide area (black = high temperature, white = low temperature). Reprinted from Serra et al. (1998).

area, pain thresholds are lowered and pain magnitude estimations are increased for punctate mechanical stimuli. For heat hyperalgesia, threshold values are little changed, but heat hyperalgesia is evident for suprathreshold stimuli. The broad area of heat hyperalgesia can be delineated only by delivering stimuli well above pain threshold. Increased pain response to heat stimuli in the area of secondary hyperalgesia was unambiguously described by Hardy et al. (1952).

The most striking findings of experiments by Serra et al. (1993, 1994b, 1998) are that the area of punctate mechanical hyperalgesia precisely matches the area of heat hyperalgesia, and that both match the very large area of flare. Such matching was well described by Lewis (1935–1936) and has significant implications. Even if nociceptive input to the dorsal horn might follow some somatotopic order (Bullit 1991), such input, if pathogenetic, could not be so accurate as to result in sensitization of precisely those dorsal horn neurons whose receptive fields match a remote local vascular process of the skin. It is more logical to envisage this vascular-sensory matching as the consequence of related mechanisms resolved at a peripheral level. However, it still remains to be established how flare and hyperalgesia are linked.

Although the common C-polymodal nociceptor does not change its properties in the area of secondary hyperalgesia (Baumann et al. 1991; LaMotte et al. 1992; Schmelz et al. 1996), this need not imply that secondary hyperalgesia cannot be due to sensitization of peripheral units. Recently discovered "silent" C or Aδ nociceptor units that become active during inflammation (Davis et al. 1993; Schmelz et al. 2000) might be likely subsets of peripheral nociceptors responsible for signaling secondary hyperalgesia. To the best of our knowledge the behavior of these units has not been reported in areas of secondary hyperalgesia. A previous study (Serra et al. 1993) and a recent study in human volunteers (J. Serra et al., unpublished observations) identified peripheral units fulfilling the criteria for "silent" nociceptors whose receptors become sensitized in the area of secondary hyperalgesia. They engage in spontaneous activity and display significant reduction of receptor threshold or enhanced firing in response to mechanical or heat stimuli. This type of "silent" nociceptor, which becomes sensitized during inflammation, probably contributes to the pathophysiology of secondary hyperalgesia. Injection of capsaicin aimed at the receptive field of primary nociceptor endings within human skeletal muscle may also sensitize those nociceptors (Simone et al. 1992).

In summary, peripheral nociceptors undoubtedly play a critical primary role in determining neuropathic pains in humans, and it will suit patients if science and industry prioritize research on primary nociceptor malfunction and its treatment.

ACKNOWLEDGMENT

Many thanks to Dr. Cristina Quiles for her encouragement and constant support in the creation of this chapter.

REFERENCES

Adriaensen H, Gybels J, Handwerker HO, Van Hees J. Response properties of thin myelinated (A-δ) fibers in human skin nerves. *J Neurophysiol* 1983; 49:111–122.

Adrian ED. The effects of injury on mammalian nerve fibres. *Proc R Soc Lond* 1930; 106:596–618.

Ali Z, Meyer RA, Campbell JN. Secondary hyperalgesia to mechanical but not to heat stimuli following a capsaicin injection in hairy skin. *Pain* 1996; 68:401–411.

Baker M, Bostock H. Ectopic activity in demyelinated spinal root axons of the rat. *J Physiol* 1992; 451:539–552.

Baumann TK, Simone DA, Shain CN, LaMotte RH. Neurogenic hyperalgesia: the search for the primary cutaneous afferent fibers that contribute to capsaicin-induced pain and hyperalgesia. *J Neurophysiol* 1991; 66:212–227.

Bayliss WM. On the origin from the spinal cord of the vasodilator fibres of the hind limb, and the nature of these fibres. *J Physiol* 1901; 26:173–209.

Bergmans J. *The Physiology of Single Human Nerve Fibres.* University of Louvain, 1970.

Beric A. Transcranial electrical and magnetic stimulation. *Adv Neurol* 1993; 63:29–42.

Bharali LA, Lisney SJ. The relationship between unmyelinated afferent type and neurogenic plasma extravasation in normal and reinnervated rat skin. *Neuroscience* 1992; 47:703–712.

Boivie J, Leijon G, Johansson I. Central post-stroke pain—a study of the mechanisms through analyses of the sensory abnormalities. *Pain* 1989; 37:173–185.

Bonica JJ. Causalgia and other reflex sympathetic dystrophies. In: Bonica JJ, Liebeskind JC, Albé-Fessard DJ (Eds). *Proceedings of the Second World Congress on Pain,* Advances in Pain Research and Therapy, Vol. 3. New York: Raven Press, 1979, pp 141–166.

Bostock H, Gafe P. Activity-dependent excitability changes in normal and demyelinated rat spinal root axons. *J Physiol* 1985; 365:229–257.

Bostock H, Burke D, Hales JP. Differences in behaviour of sensory and motor axons following release of ischemia. *Brain* 1994; 117:225–234.

Brain SD, Escott KJ. Calcitonine-gene related peptide. *Agents Actions* 1994; 41:C262–263.

Bullit E. Somatotopy of spinal nociceptive processing. *J Comp Neurol* 1991; 321:279–290.

Burchiel K. Abnormal impulse generation in focally demyelinated trigeminal roots. *J Neurosurg* 1980; 53:674–683.

Campbell JN, Meyer RA. Sensitization of unmyelinated nociceptive afferents in monkey varies with skin type. *J Neurophysiol* 1983; 49:98–110.

Campero M, Ochoa J, Pubols L. Receptive fields of hyperalgesia confined to districts of injured nerves; fields "expand" in "RSD" without nerve injury. *Soc Neurosci Abstracts* 1992; 18:287.

Campero M, Serra J, Ochoa J. Stimulus-response properties of C polymodal nociceptors activated by noxious low temperature in humans. *J Physiol* 1996, 497:565–572.

Campero M, Serra J, Marchettini P, Ochoa JL. Ectopic impulse generation and autoexcitation in single myelinated afferent fibers in patients with peripheral neuropathy and positive sensory symptoms. *Muscle Nerve* 1998; 21:1661–1667.

Chapman LF, Ramos AO, Goodell H. Neurohumoral features of afferent fibers in man. *Arch Neurol* 1961; 4:617–650.

Cline M, Ochoa JL. Chronically sensitized C nociceptors in skin: patient with hyperalgesia, hyperpathia and spontaneous pain. *Soc Neurosci Abstracts* 1986; 12:331.

Cline MA, Ochoa JL, Torebjörk HE. Chronic hyperalgesia and skin warming caused by sensitized C nociceptors. *Brain* 1989; 112:621.

Coderre TJ, Katz J. Peripheral and central hyperexcitability: differential signs and symptoms in persistent pain. *Behav Brain Sci* 1997; 20:404–419.

Craig AD, Bushnell MC. The thermal grill illusion: unmasking the burn of cold pain. *Science* 1994; 265:252–255.

Culp WJ, Ochoa JL, Cline MA, Dotson R. Heat and mechanical hyperalgesia induced by capsaicin: cross modality threshold modulation in human C nociceptors. *Brain* 1989; 112:1317.

Davis KD, Meyer RA, Campbell JN. Chemosensitivity and sensitization of nociceptive afferents that innervate the hairy skin of monkey. *J Neurophysiol* 1993; 69:1071.

Derbyshire SW, Jones AK, Devani P, et al. Cerebral responses to pain in patients with atypical facial pain measured by positron emission tomography. *J Neurol Neurosurg Psychiatry* 1994; 57:1166–1172.

Devor M. The pathophysiology of damaged peripheral nerves. In: Wall PD, Melzack R (Eds). *Textbook of Pain*. Edinburgh: Churchill Livingstone, 1994, pp 79–100.

Dickenson AH, Sullivan AF. Peripheral origins and central modulation of subcutaneous formalin-induced activity of rat dorsal horn neurones. *Neurosci Lett* 1987; 16:207–211.

Dubner R. Pain and hyperalgesia following tissue injury: new mechanisms and new treatment. *Pain* 1991; 44:213–214.

Evans JA. Reflex sympathetic dystrophy. *Surg Clin North Am* 1946; 26:780–790.

Foerster O. The dermatomes in man. *Brain* 1933; 56:1–39.

Gasser HS. Changes in nerve potentials produced by rapidly repeated stimuli and their relation to the responsiveness of nerve to stimulation. *Am J Physiol* 1935; 111:35–50.

Gee MD, Lynn B, Cotsell B. Activity-dependent slowing of conduction velocity provides a method for identifying different functional classes of C-fibre in the rat saphenous nerve. *Neuroscience* 1996; 73:667–675.

Grafe P, Quasthoff S, Grosskreutz J, Alzheimer C. Function of the hyperpolarization-activated inward rectification in nonmyelinated peripheral rat and human axons. *J Neurophysiol* 1997; 77:421–426.

Hallin RG, Torebjörk HE. Methods to differentiate electrically induced afferent and sympathetic C unit responses in human cutaneous nerves. *Acta Physiol Scand* 1974; 92:318–331.

Hallin RG, Torebjörk HE. Studies on cutaneous A and C fibre afferents, skin nerve blocks and perception. In: Zottermann Y (Ed). *Sensory Functions of the Skin in Primates, with Special Reference to Man*, Wennert-Gren International Symposium, Vol. 27. Oxford: Pergamon Press, 1976, pp 137–149.

Hardy JD, Wolff HG, Goodell H. *Pain Sensations and Reactions*. Baltimore: Williams & Wilkins, 1952.

Head H, Sherren J. The consequences of injury to the peripheral nerves in man. *Brain* 1905; 28:1–224.

Helme RD, McKernan S. Neurogenic flare responses following topical application of capsaicin in humans. *Ann Neurol* 1985; 18:505–509.

Hinsey JC, Gasser HS. The component of the dorsal root mediated vasodilatation and the Sherrington contracture. *Am J Physiol* 1930; 92:679–689.

Iadarola MJ, Berman KF, Zeffiro TA, et al. Neural activation during acute capsaicin-evoked pain and allodynia assessed with PET. *Brain* 1998; 121:931–947.

Jackson JH. Evolution and dissolution of the nervous system (Croonian Lecture). In: *Selected Writings of John Hughlings Jackson*, Vol. 2. London: Hodder and Stoughton, 1932.

Kenins P. Electrophysiological and histological studies of vascular permeability after antidromic sensory nerve stimulation. In: Chahl LA, Szolcsányi J, Lembek F (Eds). *Antidromic Vasodilatation and Neurogenic Inflammation*. Budapest: Akadémiae Kiadó, 1984, pp 175–191.

LaMotte RH, Thalhammer JG. Response properties of high-threshold cutaneous cold receptors in the primate. *Brain Res* 1982; 244:279–287.

LaMotte RH, Thalhammer JG, Torebjörk H-E, Robinson CJ. Peripheral neural mechanisms of cutaneous hyperalgesia following mild injury by heat. *J Neurosci* 1982; 2:765–781.

LaMotte RH, Thalhammer JG, Robinson CJ. Peripheral neural correlates of magnitude of cutaneous pain and hyperalgesia: a comparison of neural events in monkey with sensory events in humans. *J Neurophysiol* 1983; 50:1–26.

LaMotte RH, Shain CN, Simone DA, Tsai, E-FP. Neurogenic hyperalgesia: psychophysical studies of underlying mechanisms. *J Neurophysiol* 1991; 66:190–211.

LaMotte RH, Lundberg LER, Torebjörk H-E. Pain, hyperalgesia and activity in nociceptive C units in humans after intradermal injection of capsaicin. *J Neurophysiol* 1992; 448:749.

Langley JN. *The Autonomic Nervous System.* London: Cambridge University Press, 1921.

Langley JN. Antidromic action. Part I. *J Physiol* 1923; 57:428–446.

Lewis T. *The Blood Vessels of the Human Skin and Their Responses.* London: Shaw and Sons, 1927.

Lewis T. Experiments relating to cutaneous hyperalgesia and its spread through somatic nerves. *Clin Sci* 1935–1936; 2:373–421.

Lewis T. *Vascular Disorders of Limb Described for Practitioners and Students.* New York: Macmillan, 1936.

Lewis T. The nocifensor system of nerves and its reactions. Lecture II. *BMJ* 1937; 1:491–494.

Lewis T. *Pain.* London: MacMillan Press, 1942.

Lindblom U, Verrillo RT. Sensory functions in chronic neuralgia. *J Neurol Neurosurg Psychiatry* 1979; 42:422–435.

Liu CN, Wall PD, Ben-Dor E, et al. Tactile allodynia in the absence of C-fiber activation: altered firing properties of DRG neurons following spinal nerve injury. *Pain* 2000; 85:503–521.

Livingston WK. In: *Pain Mechanisms.* New York: Macmillan, 1947.

Lynn B. The fibre composition of cutaneous nerves and the classification and response properties of cutaneous afferents, with particular reference to nociception. *Pain Rev* 1994; 1:172–183.

Macefield G, Gandevia SC, Burke D. Perceptual responses to microstimulation of single afferents innervating joints, muscles and skin of the human hand. *J Physiol* 1990; 429:113–129.

MacKenzie RA, Burke D, Skuse NF, Lethlean K. Fibre function and perception during cutaneous nerve block. *J Neurol Neurosurg Psychiatry* 1975; 38:865–873.

Marchettini P, Simone DA, Caputi G, Ochoa JL. Pain from excitation of identified muscle nociceptors in humans. *Brain Res* 1996; 740:109–116.

Merskey H, Bogduk N. *Classification of Chronic Pain: Description of Chronic Pain Syndromes and Definition of Pain Terms.* Seattle: IASP Press, 1994.

Meyer RA, Campbell JN, Raja SN. Hyperalgesia following peripheral nerve injury. In: Pubols LM, Sessle BJ (Eds). *Effects of Injury on Trigeminal and Spinal Somatosensory Systems.* New York: Allan R. Liss, 1987, pp 383–388.

Meyer RA, Cohen RH, Davis KD, Treede R-D, Campbell JN. Evidence for cutaneous afferents that are insensitive to mechanical stimuli. In: *Proceedings of the VIth World Congress on Pain.* Amsterdam: Elsevier Science, 1991, pp 71–75.

Nordin M, Nyström B, Wallin U, Hagbarth KE. Ectopic sensory discharges and paresthesias in patients with disorders of peripheral nerves, dorsal roots and dorsal columns. *Pain* 1984; 20:231–245.

Nyström B, Hagbarth KE. Microelectrode recordings from transected nerves in amputees with phantom limb pain. *Neurosci Lett* 1981; 27:211–216.

Ochoa J. Pain and paresthesia from neuropathy: intraneural microrecordings and microstimulation studies and a proposed strategy for pathophysiological assessment. In: Delwaide PJ (Ed). *Clinical Neurophysiology in Peripheral Neuropathies.* Amsterdam: Elsevier Science, 1985.

Ochoa JL. The newly recognized painful ABC syndrome: thermographic aspects. *Thermology* 1986; 2:65.

Ochoa JL, Torebjörk HE. Paresthesiae from ectopic impulse generation in human sensory nerves. *Brain* 1980; 103:835–853.

Ochoa J, Torebjörk E. Sensations evoked by intraneural microstimulation of single mechanore-ceptor units innervating the human hand. *J Physiol* 1983; 342:633–654.

Ochoa JL, Torebjörk K-E. Sensations evoked by intraneural microstimulation of C nociceptor fibres in human skin nerves. *J Physiol* 1989; 415:583–599.

Ochoa JL, Yarnitsky D. Mechanical hyperalgesias in neuropathic pain patients: dynamic and static subtypes. *Ann Neurol* 1993; 33:465.

Ochoa JL, Yarnitsky D. The triple cold "CCC": cold hyperalgesia, cold hypoesthesia and cold skin in peripheral nerve disease. *Brain* 1994; 117:185–197.

Ochoa JL, Comstock WJ, Marchettini P, Nizamuddin G. Intrafascicular nerve stimulation elicits regional skin warming that matches the projected field of evoked pain. In: Schmidt RF, Schaible H-G, Vahle-Hinz C (Eds). *Fine Afferent Nerve Fibers and Pain*. Weinheim: VCH, 1987, pp 476–479.

Ochoa J, Bostock H, Serra J, Campero M, Oger J. Painful neuropathy attributable to human C nociceptors turned hyperexcitable through autoimmune disruption of the VR1 membrane receptor. *Peripheral Nerve Society Abstract Book*, Austria, 2001, in press.

Raja SN, Campbell JN, Meyer RA. Evidence for different mechanisms of primary and secondary hyperalgesia following heat injury to the glabrous skin. *Brain* 1984; 107:1179–1188.

Ritchie JM, Straub RW. The hyperpolarization which follows activity in mammalian non-medullated fibres. *J Physiol* 1957; 136:80–97.

Saumet JL, Chery-Croze S, Duclaux R. Response of cat skin mechanothermal nociceptors to cold stimulation. *Brain Res Bull* 1985; 15:529–532.

Schmidt R, Schmelz M, Forster C, et al. Novel classes of responsive and unresponsive c nociceptors in human skin. *J Neurosci* 1995; 15:333–341.

Schmelz M, Forster C, Schmidt R, et al. Delayed responses to electrical stimuli reflect C-fiber responsiveness in human microneurography. *Exp Brain Res* 1995; 104:331–336.

Schmelz M, Schmidt R, Ringkamp M, et al. Limitation of sensitisation to injured parts of receptive fields in human skin C-nociceptors. *Exp Brain Res* 1996; 109:141–147.

Schmelz M, Schmidt R, Bickel A, Handwerker HO, Torebjörk HE. Specific C-receptors for itch in human skin. *J Neurosci* 1997; 17:8003–8008.

Schmelz M, Schmid(t?) R, Handwerker HO, Torebjörk HE. Encoding of burning pain from capsaicin-treated human skin in two categories of unmyelinated nerve fibres. *Brain* 2000; 123:560–571.

Serra J, Campero M, Ochoa J. "Secondary" hyperalgesia (capsaicin) mediated by C-nociceptors. *Soc Neurosci Abstracts* 1993; 19:965.

Serra J, Campero M, Ochoa JL. Common peripheral mechanism for neurogenic flare and hyperalgesia (capsaicin) in human skin. *Muscle Nerve* 1994a; (Suppl 1):S250

Serra J, Campero M, Ochoa JL. Mechanisms of neurogenic flare in human skin. *J Neurol* 1994b; 241, S34.

Serra J, Campero M, Ochoa J. Sensitization of "silent" C-nociceptors in areas of secondary hyperalgesia (SH) in humans. *Neurology* 1995; 45:A365.

Serra J, Campero M, Ochoa J. Flare and hyperalgesia after intradermal capsaicin injection in human skin. *J Neurophysiol* 1998; 80:2801–2810.

Serra J, Campero M, Ochoa J, Bostock H. Activity-dependent slowing of conduction differenti-ates functional subtypes of C fibres innervating human skin. *J Physiol* 1999; 515:799–811.

Simone DA, Baumann TK, LaMotte RH. Dose-dependent pain and mechanical hyperalgesia in humans after intradermal injection of capsaicin. *Pain* 1989; 38:99–107.

Simone DA, Sorkin LS, Oh U, et al. Neurogenic hyperalgesia: central neural correlates in responses of spinothalamic tract neurons. *J Neurophysiol* 1991; 66:228–246.

Simone D, Caputi G, Marchettini P, Ochoa J. Cramping pain and deep hyperalgesia following intramuscular injection of capsaicin. *Soc Neurosci Abstracts* 1992; 18:134.

Sinclair D. The major theories. In: Sinclair D (Ed). *Cutaneous Sensation*. London: Oxford University Press, 1967, pp 3–18.

Stricker S. Untersuchungen über die Geffässnerven-Wurzeln des Ischiadicus. *Sitzungsberitche der Kaiserlichen Akademie Wissenchaften (Wien)* 1876; 3:173.

Szolcsányi J, Pintér E, Pethö G. Role of unmyelinated afferents in regulation of microcirculation and its chronic distortion after trauma and damage. In: Jänig W, Schmidt RF (Eds). *Reflex Sympathetic Dystrophy, Pathophysiological Mechanisms and Clinical Implications.* Weinheim: VCH, 1992, pp 245–261.

Tal M, Wall PD, Devor M. Myelinated afferent fiber types that become spontaneously active and mechanosensitive following nerve transection in the rat. *Brain Res* 1999; 824:218–223.

Talbot JD, Marrett S, Evans AC, et al. Multiple representations of pain in human cerebral cortex. *Science* 1991; 251:1355–1358.

Thalhammer JG, Raymond SA, Popitz-Bergez FA, Strichartz GR. Modality-dependent modulation of conduction by impulse activity in functionally characterized single cutaneous afferents in the rat. *Somatosens Motor Res* 1994; 11:242–257.

Torebjörk HE, Hallin RG. Identification of afferent c units in intact human skin nerves. *Brain Res* 1974; 67:387–403.

Torebjörk HE, Ochoa JL. New method to identify nociceptor units innervating glabrous skin of the human hand. *Exp Brain Res* 1990; 81:509.

Torebjörk HE, LaMotte RH, Robinson CJ. Peripheral neural correlates of magnitude of cutaneous pain and hyperalgesia: simultaneous recordings in humans of sensory judgments of pain and evoked responses in nociceptors with C-fibers. *J Neurophysiol* 1984; 51:325–339.

Torebjörk HE, Lundberg LER, LaMotte RH. Central changes in the processing of mechanoreceptive input in capsaicin-induced secondary hyperalgesia in humans. *J Physiol* 1992; 448:765–780.

Treede RD, Kenshalo DR, Gracely RH, Jones AK. The cortical representation of pain. *Pain* 1999; 79:105–111.

Vallbo Å, Hagbarth KE. Microelectrode recordings from human peripheral nerves. In: Desmedt JE (Ed). *New Developments in Electromyography and Clinical Neurophysiology,* Vol. 2. Basel: Karger, 1973, pp 67–84.

Van Hees J, Gybels J. C nociceptor activity in human nerve during painful and non painful skin stimulation. *J Neurol Neurosurg Psychiatry* 1981; 44:600–607.

Wall PD. The painful consequences of peripheral injury. *J Hand Surg* 1984; 9:37–39.

Wall PD, Devor M. Sensory afferent impulses originate from the dorsal root ganglia as well as from the periphery in normal and nerve injured rats. *Pain* 1983; 17:321–339.

Wall PD, Melzack R. In: *Textbook of Pain.* Edinburgh: Churchill Livingstone, 1994.

Waxman SG. Normal and abnormal axonal properties. In: Asbury AK, McKhann GM, McDonald WI (Eds). *Diseases of the Nervous System. Clinical Neurobiology.* Philadelphia: W.B. Saunders, 1986, pp 36–56.

Weidner C, Schmelz M, Schmidt R, et al. Functional attributes discriminating mechano-insensitive and mechano-responsive c nociceptors in human skin. *J Neurosci* 1999; 15:10184–10190.

Woolf CJ, Thompson SWN. The induction and maintenance of central sensitization is dependent on N-methyl-D-aspartic receptor activation; implications for the treatment of post-injury pain hypersensitivity states. *Pain* 1991; 44:293–300.

Yarnitsky D, Ochoa JL. Release of cold-induced burning pain by block of cold-specific afferent input. *Brain* 1990; 113:893–902.

Yarnitsky D, Simone D, Dotson R, Cline M, Ochoa J. Single C nociceptor responses and psychophysical parameters of evoked pain: effect of rate of rise of heat stimuli in humans. *J Physiol* 1992; 450:581–592.

Correspondence to: Jordi Serra, MD, Neuropathic Pain Unit, Clinica Sagrada Familia, c. Torras i Pujalt 1, 08023 Barcelona, Spain. Fax: 34-93-4176404; email: jserrac@meditex.es.

Neuropathic Pain: Pathophysiology and Treatment,
Progress in Pain Research and Management, Vol. 21,
edited by Per T. Hansson, Howard L. Fields, Raymond G.
Hill, and Paolo Marchettini, IASP Press, Seattle, © 2001.

5

Central Nervous System Mechanisms of Pain in Peripheral Neuropathy

Anthony H. Dickenson, Elizabeth A. Matthews, and Rie Suzuki

Department of Pharmacology, University College London, London, United Kingdom

Neuropathic pain syndromes are sensory disorders that arise from changes resulting from damage or dysfunction of neuronal pathways, peripheral or central. Anticonvulsants are used to treat epilepsy and pain, which both result from excessive neuronal activity. In the case of epilepsy, the therapy controls central neuronal activity (Upton 1994). By contrast, in neuropathic pain, both the causal mechanisms and the targets for drugs are likely to involve both peripheral nerves and central neurons. Somewhat paradoxically, after damage to nerves or neurons any resultant neuropathic pain is often characterized by both positive (abnormal spontaneous or evoked sensations) and negative symptoms (sensory deficits). Intuitively, only the latter might be expected, because damage to other sensory systems such as the visual or auditory system invariably results in sensory loss. Not only can ongoing pain occur in areas of sensory loss, probably associated with peripheral processes at the site of injury, but a range of natural stimuli may evoke painful or unpleasant sensations of dysesthesia, allodynia, and hyperalgesia (Fields and Rowbotham 1994; Hansson and Kinnman 1996; Gottrup et al. 1998). Counterparts of these sensations can be studied in animal models (Bennett 1994; Zeltser and Seltzer 1994). These positive symptoms are likely to result from central changes involving neurons that are still connected to the periphery. Thus evoked pain may occur when remaining intact peripheral nerves impact upon hypersensitive spinal neurons (Fig. 1). The finding that neuropathic pain has both central and peripheral causes is relevant to the mode of action of anticonvulsants. This chapter will center on the evidence for central changes following nerve injury. The clinical aspects of

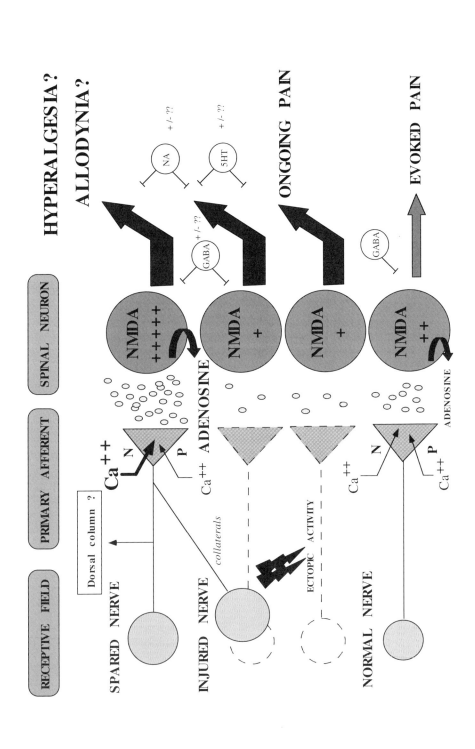

anticonvulsant drugs used for neuropathic pain have been reviewed elsewhere (McQuay et al. 1995; Sindrup and Jensen 1999; see Chapter 10 of this
volume).

The basic mechanistic studies in animals and the range of causes in
humans suggest that different pain states and symptoms may have different
underlying mechanisms. Whether allodynia, hyperalgesia, and ongoing pain
can be related to particular mechanisms remains unclear, but it is likely that
drugs with central actions will prove effective against a number of these
symptoms.

MECHANISMS OF PAIN AFTER NERVE INJURY

PERIPHERAL EVENTS

Several models of nerve injury involving manipulation of peripheral
nerves in the rat (Bennett 1994; Zeltser and Seltzer 1994), together with
careful human studies, demonstrate that neuropathic pain is the culmination
of a number of changes in the peripheral nervous system (Gracely et al.
1992). Studies after nerve section suggest that the generation of ectopic
discharges within the neuroma and the dorsal root ganglia (DRG) contribute
to these changes (Devor et al. 1992). After partial denervation in the chronic
constriction injury (CCI) model, high-frequency spontaneous activity originating in the DRG targets the spinal neurons via injured A fibers. Both large
and small fibers and DRG contribute to the behavioral responses associated
with the selective (L5/L6) spinal nerve ligation (SNL) model. A clinical
study showed that the loss of cutaneous innervation in a postherpetic neuralgia patient was inversely related to the severity of allodynia, suggesting
that surviving primary afferent nociceptors with spontaneous activity are
important for the pain and allodynia associated with this condition
(Rowbotham et al. 1996b).

All these findings suggest changes in transduction processes at and
around the site of damage. Recent advances in our knowledge of sodium
channel plasticity in different pain models will shed much light on the factors that govern the effectiveness of agents such as carbamazepine (Fields et
al. 1997; Burchiel 1998), mexiletine, and local anesthetics that act on these
substrates at the peripheral level, and may lead to the production of new
therapeutic agents (Waxman 1999; see Chapter 2). The efficacy of topical

←— **Fig. 1.** The potential mechanisms by which peripheral nerve damage causes changes
in the central processing of sensory information, together with the channel and trans-
mitter/receptor mechanisms that are subject to plasticity.

lidocaine applied to the painful area in patients supports the idea that peripheral actions are of key importance (Rowbotham et al. 1996a). However, for
pain to be sensed, these peripheral alterations must be transmitted, and secondary changes within the spinal cord appear to be critical.

CENTRAL EVENTS

Few electrophysiological studies have investigated spinal neurons in
nerve injury models. After SNL, nociceptive neurons with de novo spontaneous activity had lowered thresholds to mechanical stimuli, yet their magnitude of responses was decreased (Chapman et al. 1998) and their mechanical receptive fields were enlarged (Suzuki et al. 2000b). It is still unclear
how these changed peripheral and central neuronal responses contribute to
the resultant pain states, although the combination of both increased and
decreased responses fits well with the clinical profile of pain or allodynia
together with sensory deficits after nerve injury. However, given that neuropathic pain arises from damage to nervous pathways, sensory deficits are to
be expected. In the Seltzer and Bennett models of peripheral neuropathy,
partial section of the nerve and loose ligation lead to a loss of afferent input.
In the SNL model, ligation of L5 and L6 spinal nerves almost completely
abolishes input into these segments, but even in the spinal cord segment L4
there could be a deficit of about 35% in terms of afferent input; this is
estimated to be the contribution of adjacent unmyelinated nerves to a segment (Besse et al. 1991). Therefore, the findings of no dramatic increases in
spinal neuronal activity in all three models must be considered in terms of
central compensations for the loss of input.

It is likely that central sensitization of spinal nociceptive neurons induced by the initial injury, by ongoing pathology, and/or by ectopic activity
in injured fibers is an important aspect of nerve injury pain (Woolf and
Mannion 1999). Good evidence indicates that long-term potentiation (LTP),
first described in the brain, also can be induced in the spinal cord (Randic et
al. 1993); adaptive or learning processes in spinal neurons thus might underlie the hyperalgesia and allodynia seen in neuropathic pain patients. Recordings of single wide-dynamic-range neurons in the rat spinal dorsal horn
show that both peripheral electrical and natural conditioning stimulation
induce a long-term increase in evoked neuronal firing over periods of 3–6
hours in normal rats. The same conditioning stimulation fails to do so in
neuropathic rats (Rygh et al. 2000). It could be argued that this lack of any
increase in the firing responses after conditioning stimulation resulted either from a preexisting elevated level of excitability in the cord or from

reduced input to the cord after neuropathy. Findings that the threshold for activating C fibers was significantly lower and that the baseline C-fiber-evoked response tended to be higher in rats with peripheral neuropathy support the idea of preexisting central sensitization of the neurons studied. Hence, a further increase in the firing responses would be difficult to induce by conditioning the spinal cord with tetanic stimulation of the sciatic nerve.

The failure to show C-fiber LTP in neuropathic rats cannot be explained simply by reduced input arriving into the spinal cord during conditioning because the increase in blood pressure and heart rate during conditioning was almost exactly the same in both groups, despite the reduced peripheral input through the partially ligated sciatic nerve. Thus, if the activation of autonomic function is normal in the nerve-injured animals and yet LTP in the second-order neurons is much reduced, the most likely explanation is that an LTP-like activity has already been induced, possibly in the early period after nerve ligation, so that further increases are not attainable. This theory would suggest that spinal excitability is increased by nerve injury, which restores spinal responses to peripheral stimuli to compensate for the reduced afferent input. In addition, we have observed an enlargement of neuronal receptive fields to innocuous mechanical stimuli after peripheral nerve injury (Suzuki et al. 2000b). Receptive field reorganization is an established characteristic of neuronal plasticity following nerve injury. If receptive field size increases, then for any given stimulus, a greater number of spinal neurons will be recruited, leading to a greater afferent input and possibly enhancing pain transmission (Suzuki et al. 2000b).

These experimental observations, together with consideration of the symptoms of neuropathic pain, suggest that evoked pains may arise from central compensations for the loss of normal sensory inputs. Ongoing peripheral activity may well produce an ongoing level of transmitter release in the spinal cord, which may, in turn, favor hyperexcitability of responses to subsequent evoked stimuli. Peripheral stimuli may themselves evoke greater release of primary afferent transmitters if there is plasticity in calcium channel function, because these channels are the keys to transmitter release. Behavioral studies have shown that activation of *N*-methyl-D-aspartate (NMDA) receptors is required for both the induction and maintenance of pain-related behaviors (Bennett 1994). Thus, in neuropathic pain it is likely that aberrant peripheral activity is amplified and enhanced by spinal mechanisms mediated by NMDA receptors and by other receptors. As the operation of the NMDA receptor or channel critically depends on the underlying level of excitability, spinal neurons are probably hyperactive and may overcompensate for much of the peripheral nerve damage (Dickenson 1997).

This overcompensation, together with an enlargement of neuronal receptive fields, could form the neuronal basis for the mechanisms underlying the behavioral manifestations of allodynia, hyperalgesia, and spontaneous pain following neuropathy.

One suggested mechanism for these manifestations is that structural changes occur (Woolf et al. 1992), as discussed in a recent review (Suzuki and Dickenson 2000). The idea that Aβ-fiber sprouting into the dorsal horn is a basis for allodynia is an interesting one. Rewiring of the spinal cord would suggest that pharmacological therapy would be ineffective against allodynia because anatomical changes would be unlikely to be reversed by a drug. Another issue is that behavioral allodynia occurs before the reorganization of the afferents, so that the phenomena may contribute to the maintenance of long-term allodynia but not its induction. Furthermore, electrophysiological recordings of spinal neurons in SNL rats show no marked alterations in the magnitude or pattern of the Aβ-fiber-evoked response (Chapman et al. 1998). Additionally, drugs that exert antiallodynic effects behaviorally often have little effect on the Aβ-fiber-evoked response in electrophysiological studies, although other neuronal measures such as the spontaneous activity and mechanical evoked response appear to be markedly reduced.

CHANGES IN TRANSMITTER RELEASE

The role of high-voltage-activated Ca^{2+} channels in sensory perception has been extensively investigated. Behavioral and electrophysiological nociceptive studies in animal models of acute and persistent tissue damage and neuropathic pain have established the antinociceptive abilities of antagonists specific for L-, N- and P/Q-type Ca^{2+} channels, highlighting the differential role each subtype plays in nociception, often depending on the nature of the pain state (Vanegas and Schaible 2000). High-voltage-activated Ca^{2+} channels, consisting of a pore-forming α_1 subunit and modulatory accessory subunits, β_2, $\alpha_2\delta$, and γ (Walker and De Waard 1998), are widely expressed throughout the brain and spinal cord (Gohil et al. 1994). Activated by relatively strong membrane depolarization, they permit Ca^{2+} influx in response to action potentials. Consequential secondary actions include neurotransmitter release. These channels thus provide a major link between neuronal excitability and synaptic transmission.

N- and P-type voltage-dependent calcium channels (VDCCs) are sensitive to block by ω-conotoxin GVIA and ω-agatoxin IVA, respectively (Olivera et al. 1994), and are widely expressed throughout the brain and spinal cord (Gohil et al. 1994). The N-type channel is concentrated in laminae I and II of the superficial dorsal horn, where nociceptive primary afferents synapse (Gohil et al. 1994). In vitro studies have demonstrated that calcium ion influx through N- and P-type VDCCs is required for depolarization-coupled neurotransmitter release (Miljanich and Ramachandran 1995).

The spinal N-type VDCC appears to be the predominant isoform involved in the pre- and postsynaptic processing of sensory nociceptive information. Tactile allodynia in the SNL model is blocked by intrathecal N-type blockers, SNX-111, -239 and -159, which have no effect when administered intravenously or regionally to the nerve. ω-Agatoxin-IVA and SNX-230 (a synthetic P/Q-type selective conopeptide homologue) are inactive in this condition (Chaplan et al. 1994; Bowersox et al. 1996). In another model of nerve injury, SNX-111 and -124 reduced heat hyperalgesia and mechanoallodynia when delivered directly to the site of injury (Xiao and Bennett 1995). Mechanical hyperalgesia in rats with partial nerve ligation was reduced by subcutaneous injection of SNX-111 into the receptive field, whereas SNX-230 had no effect; neither compound had any effect in control animals (White and Cousins 1998). Complementing these behavioral studies, Matthews and Dickenson (2001) used in vivo electrophysiology to show an enhanced ability of ω-conotoxin GVIA to inhibit evoked neuronal responses after the establishment of neuropathy. We showed that N-type VDCCs are important for the transmission of low- and high-threshold mechanical and thermal stimuli onto dorsal horn neurons. Compensatory increases in peripheral and/or spinal neuronal activity after neuropathy may enhance the functional role of N-type VDCCs, increasing neurotransmitter release and membrane depolarization (Smith and Augustine 1988) and thus promoting spinal mechanisms of hyperexcitability that contribute to the ensuing neuropathic syndromes. Additionally, expression of the N-type VDCC α_{1B} subunit is increased in small DRG cells and in lamina II of the spinal cord after neuropathy (Cizkova et al. 1999), and mRNA and protein for the auxiliary $\alpha_2\delta$ subunit of VDCCs also are upregulated in the ipsilateral DRG and spinal cord of SNL rats (Luo et al. 1999). Nerve terminals throughout the dorsal horn are immunoreactive for N-type VDCCs, often correlating with the presence of substance P originating from primary afferents (Westenbroek et al. 1998).

In a clinical study, SNX-111 delivered intrathecally to chronic neuropathic pain patients produced some pain relief (Brose et al. 1997). However, pharmacological targeting of these channels with toxin antagonists as a potential therapy for chronic pain is hindered by the adverse systemic side effects (Penn and Paice 2000) and by the inconvenient spinal route of administration.

The antiepileptic drug gabapentin has analgesic efficacy in patients with postherpetic neuralgia (Rowbotham et al. 1998) and diabetic polyneuropathy (Backonja et al. 1998). Despite being a γ-aminobutyric acid (GABA) analogue, it binds to the auxiliary $\alpha_2\delta$ subunit of VDCCs (Taylor et al. 1998), where it is assumed to act as an antagonist. Gabapentin's efficacy may highlight the importance of VDCCs as targets in pain control. It is difficult to envisage how interactions of gabapentin with the ubiquitous $\alpha_2\delta$ subunits can result in specific therapeutic effects. However, DRG cells express at least two distinct forms of the $\alpha_2\delta$ subunit that differ from those in the spinal cord and brain (Luo 2000). Agents that act on VDCCs thus may have tissue-specific effects.

P-type VDCCs appear to be implicated in the initiation of a facilitated pain state, especially inflammation, with a limited role in the maintenance of neuropathy. In animal studies, ω-agatoxin IVA given prior to the application of capsaicin (Sluka 1997) or carrageenan (Sluka 1998) prevents the development of hyperalgesia. In vivo electrophysiology utilizing the formalin response demonstrated that ω-agatoxin IVA only inhibited neuronal responses in the second phase (Diaz and Dickenson 1997), for which NMDA-receptor activity is critical, yet after the establishment of neuropathy ω-agatoxin IVA had its most marked effects on NMDA-receptor-mediated events, in a profile no different from that in control animals (Matthews and Dickenson 2001b). The P-type channel appears to be linked selectively to NMDA-receptor-mediated events.

Immunolocalization has demonstrated the presence of P/Q-type VDCCs primarily on the nerve terminals of dorsal horn neurons in laminae II–VI, but unlike N-type channels, they are rarely found in neurons that contain substance P (Westenbroek et al. 1998). Intriguingly, this finding may indicate that N-type channels regulate the release of neurotransmitters, including glutamate, from peptide-containing C fibers, whereas P-type channels could possibly be localized to nonpeptide, IB4-positive neurons. Furthermore, both N- and P-type VDCCs occur in the deeper laminae of the dorsal horn, suggesting localization on terminals of large fibers and spinal neurons.

In addition to high-voltage-activated Ca^{2+} channels, kinetically distinct low-voltage-activated Ca^{2+} channels, or T-type channels, also exist both in neuronal and non-neuronal cells. These channels are activated at voltages near the resting membrane potential (Huguenard 1996). Due to their unique biophysical characteristics, T-type channels alone cannot support neurotransmission, but they may help regulate cell excitability. The α_{1G}, α_{1H}, and α_{1I} subunits have been cloned (Lee et al. 1999). In situ hybridization studies have detected these channels in the dorsal horn of the spinal cord and sensory ganglia (Talley et al. 1999). Further, T-type currents have been recorded in primary sensory neurons (Todorovic and Lingle 1998) and in some superficial rat dorsal horn neurons (Ryu and Randic 1990). Unlike investigations of the high-voltage-activated Ca^{2+} channels, studies of the involvement of T-type channels in pain-related central sensitization have been hindered by a scarcity of specific pharmacological agents. Given that antiepileptic drugs that target neuronal hyperexcitability have been proven effective in treating various forms of neuropathic pain (McQuay et al. 1995), the anticonvulsant ethosuximide, a relatively specific T-type channel antagonist (Kostyuk et al. 1992), was used in the first electrophysiological study to address the role of low-voltage-activated T-type Ca^{2+} channels in the spinal processing of sensory information after nerve injury (Matthews and Dickenson 2001a). Ethosuximide inhibited evoked rat dorsal horn neuronal responses in a manner unaltered after nerve injury, indicating some role for T-type Ca^{2+} channels in sensory transmission. Blocking these channels would reduce the underlying level of neuronal excitability, making it less likely that threshold levels of membrane depolarization could be achieved. Postsynaptically, NMDA-receptor activation would be reduced, as would the consequential development of central sensitization.

The lack of difference in the effects of ethosuximide after the establishment of neuropathy is surprising because neuronal hyperexcitability is a key underlying factor. Interestingly, SNL increases the prevalence of subthreshold membrane potential oscillations in DRG neurons, which augments ectopic discharge (Liu et al. 2000). It seems reasonable to postulate a role for T-type Ca^{2+} channels in this underlying oscillatory behavior, which may imply increased activity via T-type channels in the remaining afferents that would restore the level of excitability to that of the non-injured situation.

In animal studies, the roles of L-, N-, P-, and T-type calcium channels can be discerned by the use of selective drugs. L-type channels seem to play little role in neuronal responses, but even if they did, their important role in vascular control would minimize their therapeutic profile. In the models of neuropathy, a comparison of the effects of the calcium-channel-blocking drugs has revealed that N-type channels exhibit plasticity, whereas the roles of P- and T-type channels are unchanged. If the therapeutic effects of gabapentin are mediated through calcium channels, then the N-type channels seem the likely target.

NMDA RECEPTORS

Increased N-type VDCC activity means increased transmitter release after nerve injury, thus spinal neurons will be exposed to greater levels of transmitter and postsynaptic neurons will be more likely to be activated.

In recent years, attention has focused on glutamate's action on the NMDA receptor as a pivotal event in the transmission of persistent pain. NMDA-receptor antagonists have been tested as potential therapies for neuropathic pain states, based on earlier results from animal studies (Davar et al. 1991; Seltzer et al. 1991). Evidence suggests that NMDA receptors are involved in the induction and maintenance of certain pathological pain states, possibly by sensitizing dorsal horn neurons (Dickenson 1995; Kristensen and Gordh 1997). NMDA receptors have been implicated in the phenomenon of wind-up and in related changes, such as spinal hyperexcitability, that enhance and prolong sensory transmission (Seltzer et al. 1991; Dickenson 1995; Kristensen and Gordh 1997). Persistent injury states such as neuropathy may produce a prolonged activation of the NMDA receptor subsequent to a sustained afferent input that causes a relatively small, but continuous increase in the levels of glutamate and enhances the evoked release of the amino acid. These effects have been reported in the ipsilateral dorsal horn of CCI rats (Kawamata and Omote 1996), and there is evidence that glutamate receptors are upregulated after nerve injury (Harris et al. 1996; Croul et al. 1998; Popratiloff et al. 1998). Ectopic impulse generation in peripheral nerves and in DRG, alterations in the phenotype of damaged nerves, and loss of inhibitory GABA controls (Fields and Rowbotham 1994; Jensen 1996; Suzuki and Dickenson 2000) may all contribute to greater activation of the NMDA-receptor-channel complex. In support of these findings, the systemic administration of two clinically licensed NMDA-receptor antagonists, memantine and ketamine, was highly effective in inhibiting a wide range of evoked neuronal responses (of low and high intensity) 2 weeks after nerve injury (Suzuki et al. 2001a). Overall, the inhibitory effects of these antagonists tended to be greater in nerve-injured rats, which may reflect a greater contribution of the NMDA-receptor system to neuronal activity following neuropathy, possibly as a component of the suggested central compensations (Suzuki et al. 2001a).

Numerous clinical studies have reported the use of NMDA-receptor antagonists in various neuropathic pain states (Sang 2000), including phantom limb pain (Stannard and Porter 1993), postamputation stump pain (Nikolajsen et al. 1997), and postherpetic neuralgia (Eide et al. 1994, 1995). The main drawback of most NMDA-receptor antagonists, such as ketamine, is their severe side-effect profile at therapeutic doses. NMDA receptors are ubiquitous and are implicated in sensory perception, cognition, and consciousness, hence their antagonists will inevitably result in unwanted psychotropic effects. Interestingly, memantine, an NMDA-receptor antagonist used to treat Parkinson's disease and spasticity, may have a lower side-effect profile and has therefore received considerable attention as a potential therapy for neuropathic pain states (Parsons et al. 1999).

Although both ketamine and memantine block the NMDA receptor via the same mechanism (open channel block), the different tolerability of these agents may relate to the characteristics of their voltage- and use-dependent channel block. Ketamine will block physiological as well as pathological activation of the NMDA receptor because its block is not highly dependent on synaptic activity. In addition, because of its slow unblocking kinetics, it will not leave the channel within the time course of a normal NMDA-receptor-mediated excitatory postsynaptic potential. By contrast, memantine, with weak use dependency and rapid unblocking kinetics, will rapidly leave the channel upon transient physiological activation, while blocking the sustained activation during pathological conditions. Memantine should therefore preferentially act to block channels in active neurons and effectively reduce pathological synaptic activation of neuropathic pain states. Clinical data are sparse on the use of memantine in treating neuropathic pain conditions, although one study has reported it to be ineffective (Eisenberg et al. 1998). Amantadine, a related drug, attenuates both spontaneous and evoked pain in neuropathic patients (Eisenberg and Pud 1998; Pud et al. 1998); further clinical trials, employing sufficient dose escalation, are needed to assess the therapeutic potential of this drug in chronic pain states. However, memantine may offer an alternative approach to the long-term treatment of neuropathic pain states, with the potential of analgesia with few adverse effects.

A final approach to the modulation of NMDA-receptor-mediated activity would rely on the synthesis of subtype-selective drugs that target certain NMDA receptors. In this respect the NR2B receptor appears promising from animal studies (see Carpenter and Dickenson 2001). Combinations of the different NR2 subunits and NR1 splice variants generate a wide diversity of receptor types, which differ in physiological and pharmacological properties and in their sensitivity to glutamate and antagonists Ifenprodil is a noncompetitive NMDA-receptor antagonist, selective for receptors containing the NR2B subunit. A recent study showed a restricted distribution of the NR2B subunit protein in the rat lumbar spinal cord, with moderate labeling in the superficial dorsal horn. Two selective NR2B antagonists, (+/–)-CP-101,606 and (+/–)-Ro 25-6981, caused no motor impairment or stimulation, even at doses far in excess of those required to inhibit allodynia in neuropathic rats. These findings demonstrate that NR2B-selective antagonists may have clinical utility for pain conditions, with a reduced side-effect profile compared to existing NMDA-receptor antagonists (Boyce et al. 1999).

CENTRAL INHIBITIONS

GABA is the most abundant inhibitory neurotransmitter in the central nervous system and plays roles in the control of the pathways that transmit sensory events, including nociception. GABAergic interneurons can be found in nearly all layers of the spinal cord, with the highest concentrations in Lissauer's tract and laminae I–III (Dickenson et al. 1997). Evidence suggests that both GABA and glycinergic interneurons are preferentially associated with the control of low-threshold afferent input to the spinal cord. For example, intrathecal administration of the $GABA_A$-receptor antagonist bicuculline or the glycine receptor antagonist strychnine produces segmentally localized tactile allodynia-like behavior in conscious rats (see Kontinen and Dickenson 2000). These studies indicate a tonic GABAergic and glycinergic inhibition of low-threshold afferents innervating mechanoreceptors in normal rats. Thus, reduced activity in these spinal inhibitory systems could result in mechanical allodynia.

Changes in the inhibitory activity mediated by these two transmitters are hence of interest in the development of neuropathic pain, where mechanical allodynia is present in subgroups of patients. GABA immunoreactivity in the dorsal horn of the spinal cord decreases after partial injury of a sciatic nerve (Ibuki et al. 1997), and transection of the sciatic nerve significantly reduces the number of GABA-immunoreactive cells in the dorsal horn of the rat spinal cord (Castro-Lopes et al. 1993). Overall, these findings suggest that a decrease in GABAergic tone in the spinal cord may underlie the allodynia seen in these models. However, these decreases could be interpreted as resulting from increased release of the amino acid, and in fact higher concentrations of GABA have been measured in the dorsal quadrant of the spinal cord ipsilateral to the nerve injury (Satoh and Omote 1996). Much less is known about the changes in the glycinergic system after nerve injuries, although increased glycine levels have been reported (Satoh and Omote 1996). Interestingly, a recent report has shown a significant increase in the ratio of aspartate to GABA and glycine in the spinal dorsal horn of neuropathic patients, suggesting an imbalance in the levels of excitatory and inhibitory amino acids in this chronic pain state (Mertens et al. 2000).

Midazolam reduces C-fiber-evoked firing significantly more in SNL rats than in controls and significantly reduces Aδ-fiber-evoked activity in SNL rats, but not in normal and sham-operated rats (Kontinen and Dickenson 2000). Benzodiazepines such as midazolam increase the probability that GABA will open the chloride channel associated with the $GABA_A$ receptor and so induce neuronal inhibition. Thus, because the effects of midazolam depend on the level of GABA activity, the same dose of the benzodiazepine would be more effective when GABA transmission is enhanced (Kontinen and Dickenson 2000). Enhanced transmission of GABA could result from an increase in the levels or release of GABA itself, or alternatively from an upregulation of the receptor as a result of a possible decrease in GABA levels due to morphological changes induced by nerve injury.

ADENOSINE

There is a growing interest in developing therapeutic agents that recruit adenosine systems for the treatment of neuropathic pain. Numerous clinical and animal studies have reported adenosine analogues to be effective against neuropathic pain (Karlsten et al. 1992; Sollevi et al. 1995; Lee and Yaksh 1996; Cui et al. 1997). Although little is known regarding the mechanisms behind these effects, the direct and indirect manipulation of the adenosine system may prove to be a useful approach in producing spinally mediated antinociception.

Adenosine receptors play an important inhibitory role in the development and maintenance of central sensitization of spinal dorsal horn neurons (Sumida et al. 1998). Studies have suggested a possible interaction between adenosine and glutamate in the spinal cord (Dolphin and Prestwich 1985) and between NMDA-receptor activation and adenosine release elsewhere in the brain (Craig and White 1992). These studies have implicated the A1 receptor in indirectly controlling the spinal NMDA polysynaptic nociceptive pathway, a mechanism that may contribute to adenosine-mediated antinociception at the spinal level (Reeve and Dickenson 1995a,b). A greater degree of NMDA-receptor activation after nerve injury could therefore lead to a greater release of adenosine, which in turn could eventually deplete the purine. It could then be envisaged that any disruption of the endogenous purinergic tone as a result of nerve injury could affect spinal nociceptive transmission and contribute to facilitated sensory transmission (hyperalgesia) and miscoding of innocuous information (allodynia).

Based on electrophysiological recordings of spinal dorsal horn neurons, we have previously shown that N6-cyclopentyladenosine (CPA), an adenosine A1 receptor agonist, is effective in inhibiting the evoked neuronal responses to noxious and innocuous peripheral stimuli (Suzuki et al. 2000a). These inhibitions were significantly greater following nerve injury in the SNL model, and a leftward shift was observed in the dose-response curves. Similarly, the administration of ABT-702, a novel selective adenosine kinase inhibitor (Jarvis et al. 2000) that protects adenosine from breakdown by endogenous enzymes, had greater effectiveness on the neuronal responses after nerve injury (Suzuki et al. 2001b). The use of adenosine metabolism inhibitors allows the site- and state-selective recruitment of the endogenous adenosine system, so this approach could potentially minimize side effects; when administered in areas of the central nervous system where adenosine is released, it could be a more favorable therapy than direct-acting adenosine agonists.

These results suggest an enhanced role of adenosine in this chronic pain state, which may reflect an increased release of the purine in the spinal cord or alternatively, an upregulation of A1 receptors. Taken together, these results suggest that the direct and indirect manipulation of the adenosine receptor system may be a useful approach in treating neuropathic pain states. The leftward shift in the dose-response curves for CPA and ABT-702 after neuropathy favors the use of lower doses of the drug in this pain state so as to minimize side effects.

BRAIN MECHANISMS

The final resolution of the signals arising in the periphery occurs at the highest centers of the brain and is likely to reflect activity in multiple areas. This divergence of information makes elucidation of mechanisms difficult, but brainstem mechanisms relevant to neuropathic pain are better defined.

Clear clinical evidence attests to the effectiveness of antidepressants in the treatment of neuropathic pain (see Chapter 9). Although their actions may have peripheral components, including sympathetic effects, their primary mode of action is more likely to be through interactions with pathways running to the spinal cord from 5-HT and noradrenergic nuclei of the brainstem and midbrain, including the raphe nuclei, the periaqueductal gray matter, and the locus ceruleus (Millan 1999). Because the older, less selective drugs are more effective in relieving neuropathic pain, the antidepressants are likely to exert their effects due to increased synaptic levels of these monoamines resulting from a block of their uptake. The relative roles of the 5-HT receptors in the spinal cord are unknown, but the spinal targets for the norepinephrine released from descending pathways are the α_2 receptors, which have similar actions and distribution to the opioid receptors. Sedation and hypotension with α_2 agonists presently limit their use as analgesics. It is unclear whether the antidepressants are interacting with altered monoamine controls induced by nerve injury (Satoh and Omote 1996) or whether they are simply increasing monoamine levels in a constitutive system.

With regard to allodynia, the bulk of the low-threshold afferent fibers traverse the dorsal columns to terminate in the brainstem, circumventing the spinal cord. It is therefore surprising that little is known regarding the potential plasticity of the dorsal column nuclei such as the gracile nucleus. Other than reports of an expression of the precursor for substance P in the dorsal column nuclei after nerve transection (Noguchi et al. 1995), little it is known about the functional aspects of these brainstem nuclei in neuropathic pain. However, a noteworthy behavioral study shows that temporary block of the gracile nucleus abolishes allodynia in rats (Sun et al. 2001). Further investigations are warranted.

CONCLUSIONS

"What goes up can come down" applies to neuronal activity. Although the peripheral mechanisms of neuropathic pain are clearly the cause of much of the ensuing chaos, many of the drugs that act on peripheral substrates, by merit of being excitability blockers, have narrow therapeutic windows. This situation may well improve if the characterization of the novel sodium channels described at and around the sites of injury lead to therapeutic advances as a result of the synthesis of more selective channel blockers lacking cardiac and brain side effects.

Many of the other drugs that are effective in patients and in animals seem to produce their effects through central targets, although for many, the exact mechanisms remain unclear. However, the effects of gabapentin seem to be mediated through the modulation of calcium channels on central terminals of sensory neurons, and antidepressants are also likely to be influencing the spinal and brainstem terminals of monoamine pathways. Together with the effectiveness of ketamine and other NMDA-receptor antagonists (although not without problematic side effects) and the ability of adenosine to reduce the symptoms of nerve injury, these findings suggest that peripheral damage induces central spinal plasticity of several voltage-gated and ligand-gated ion channels. Further changes at higher centers may ensue. The evoked allodynia and hyperalgesia can only occur from activity in neuronal pathways where the peripheral fibers are still able to contact and excite central neurons. We suggest that these altered central systems, driven by the peripheral changes, are responsible for the evoked pains that accompany nerve injury. This framework allows for drugs with peripheral or central actions to be effective against neuropathic pain. The clinical data so far do not show that different drugs have clearly discernible differences in their effects on various types of neuropathic pain (McQuay et al. 1995; Sindrup and Jensen 1999), although some differentiation has been seen with gabapentin (Attal et al. 1998). Whether a mechanism-based classification

Table I

The effectiveness of various established therapeutic agents in the spinal nerve ligation model of neuropathy using recordings of spinal dorsal horn neurons; the ability of the drugs to reduce various neuronal measures was quantified using a wide range of peripheral stimuli

Drug	Spontaneous Activity Ongoing Pain	Evoked Activity		
		Mechanical Stimuli		Thermal Stimuli
		Noxious von Frey Mechanical Hyperalgesia	Innocuous von Frey Allodynia	Noxious Heat Thermal Hyperalgesia
Gabapentin	Effective	Effective	Effective	Effective
Carbamazepine	Effective	Effective	Effective	Not tested
Intrathecal morphine	Effective	Effective	Effective	Effective
NMDA-receptor antagonist (ketamine)	Effective	Effective	Effective	Effective
N-type calcium channel blocker (ω-conotoxin)	Effective	Effective	Effective	Effective
Adenosine A1 receptor agonist (CPA)	Not tested	Effective	Effective	Effective
Adenosine kinase inhibitor (ABT-702)	Not tested	Effective	Effective	Effective

will be possible (Woolf 1998) remains to be seen. Sensory testing (Hansson and Kinnman 1996; Gottrup et al. 1998) of many patients will be necessary to quantify particular symptoms and then to gauge drug effects on these symptoms in different neuropathic pain states. However, the modes of action of the drugs with central actions such as attenuation of transmitter release and reduction of central hypersensitivity, together with the degree of convergence of peripheral inputs onto central neurons, would make any highly selective effects on particular symptoms appear unlikely. Table I lists the effects of a number of established therapeutic agents in the SNL model of neuropathy where we have quantified the responses of spinal neurons to a wide range of stimuli. The results are similar to those found overall in a number of behavioral studies that generally have focused on single modalities of stimuli. The key point is that drugs acting to alter transmitter release (gabapentin), NMDA-receptor excitability (ketamine), central GABA controls (benzodiazepines), opioid systems (morphine), and adenosine and monoamine controls (antidepressants) would not be expected to selectively target single modalities. An exception could be that the inhibitory controls, where presynaptic actions occur, could by virtue of the receptor location differentially modulate different fiber inputs. Given that the drugs used in neuropathic pain target many of the key mechanisms at central and peripheral sites, one of the major clinical issues with these drugs may simply be their tolerability. Improved knowledge of the changes induced by nerve injury will allow a rational approach to effective treatment.

ACKNOWLEDGMENTS

Work in the laboratory was supported by the Wellcome Trust, MRC, and the European Commission.

REFERENCES

Attal N, Brasseur L, Parker F, Chauvin M, Bouhassira D. Effects of gabapentin on the different components of peripheral and central neuropathic pain syndromes: a pilot study. *Eur Neurol* 1998; 40:191–200.

Backonja M, Beydoun A, Edwards K, et al. Gabapentin for the symptomatic treatment of painful neuropathy in patients with diabetes mellitus: a randomised controlled trial. *JAMA* 1998; 280:1831–1836.

Bennett G. Neuropathic pain. In: Wall P, Melzack R (Eds). *Textbook of Pain*, 3rd ed. London: Churchill Livingstone, 1994, pp 201–224.

Besse D, Lombard MC, Besson JM. Autoradiographic distribution of mu, delta and kappa opioid binding sites in the superficial dorsal horn, over the rostrocaudal axis of the rat spinal cord. *Brain Res* 1991; 548:287–291.

Bowersox SS, Gadbois T, Singh T, et al. Selective N-type neuronal voltage-sensitive calcium channel blocker, SNX-111, produces spinal antinociception in rat models of acute, persistent and neuropathic pain. *J Pharmacol Exp Ther* 1996; 279:1243–1249.

Boyce S, Wyatt A, Webb J, et al. Selective NMDA NR2B antagonists induce antinociception without motor dysfunction: correlation with restricted localisation of NR2B subunit in dorsal horn. *Neuropharmacology* 1999; 38:611–623.

Brose WG, Gutlove DP, Luther RR, Bowersox SS, McGuire D. Use of intrathecal SNX-111, a novel, N-type, voltage-sensitive, calcium channel blocker, in the management of intractable brachial plexus avulsion pain. *Clin J Pain* 1997; 13:256–259.

Burchiel K. Carbamazepine inhibits spontaneous activity in experimental neuromas. *Exp Neurol* 1998; 102:249–253.

Carpenter KJ, Dickenson AH. Amino acids are still as exciting as ever. *Curr Opin Pharmacol* 2001; 1:57–61.

Castro-Lopes JM, Tavares I, Coimbra A. GABA decreases in the spinal cord dorsal horn after peripheral neurectomy. *Brain Res* 1993; 620:287–291.

Chaplan SR, Pogrel JW, Yaksh TL. Role of voltage-dependent calcium channel subtypes in experimental tactile allodynia. *J Pharmacol Exp Ther* 1994; 269:1117–1123.

Chapman V, Suzuki R, Dickenson AH. Electrophysiological characterization of spinal neuronal response properties in anaesthetized rats after ligation of spinal nerves L5–L6. *J Physiol* 1998; 507:881–894.

Cizkova D, Marsala M, Stauderman K, Yaksh T. Calcium channel α1B subunit in spinal cord/DRG of normal and nerve-injured rats. *Abstracts: 9th World Congress on Pain.* Seattle: IASP Press, p 134.

Craig CG, White TD. Low-level N-methyl-D-aspartate receptor activation provides a purinergic inhibitory threshold against further N-methyl-D-aspartate-mediated neurotransmission in the cortex. *J Pharmacol Exp Ther* 1992; 260:1278–1284.

Croul S, Radzievsky A, Sverstiuk A, Murray M. NK1, NMDA, 5HT1a, and 5HT2 receptor binding sites in the rat lumbar spinal cord: modulation following sciatic nerve crush. *Exp Neurol* 1998; 154:66–79.

Cui JG, Sollevi A, Linderoth B, Meyerson BA. Adenosine receptor activation suppresses tactile hypersensitivity and potentiates spinal cord stimulation in mononeuropathic rats. *Neurosci Lett* 1997; 223:173–176.

Davar G, Hama A, Deykin A, Vos B, Maciewicz R. MK-801 blocks the development of thermal hyperalgesia in a rat model of experimental painful neuropathy. *Brain Res* 1991; 553:327–330.

Devor M, Wall PD, Catalan N. Systemic lidocaine silences ectopic neuroma and DRG discharge without blocking nerve conduction. *Pain* 1992; 48:261–268.

Diaz A, Dickenson AH. Blockade of spinal N- and P-type, but not L-type, calcium channels inhibits the excitability of rat dorsal horn neurons produced by subcutaneous formalin inflammation. *Pain* 1997; 69:93–100.

Dickenson AH. Spinal cord pharmacology of pain. *Br J Anaesth* 1995; 75:193–200.

Dickenson AH. NMDA receptor antagonists: interactions with opioids. *Acta Anaesthesiol Scand* 1997; 41:112–115.

Dickenson AH, Chapman V, Green GM. The pharmacology of excitatory and inhibitory amino acid-mediated events in the transmission and modulation of pain in the spinal cord. *Gen Pharmacol* 1997; 28:633–638.

Dolphin AC, Prestwich SA. Pertussis toxin reverses adenosine inhibition of neuronal glutamate release. *Nature* 1985; 316:148–150.

Eide PK, Jorum E, Stubhaug A, Bremnes J, Breivik H. Relief of post-herpetic neuralgia with the N-methyl-D-aspartic acid receptor antagonist ketamine: a double-blind, cross-over comparison with morphine and placebo. *Pain* 1994; 58:347–354.

Eide PK, Stubhaug A, Oye I, Breivik H. Continuous subcutaneous administration of the N-methyl-D-aspartic acid (NMDA) receptor antagonist ketamine in the treatment of post-herpetic neuralgia. *Pain* 1995; 61:221–228.

Eisenberg E, Pud D. Can patients with chronic neuropathic pain be cured by acute administration of the NMDA receptor antagonist amantadine?. *Pain* 1998; 74:337–339.

Eisenberg E, Kleiser A, Dortort A, Haim T, Yarnitsky D. The NMDA (*N*-methyl-D-aspartate) receptor antagonist memantine in the treatment of postherpetic neuralgia: a double blind, placebo-controlled study. *Eur J Pain* 1998; 2:321–327.

Fields HL, Rowbotham MC. Multiple mechanisms of neuropathic pain: a clinical perspective. In: Gebhart G, Hammond DL, Jensen TS (Eds). *Proceedings of the 7th World Congress on Pain,* Progress in Pain Research and Management, Vol. 2. Seattle: IASP Press, 1994, pp 437–454.

Fields H, Rowbotham M, Devor M. Excitability blockers: anticonvulsants and low concentration local anesthetics in the treatment of chronic pain. In: Dickenson A, Besson J (Eds). *The Pharmacology of Pain,* Handbook of Experimental Pharmacology, Vol. 130. Heidelberg: Springer, 1997, pp 93–116.

Gohil K, Bell JR, Ramachandran J, Miljanich GP. Neuroanatomical distribution of receptors for a novel voltage-sensitive calcium-channel antagonist, SNX-230 (omega-conopeptide MVIIC). *Brain Res* 1994; 653:258–266.

Gottrup H, Nielsen J, Nielsen L, Jensen T. The relationship between sensory thresholds and mechanical hyperalgesia in nerve injury. *Pain* 1998; 75:321–329.

Gracely RH, Lynch SA, Bennett GJ. Painful neuropathy: altered central processing maintained dynamically by peripheral input. *Pain* 1992; 51:175–194.

Hansson P, Kinnman E. Unmasking neuropathic pain mechanisms in a clinical perspective. *Pain Rev* 1996; 3:272–292.

Harris JA, Corsi M, Quartaroli M, Arban R, Bentivoglio M. Upregulation of spinal glutamate receptors in chronic pain. *Neuroscience* 1996; 74:7–12.

Huguenard JR. Low-threshold calcium currents in central nervous system neurons. *Annu Rev Physiol* 1996; 58:329–348.

Ibuki T, Hama AT, Wang XT, Pappas GD, Sagen J. Loss of GABA-immunoreactivity in the spinal dorsal horn of rats with peripheral nerve injury and promotion of recovery by adrenal medullary grafts. *Neuroscience* 1997; 76:845–858.

Jarvis M, Yu H, Kohlhaas K, et al. ABT-702, A novel orally effective adenosine kinase inhibitor analgesic with anti-inflammatory properties: I. In vitro characterization and acute antinociceptive effects in the mouse. *J Pharmacol Exp Ther* 2000; 295:1156–1164.

Jensen T. Mechanisms of neuropathic pain. In: Campbell JN (Ed). *Pain 1996: An Updated Review.* Seattle: IASP Press, 1996, pp 77–88.

Karlsten R, Gordh T, Post C. Local antinociceptive and hyperalgesic effects in the formalin test after peripheral administration of adenosine analogues in mice. *Pharmacol Toxicol* 1992; 70:434–438.

Kawamata M, Omote K. Involvement of increased excitatory amino acids and intracellular Ca2+ concentration in the spinal dorsal horn in an animal model of neuropathic pain. *Pain* 1996; 68:85–96.

Kontinen V, Dickenson A. Effects of midazolam in the spinal nerve ligation model of neuropathic pain in rats. *Pain* 2000; 85:425–431.

Kostyuk PG, Molokanova EA, Pronchuk NF, Savchenko AN, Verkhratsky AN. Different action of ethosuximide on low- and high-threshold calcium currents in rat sensory neurons. *Neuroscience* 1992; 51:755–758.

Kristensen J, Gordh T. Modulation of NMDA receptor function for pain treatment. In: Yaksh T, Lynch C, Zapol W, et al. (Eds). *Anesthesia: Biologic Foundations.* Philadelphia: Lippincott-Raven, 1997, pp 943–952.

Lee JH, Daud AN, Cribbs LL, et al. Cloning and expression of a novel member of the low voltage-activated T-type calcium channel family. *J Neurosci* 1999; 19:1912–1921.

Lee YW, Yaksh TL. Pharmacology of the spinal adenosine receptor which mediates the antiallodynic action of intrathecal adenosine agonists. *J Pharmacol Exp Ther* 1996; 277:1642–1648.

Liu C-N, Michaelis M, Amir R, Devor M. Spinal nerve injury enhances subthreshold membrane potential oscillations in DRG neurons: relation to neuropathic pain. *J Neurophysiol* 2000; 84:205–215.

Luo Z. Rat dorsal root ganglia express distinctive forms of the alpha 2 calcium channel subunit. *Neuroreport* 2000; 11:3449–3452.

Luo ZD, Higuera ES, Stauderman KA, Williams ME, Chaplan SR. Regulation of α2δ calcium channel subunit in dorsal root ganglia and spinal cord of rats with tactile allodynia. *Abstracts: 9th World Congress on Pain.* Seattle: IASP Press, 1999, p 7.

Matthews E, Dickenson A. Effects of ethosuximide, a T-type calcium channel blocker, on dorsal horn neuronal responses in rats. *Eur J Pharmacol* 2001a; in press.

Matthews E, Dickenson A. Effects of spinally delivered N- and P-type voltage-dependent calcium channel antagonists on dorsal horn neuronal responses in a rat model of neuropathy. *Pain* 2001b; in press.

McQuay H, Carroll D, Jadad AR, Wiffen P, Moore A. Anticonvulsant drugs for management of pain: a systematic review. *BMJ* 1995; 311:1047–1052.

Mertens P, Ghaemmaghami C, Bert L, et al. Amino acids in spinal dorsal horn of patients during surgery for neuropathic pain or spasticity. *Neuroreport* 2000; 11:1795–1798.

Miljanich GP, Ramachandran J. Antagonists of neuronal calcium channels: structure, function, and therapeutic implications. *Annu Rev Pharmacol Toxicol* 1995; 35:707–734.

Millan MJ. The induction of pain: an integrative review. *Prog Neurobiol* 1999; 57:1–164.

Nikolajsen L, Hansen PO, Jensen TS. Oral ketamine therapy in the treatment of postamputation stump pain. *Acta Anaesthesiol Scand* 1997; 41:427–429.

Olivera BM, Miljanich GP, Ramachandran J, Adams ME. Calcium channel diversity and neurotransmitter release: the omega-conotoxins and omega-agatoxins. *Annu Rev Biochem* 1994; 63:823–867.

Parsons CG, Danysz W, Quack G. Memantine is a clinically well tolerated *N*-methyl-D-aspartate (NMDA) receptor antagonist-a review of preclinical data. *Neuropharmacology* 1999; 38:735–767.

Penn RD, Paice JA. Adverse effects associated with the intrathecal administration of zinconotide. *Pain* 2000; 85:291–296.

Popratiloff A, Weinberg RJ, Rustioni A. AMPA receptors at primary afferent synapses in substantia gelatinosa after sciatic nerve section. *Eur J Neurosci* 1998; 10:3220–3230.

Pud D, Eisenberg E, Spitzer A, et al. The NMDA receptor antagonist amantadine reduces surgical neuropathic pain in cancer patients: a double blind, randomized, placebo controlled trial. *Pain* 1998; 75:349–354.

Randic M, Jiang MC, Cerne R. Long-term potentiation and long-term depression of primary afferent neurotransmission in the rat spinal cord. *J Neurosci* 1993; 13:5228–5241.

Reeve AJ, Dickenson AH. Electrophysiological study on spinal antinociceptive interactions between adenosine and morphine in the dorsal horn of the rat. *Neurosci Lett* 1995a; 194:81–84.

Reeve AJ, Dickenson AH. The roles of spinal adenosine receptors in the control of acute and more persistent nociceptive responses of dorsal horn neurons in the anaesthetized rat. *Br J Pharmacol* 1995b; 116:2221–2228.

Rowbotham M, Davies P, Verkempinck C, Galer B. Lidocaine patch: double-blind controlled study of a new treatment method for post-herpetic neuralgia. *Pain* 1996a; 65:39–44.

Rowbotham M, Yosipovitch G, Connolly M, et al. Cutaneous innervation density in the allodynic form of postherpetic neuralgia. *Neurobiol Dis* 1996b; 3:205–214.

Rowbotham M, Harden N, Stacey B, Bernstein P, Magnus-Miller L. Gabapentin for the treatment of postherpetic neuralgia: a randomized controlled trial. *JAMA* 1998; 280:1837–1842.

Rygh L, Kontinen V, Suzuki R, Dickenson A. Different increase in C-fibre evoked responses after nociceptive conditioning stimulation in sham-operated and neuropathic rats. *Neurosci Lett* 2000; 288:99–103.

Ryu PD, Randic M. Low- and high-voltage-activated calcium currents in rat spinal dorsal horn neurons. *J Neurophysiol* 1990; 63:273–285.

Sang C. NMDA-receptor antagonists in neuropathic pain: experimental methods to clinical trials. *J Pain Symptom Manage* 2000; 19:S21–25.

Satoh O, Omote K. Roles of monoaminergic, glycinergic and GABAergic inhibitory systems in the spinal cord in rats with peripheral mononeuropathy. *Brain Res* 1996; 728:27–36.

Seltzer Z, Cohn S, Ginzburg R, Beilin B. Modulation of neuropathic pain behavior in rats by spinal disinhibition and NMDA receptor blockade of injury discharge. *Pain* 1991; 45:69–75.

Sindrup S, Jensen T. Efficacy of pharmacological treatments of neuropathic pain: an update and effect related to mechanism of drug action. *Pain* 1999; 83:389–400.

Sluka KA. Blockade of calcium channels can prevent the onset of secondary hyperalgesia and allodynia induced by intradermal injection of capsaicin in rats. *Pain* 1997; 71:157–164.

Sluka KA. Blockade of N- and P/Q-type calcium channels reduces the secondary heat hyperalgesia induced by acute inflammation. *J Pharmacol Exp Ther* 1998; 287:232–237.

Smith SJ, Augustine GJ. Calcium ions, active zones and synaptic transmitter release. *Trends Neurosci* 1988; 11:458–464.

Sollevi A, Belfrage M, Lundeberg T, Segerdahl M, Hansson P. Systemic adenosine infusion: a new treatment modality to alleviate neuropathic pain. *Pain* 1995; 61:155–158.

Stannard CF, Porter GE. Ketamine hydrochloride in the treatment of phantom limb pain. *Pain* 1993; 54:227–230.

Sumida T, Smith MA, Maehara Y, Collins JG, Kitahata LM. Spinal R-phenyl-isopropyl adenosine inhibits spinal dorsal horn neurons responding to noxious heat stimulation in the absence and presence of sensitization. *Pain* 1998; 74:307–313.

Sun H, Ren K, Zhong C, et al. Nerve injury-induced tactile allodynia is mediated via ascending spinal dorsal column projections. *Pain* 2001; 90:105–111.

Suzuki R, Dickenson A. Neuropathic pain: nerves bursting with excitement. *Neuroreport* 2000; 11:R17–R21.

Suzuki R, Gale A, Dickenson A. The inhibitory effects of the A1 adenosine receptor agonist, N6-cyclopentyladenosine on the electrical and natural evoked responses of spinal dorsal horn neurons in a rat model of mononeuropathy. *J Pain* 2000a; 1:99–110.

Suzuki R, Kontinen V, Matthews E, Dickenson A. Enlargement of receptive field size to low intensity mechanical stimulation in the rat spinal nerve ligation model of neuropathy. *Exp Neurol* 2000b; 163:408–413.

Suzuki R, Matthews E, Dickenson A. Comparison of the effects of MK-801, ketamine and memantine on responses of spinal dorsal horn neurons in a rat model of mononeuropathy. *Pain* 2001a; 91:101–109.

Suzuki R, Stanfa L, Kowaluk E, et al. The effect of ABT-702, a novel adenosine kinase inhibitor, on the responses of spinal neurons following carrageenan inflammation and peripheral nerve injury. *Br J Pharmacol* 2001b; 132:1606–1614.

Talley EM, Cribbs LL, Lee JH, et al. Differential distribution of three members of a gene family encoding low voltage-activated (T-type) calcium channels. *J Neurosci* 1999; 19:1895–1911.

Taylor CP, Gee NS, Su TZ, et al. A summary of mechanistic hypotheses of gabapentin pharmacology. *Epilepsy Res* 1998; 29:223–249.

Todorovic SM, Lingle CJ. Pharmacological properties of T-type Ca^{2+} current in adult rat sensory neurons: effects of anticonvulsant and anesthetic agents. *J Neurophysiol* 1998; 79:240–252.

Upton N. Mechanisms of action of new antiepileptic drugs: rational design and serendipitous findings. *Trends Pharmacol Sci* 1994; 12:456–463.

Vanegas H, Schaible H. Effects of antagonists to high-threshold calcium channels upon spinal mechanisms of pain, hyperalgesia and allodynia. *Pain* 2000; 85:9–18.

Walker D, De Waard M. Subunit interaction sites in voltage-dependent Ca^{2+} channels: role in channel function. *Trends Neurosci* 1998; 21:148–154.

Waxman SG. The molecular pathophysiology of pain: abnormal expression of sodium channel genes and its contributions to hyperexcitability of primary sensory neurons. *Pain* 1999; (Suppl 6): S133–S140.

Westenbroek RE, Hoskins L, Catterall WA. Localization of Ca^{2+} channel subtypes on rat spinal motor neurons, interneurons, and nerve terminals. *J Neurosci* 1998; 18:6319–6330.

White DM, Cousins MJ. Effect of subcutaneous administration of calcium channel blockers on nerve injury-induced hyperalgesia. *Brain Res* 1998; 801:50–58.

Woolf C, Mannion R. Neuropathic pain: aetiology, symptoms, mechanisms and management. *Lancet* 1999; 353:1959–1964.

Woolf CJ, Shortland P, Coggeshall RE. Peripheral nerve injury triggers central sprouting of myelinated afferents. *Nature* 1992; 355:75–78.

Woolf CJ, Bennett GJ, Doherty M, et al. Towards a mechanism-based classification of pain. *Pain* 1998; 77:227–229.

Xiao WH, Bennett GJ. Synthetic omega-conopeptides applied to the site of nerve injury suppress neuropathic pains in rats. *J Pharmacol Exp Ther* 1995; 274:666–672.

Zeltser R, Seltzer Z. A practical guide for the use of animal models in the study of neuropathic pain. In: Boivie J, Hansson P, Lindblom U (Eds). *Touch, Temperature, and Pain in Health and Disease: Mechanisms and Assessments,* Progress in Pain Research and Management, Vol. 3. Seattle: IASP Press, 1994, pp 295–338.

Correspondence to: Anthony H. Dickenson, PhD, Department of Pharmacology, University College London, Gower Street, London WC1E 6BT, United Kingdom.

Neuropathic Pain: Pathophysiology and Treatment,
Progress in Pain Research and Management, Vol. 21,
edited by Per T. Hansson, Howard L. Fields, Raymond G.
Hill, and Paolo Marchettini, IASP Press, Seattle, © 2001.

6

Tonic Descending Facilitation as a Mechanism of Neuropathic Pain

Michael H. Ossipov,[a] Josephine Lai,[a] T. Philip Malan, Jr.,[a,b]
Todd W. Vanderah,[a,b] and Frank Porreca[a,b]

*Departments of [a]Pharmacology and [b]Anesthesiology, Health Sciences Center,
University of Arizona, Tucson, Arizona, USA*

Damage to peripheral nerves from either injury or disease can cause chronic abnormal (i.e., neuropathic) pain states. Such conditions are characterized by persistent pain, spontaneous paroxysmal pain, allodynia (a condition in which normally innocuous stimuli are perceived as nociceptive), and hyperalgesia (increased sensitivity to noxious stimuli) (Payne 1986; Merskey and Bogduk 1994). Painful neuropathy is a seriously debilitating syndrome that affects millions of people, significantly diminishing their quality of life. Moreover, such pain is often resistant to common protocols for the treatment of chronic pain, including opioid analgesics. It is important to increase our understanding of the mechanisms that underlie neuropathic pain states in order to identify strategies for the development of effective therapies. Significantly, the mechanisms that initiate nerve injury pain may differ from those that are critical to maintaining it.

Several potential mechanisms have been suggested to explain neuropathic pain. Among these, increased spontaneous and persistent afferent discharge from injured nerves (Devor 1991) has been shown to result in the development of a hypersensitive state of spinal neurons ("central sensitization"). Nerve injury produces spontaneous firing of sensory nerves in rats and rabbits (Kirk 1974; Wall and Gutnick 1974). Such injury-induced spontaneous activity appears to be generated ectopically at the site of injury and at the dorsal root ganglion (DRG) of the injured or adjacent uninjured nerves (Kajander et al. 1992; Devor 1994). The ectopic sites are also believed to be associated with the generation of discharges initiated by noxious or by normally non-noxious mechanical or chemical stimuli (Devor 1994; Fields et al. 1997).

A prominent molecular basis that might explain the abnormal, repetitive firing of injured primary afferent neurons is the accumulation of sodium channels at the sites of injury, creating a lower threshold for the initiation of action potentials and the generation of ectopic impulses (e.g., the tetrodo-toxin-resistant sodium channel PN3/SNS or type III sodium channel) (England et al. 1996; Sangameswaran et al. 1996; Boucher et al. 2000; see Chapter 2). Recently, three independent studies attempted to correlate spontaneous neuronal activity with the development of enhanced sensitivity to normally innocuous mechanical stimulation after spinal nerve injury. Chung and coworkers (Han et al. 2000) measured the action potentials of afferent nerve fibers from small fascicles of L5 spinal nerve roots in rats with transections of L4, L5, and L6 spinal nerves. Spontaneous ectopic discharges were most pronounced 1 week after injury and diminished significantly over time. In a separate study, X. Liu and colleagues (2000) reported brief discharges occurring from the time of the nerve injury to 6 hours afterwards. These investigators observed the greatest spontaneous activity between 3 and 8 days after injury and found that such activity was reduced to less than half the initial frequency by 20 days. Both studies claimed a positive correlation between the rate of spontaneous discharge and neuropathic pain behaviors. However, increased sensitivity to normally innocuous mechanical stimulation (perhaps representative of tactile allodynia) and hyperalgesia to noxious thermal stimulation lasts for more than 6 weeks after L5/L6 spinal nerve ligation (SNL), despite the apparently decreasing rate of ectopic discharge (Chaplan et al. 1994; Bian et al. 1999; Malan et al. 2000). When the data obtained from the initial 3 days are excluded, no obvious correlation is seen between spontaneous activity and nociceptive behaviors (X. Liu et al. 2000). These observations suggest that the behavioral signs that characterize the neuropathic state are maintained for long periods of time despite the fact that nerve-injury-induced ectopic activity diminishes significantly within a few days after the injury. The mechanisms responsible for the initiation of the neuropathic pain condition thus are insufficient to explain the persistence of such pain.

While large-diameter myelinated Aβ fibers normally play a limited role in the processing of acute noxious signals, these fibers may take on greater significance in mediating neuropathic pain. In the uninjured condition, behavioral responses to acute nociceptive stimuli can be reduced or even abolished by the selective desensitization of small-diameter unmyelinated C fibers with capsaicin or resiniferatoxin (RTX) (Szallasi et al. 1989; Craft et al. 1993; Xu et al. 1997). Wind-up of dorsal horn units can be induced by repetitive C-fiber stimulation, and this special case of sensitization is also abolished by RTX (Xu et al. 1997). However, large fibers, which are not sensitive to RTX, appear to be important in mediating the increased sensitivity to normally innocuous probing of the paw with von Frey filaments in the nerve-injured state. In a recent study, C fibers were desensitized by systemic injections of RTX in animals with L5/L6 SNL (Ossipov et al. 1999). These animals demonstrated increased response latencies to acute thermal stimuli applied to the tail and hindpaws that were irreversible over the course of the experiment (more than 40 days) (Ossipov et al. 1999). Treatment with RTX, however, had no effect on the increased sensitivity to non-noxious mechanical stimuli observed in the nerve-injured rats (Ossipov et al. 1999), implying that these responses were not mediated by C fibers, or at least not by capsaicin-sensitive C fibers. Indeed, $A\beta$, rather than C, fibers show the greatest degree of spontaneous ectopic discharge after peripheral nerve injury (Kajander and Bennett 1992). C. Liu and colleagues (2000) found large increases in afferent discharge immediately after L5 ligation and transection, and determined that the spontaneous afferent activity was due to myelinated afferent fibers, with little or no repetitive discharge occurring in C fibers, consistent with other findings (Han et al. 2000; X. Liu et al. 2000). In fact, no evidence of C-fiber nociceptors becoming sensitive to light touch has been found after spinal nerve injury (C. Liu et al. 2000). Such observations correlate well with our own observations that sensitivity to normally innocuous mechanical stimulation increases after nerve injury, even when C fibers have been desensitized (Ossipov et al. 1999). Tal and colleagues (1999) report that touch-evoked firing in a neuroma model is transmitted through $A\beta$ afferent fibers. These studies indicate that increased sensitivity to light touch is likely to be mediated through large-diameter $A\beta$ afferent fibers (Gracely et al. 1992; C. Liu et al. 2000; X. Liu et al. 2000).

Spinal sensitization is typically attributed to increased C-fiber activity that elicits increased output of excitatory neurotransmitter release, including glutamate acting at the *N*-methyl-D-aspartate (NMDA) receptor complex (Wall and Woolf 1986). Some investigators have proposed that structural reorganization of the spinal dorsal horn may underlie increased sensitivity to normally innocuous mechanical stimulation after nerve injury (Woolf et al. 1992; Lekan et al. 1997). However, the rapid onset of behavioral signs of nerve injury pain appears inconsistent with this idea. For these reasons, discharge of large myelinated fibers may represent an important mechanism that mediates some aspects of the neuropathic pain state. Critically, these fibers may ultimately be responsible for the expression of tactile allodynia, often the most relevant and devastating characteristic of clinical neuropathic pain (Shir and Seltzer 1990; Ossipov et al. 1999). In light of these considerations, we explored the possible role of large fibers in the expression of behavioral signs of nerve injury pain. Such large sensory fibers are known to project directly, or through a postsynaptic link, to the brainstem by way of the ipsilateral dorsal columns.

ASCENDING INPUT AND SUPRASPINAL SITES IN THE MEDIATION OF EXPERIMENTAL NEUROPATHIC PAIN

Converging evidence indicates that some behavioral manifestations of sustained pain states, including neuropathic pain, are under supraspinal control. Pertovaara and colleagues demonstrated the development of secondary hyperalgesia and increased neuronal activity of wide-dynamic-range (WDR) neurons in response to light mechanical stimuli after application of mustard oil to the rat hindpaw (Mansikka and Pertovaara 1997; Pertovaara 1998). These responses were abolished by transection of the spinal cord, indicating that increased sensitivity to innocuous or noxious mechanical stimuli may require a supraspinal loop (Mansikka and Pertovaara 1997; Pertovaara 1998). When rats with experimental nerve injury pain were subjected to spinal transection at T8, their increased sensitivity to normally non-noxious mechanical, but not to noxious thermal stimuli, was abolished (Bian et al. 1998). Similarly, increased sensitivity of the tail to probing with von Frey filaments after sacral nerve ligation was abolished by spinal transection (Sung et al. 1998). The increased sensitivity to normally non-noxious mechanical stimuli resulting from either carrageenan-induced inflammation or nerve injury was also blocked by a complete transection of the spinal cord (Kauppila et al. 1998). In contrast, responses to noxious thermal stimuli were facilitated, more so in the tail than in the hindpaw (Kauppila et al. 1998). These results are consistent with previous observations that spinalization facilitates thermal nociceptive responses (Advokat 1989; Bian et al. 1998).

The variable responses to spinalization, along with the presence of motor paralysis of the hindpaws, suggested the need for additional studies employing more circumscribed lesions. We have shown that spinal hemisections performed at T8 block increased sensitivity to normally non-noxious mechanical stimuli only when the transection is ipsilateral, and not contralateral, to the experimental nerve injury (Sun et al. 2001). If the driving force promoting neuropathic pain were mediated through the anterolateral spinothalamic tract (STT), as would occur if the large-diameter Aβ fibers formed abnormal collateral sprouts synapsing with second-order neurons of the superficial laminae of the spinal cord (Woolf et al. 1992; Lekan et al. 1997), then contralateral hemisections would be expected to block such increased sensitivity to normally innocuous mechanical stimuli; however, this was not observed (Sun et al. 2001). Rather, the data suggested that afferent sensory input through large-diameter fibers may reach supraspinal sites by means of direct, and/or postsynaptic, dorsal column neurons (Bennett et al. 1984; Willis 1985; Willis and Westlund 1997). In this case, the afferent projections occur predominantly ipsilateral to afferent input, and thus spinal hemisection performed ipsilateral to SNL should block behavioral signs of neuropathic pain. This possibility was supported by observations that ablation of the dorsal columns completely blocked increased sensitivity to normally non-noxious mechanical stimuli in rats with nerve injury (Sun et al. 2001). Responses to acute noxious stimuli were not altered, and the animals displayed no signs of compromised motor activity. Most convincingly, discrete lesions limited to one-half the dorsal column also blocked increased sensitivity to normally non-noxious mechanical stimuli only when performed ipsilateral, and not contralateral, to the side of experimental nerve injury (Sun et al. 2001). Animals with sham nerve injury and with dorsal column lesions behaved normally and displayed normal sensory thresholds. Similar results come from studies using a model of bone pain. Lesions of the dorsal column blocked increased sensitivity to normally innocuous mechanical stimuli, but without altering behaviors suggestive of spontaneous pain; the investigators concluded that supraspinal input through the dorsal columns may be essential for the development of tactile-evoked pain (Houghton et al. 1997). These observations collectively support the hypothesis that ascending sensory input through the dorsal columns may drive abnormal pain.

The dorsal column postsynaptic neurons represent one of the largest somatosensory inputs to the brain; they innervate the dorsal column nuclei, including the nucleus gracilis (Bennett et al. 1983, 1984). The nucleus gracilis may act as a relay for hindpaw mechanical nociceptive input from the spinal cord through to the thalamic nuclei after peripheral nerve injury (Miki et al. 2000). The nucleus gracilis integrates nociceptive visceral and somatic inputs (Al-Chaer et al. 1997), and possibly ascending nociceptive inputs (Willis et al. 1999). The nucleus gracilis undergoes neuroplastic changes after peripheral nerve injury (Noguchi et al. 1994). Retrograde tracer studies show that chronic constriction injury (CCI) causes de novo synthesis of substance P in medium- and large-diameter DRG neurons projecting to the nucleus gracilis, which usually do not express this peptide (Noguchi et al. 1994). Furthermore, CCI also increases the sensitivity and spontaneous activity of nucleus gracilis neurons (Miki et al. 1998), and consequently, of neurons of the ventroposterolateral nucleus of the thalamus (VPL) (Miki et al. 2000). Consistent with these observations, our studies have shown that microinjection of lidocaine into the nucleus gracilis ipsilateral (but not contralateral) to the experimental nerve injury produces a time-related and reversible block of increased sensitivity to normally non-noxious mechanical stimuli, but does not affect the reduced response latencies to noxious thermal stimuli in these nerve-injured rats (Sun et al. 2001).

DESCENDING FACILITATION AND THE MEDIATION OF EXPERIMENTAL NEUROPATHIC PAIN

Input to the nucleus gracilis may be projected to rostral sites, ultimately activating descending facilitatory influences. Projections of the spinothalamic tract and the dorsal column/medial lemniscus converge on the same neurons of the ventrobasal thalamus (Ma et al. 1987). This convergence provides an anatomical basis for an interaction between light mechanical and nociceptive inputs at supraspinal centers. Nociceptive information projects to the somatosensory cortex from this region. To test the hypothesis that input to the somatosensory cortex should give rise to descending inhibitory controls, Calejesan et al. (2000) applied electrical stimulation to the anterior cingulate cortex (ACC). The unexpected result was a facilitation, rather than inhibition, of the nociceptive tail-flick reflex. This electrically evoked facilitation was blocked by microinjection of lidocaine into the rostroventromedial medulla (RVM) (Calejesan et al. 2000). Such observations suggest an anatomical basis by which sensory input ascending through the dorsal columns might subserve descending pain-modulatory systems.

Considerable evidence points to the RVM as an important source of descending modulation of nociceptive input to the spinal cord. Studies of modulatory activity of a noxious stimulus of the tail have characterized three types of cells in the RVM. Based on response characteristics to nociception and withdrawal reflexes, these cells are described as "ON" cells, "OFF" cells, and neutral cells (Fields et al. 1983; Fields and Heinricher 1985; Fields 1992). The physiological function of the neutral cells is undetermined, but they do not appear to contribute to opioid analgesia. The "OFF" cells are tonically active and pause in their firing immediately before a withdrawal response occurs to nociceptive stimuli. Mu-opioid agonists increase "OFF" cell activity and block their pause, concomitant with inhibition of withdrawal reflexes. An extensive series of experiments has determined that activation of the "OFF" cells is responsible for spinopetal inhibitory influences, producing an attenuation of nociceptive input, and thus nocifensive responses, at the level of the spinal cord (Fields et al. 1983; Fields and Heinricher 1985; Heinricher et al. 1992; Fields and Basbaum 1999). The "ON" cells accelerate their firing immediately before the nociceptive reflex occurs. These neurons are likely to be the source of descending facilitation from the RVM, possibly through both local interactions within the RVM and descending systems projecting to the spinal cord (Fields et al. 1991; Heinricher et al. 1992; Heinricher and Roychowdhury 1997). For example, tail-flick latency was reduced during periods of increased "ON"-cell activity (Heinricher et al. 1989). Manipulations that increase nociceptive responsiveness, thus indicating facilitation, also increase "ON"-cell activity. The spontaneous activity of "ON" cells increases along with facilitated nociresponsive behavior during naloxone-precipitated withdrawal (Bederson et al. 1990; Kim et al. 1990). Additionally, these actions can be blocked by microinjection of lidocaine into the RVM (Kaplan and Fields 1991). Electrical stimulation of the RVM at low intensities facilitates dorsal horn neuronal activity and the spinal nociceptive tail-flick reflex, further demonstrating the nociceptive facilitation arising from this region (Zhuo and Gebhart 1992, 1997).

While the importance of "ON" cells in the physiological modulation of acute pain is unclear, their presence suggests that inappropriate tonic discharge of these cells may represent a mechanism of chronic abnormal pain, such as that arising from nerve injury. Experimental observations support this possibility. Prolonged delivery of a noxious thermal stimulus produced increased "ON"-cell activity along with a facilitation of nociceptive reflexes (Morgan and Fields 1994). Moreover, inactivation of RVM activity with lidocaine blocked these facilitated withdrawal responses (Morgan and Fields 1994). The activation of "ON" cells by cholecystokinin (CCK)-8 microinjected into the RVM enhanced nociceptive input and attenuated the morphine-induced reduction of "ON"-cell responses to nociception (Heinricher and McGaraughty 1996). Behavioral signs of experimental neuropathic pain were produced by microinjection of CCK-8 in the RVM of uninjured rats (Kovelowski et al. 2000). Further, microinjection of the CCK_B-receptor antagonist L365,260 into the RVM blocked the increased sensitivity to both normally non-noxious mechanical and noxious thermal stimuli in nerve-injured rats (Kovelowski et al. 2000). Critically, RVM microinjection of lidocaine reversibly blocks the behavioral signs of experimental neuropathic pain (Pertovaara et al. 1996; Kovelowski et al. 2000), suggesting tonic discharge of descending facilitation arising in the RVM.

Facilitation from the RVM has been implicated in multiple pain states. Persistent nociceptive input from an injection of formalin into the hindpaw facilitates the tail-flick reflex through an NMDA-dependent action within the RVM (Wiertelak et al. 1994). Similarly, the application of mustard oil to a hindlimb increases both WDR activity and sensitivity to non-noxious stimuli, both of which are abolished by the administration of lidocaine into medullary nuclei of intact rats (Mansikka and Pertovaara 1997; Pertovaara 1998). Bilateral RVM lesions produced by the soma-selective neurotoxin ibotenic acid block thermal secondary, but not primary, hyperalgesia (Urban et al. 1999). Such observations support the concept that the RVM contributes significantly to descending facilitation of nociception, and that such facilitation may manifest behaviorally as increased sensitivity to normally non-noxious mechanical and noxious thermal stimuli induced by injury.

The RVM is considered the principal source of the descending projections of the dorsolateral funiculus (DLF) (Fields et al. 1991; Fields and Basbaum 1999). The function of the DLF as a conduit of descending inhibition from the RVM has been well established. Transection of the DLF abolishes antinociception arising from morphine or from electrical stimulation applied in the RVM (Fields et al. 1991; Fields and Basbaum 1999). In contrast, although "ON"-cell axons are clearly present in the DLF (Fields et. al. 1995), direct evidence for spinopetal facilitatory fibers from the RVM in the DLF has not been well explored. Electrical stimulation of the DLF excites dorsal horn units in lamina I (McMahon and Wall 1983, 1988). Spinal cord block confirmed that at least part of the excitation of these units was due to activation of descending fibers, and not to antidromic activation of ascending fibers (McMahon and Wall 1988). We have shown that increased sensitivity to normally non-noxious mechanical stimulation resulting from spinal nerve injury is reversed by a lesion of the DLF made ipsilateral to the nerve injury (Ossipov et al. 2000). DLF lesion contralateral to the side of the nerve injury, or sham surgery, had no effect on the behavioral manifestation of experimental neuropathic pain (Ossipov et al. 2000). Abnormal pain induced by prolonged opioid exposure was also blocked by DLF lesions or by lidocaine administered to the RVM, indicating that enhanced sensitivity to normally innocuous mechanical stimulation or to noxious thermal stimulation is mediated by descending facilitation from the RVM (Vanderah et al. 2001). Other studies have also suggested the potential importance of RVM-mediated facilitation through the ventrolateral funiculus (VLF). Facilitation of nociceptive reflexes and dorsal horn unit activity in response to noxious stimuli was blocked by lesions of the VLF, but not of the DLF (Zhuo and Gebhart 1997; Urban and Gebhart 1999). Similarly, microinjection of neurotensin into the RVM either inhibited or facilitated dorsal horn unit responses to thermal stimuli. Lesions of the DLF abolished the inhibitory effect of neurotensin, whereas VLF lesions abolished facilitation (Urban and Gebhart 1997). These studies involving VLF lesions were performed under different experimental conditions (awake, freely moving rats versus lightly anesthetized rats) and involving different mechanisms of inducing chronic pain (neuropathic versus inflammatory).

Clearly, sustained afferent input after nerve injury is likely to be required for the expression of experimental neuropathic pain. Application of lidocaine directly at the site of peripheral nerve injury produces a time-related block of increased sensitivity both to normally innocuous mechanical stimulation and to noxious thermal stimulation of the hindpaws (Malan et al. 2000). Spinal injection of NMDA antagonists to rats or mice with SNL blocks behavioral signs of neuropathic pain, presumably by reducing the consequences of increased afferent input (Chaplan et al. 1997; Wegert et al. 1997; Wang et al. 2001). Furthermore, spinal nerve injury diminishes the antinociceptive activity of intrathecal morphine, which may reflect an increase in required dose to compensate for facilitation of nociception (Ossipov et al. 1995a). This possibility is supported by the fact that the antinociceptive action of spinal morphine was restored by bupivacaine at the site of injury (Ossipov et al. 1995b). Further, lidocaine at the site of spinal nerve injury restored the diminished ability of morphine, administered to the periaqueductal gray, to suppress the tail-flick response in rats with SNL (Kovelowski et al. 2000). These findings also indicate that injury to afferent fibers in the hindlimb elicits plasticity of the central nervous system at rostral sites such as the midbrain. Similarly, persistent afferent input arising from peripheral nerve injury is likely to elicit neuroplastic changes within the RVM, resulting in tonic discharge of descending pain facilitation pathways. The demonstration of tonic facilitation arising from the RVM suggests that some of the changes seen in the spinal cord after nerve injury result from activation of descending modulation, independent of sustained primary afferent input to the spinal dorsal horn. Of particular interest is the observation that the expected increase in the expression of dynorphin in the spinal cord after SNL is prevented by lesions of the DLF (T.W. Vanderah and F. Porreca, unpublished observations).

SPINAL DYNORPHIN AND EXPERIMENTAL NEUROPATHIC PAIN

Considerable evidence supports the concept that dynorphin is pronociceptive. States of chronic inflammation and peripheral nerve injury that are accompanied by manifestations of abnormal pain, including spontaneous pain, and by increased sensitivity to normally non-noxious and noxious stimuli (i.e., allodynia and hyperalgesia), arc also associated with increased levels of dynorphin mRNA or protein (Kajander et al. 1990; Draisci et al. 1991; Dubner and Ruda 1992). Dynorphin-like immunoreactivity and prodynorphin mRNA levels are substantially elevated in the spinal cord perfusate of polyarthritic rats (Pohl et al. 1997). Increased sensitivity to normally innocuous mechanical and noxious thermal stimuli following spinal nerve injury is reversed by spinal injection of dynorphin antiserum (Malan et al. 2000; Wang et al. 2001). Similarly, after cryoneurolytic disruption of the sciatic nerve that elevated spinal dynorphin levels, the associated pain behaviors were blocked by spinal administration of dynorphin antiserum (Wagner et al. 1993; Wagner and Deleo 1996). Conversely, in uninjured rats and mice, a single spinal injection of dynorphin, or its non-opioid des-Tyr fragments, produced long-lasting increased sensitivity to normally innocuous mechanical stimuli (Vanderah et al. 1996; Laughlin et al. 1997).

Evidence supports a functional link between dynorphin and NMDA-receptor activity. Blockade of NMDA-receptor activity protects against dynorphin-induced hindlimb paralysis (Bakshi and Faden 1990; Bakshi et al. 1992; Long et al. 1994), loss of tail-flick reflex (Caudle and Isaac 1988; Stewart and Isaac 1991), and increased sensitivity to normally non-noxious mechanical stimuli (Vanderah et al. 1996). Electrophysiological studies have suggested both an inhibitory (Chen et al. 1995) and an excitatory (Lai et al. 1998) action of dynorphin at the NMDA-receptor complex. We demonstrated a direct, high-affinity inhibitory binding site for dynorphin at the NMDA receptor (Tang et al. 1999). Dynorphin's ability to increase calcium accumulation in isolated cortical cells by a mechanism not mediated through opioid or NMDA receptors suggests a novel excitatory action (Tang et al. 2000). Clearly, dynorphin acts either directly or indirectly to stimulate NMDA-receptor activity, although the precise mechanism is uncertain.

Spinal dynorphin content is substantially elevated after experimental injury to spinal nerves, with maximal levels of dynorphin occurring as late as post-injury day 10 (Malan et al. 2000; Wang et al. 2001). In contrast, behavioral signs of abnormal pain occur within 2 days (Bian et al. 1999; Malan et al. 2000; Wang et al. 2001), suggesting that elevation of spinal dynorphin is not important in the initial stages of nerve injury pain. This proposal is supported by the observation that in mice tested within 2 days of SNL, increased sensitivity to normally innocuous mechanical stimuli was reversed by spinal injections of the NMDA antagonist MK-801, but not by antiserum to dynorphin. In contrast, on the 10th day after SNL, spinal injections of both MK-801 and antiserum to dynorphin blocked signs of neuropathic pain, indicating that spinal dynorphin was elevated at that time (Wang et al. 2001). Furthermore, mice with deletions of the prodynorphin gene developed behavioral signs of neuropathic pain within 2 days of experimental nerve injury, and these signs were blocked by MK-801. These behavioral signs of experimental neuropathic pain spontaneously resolved, returning to baseline levels in the prodynorphin knockout mice by post-injury day 10; in contrast, wild-type litter-mates maintained enhanced sensitivity to normally non-noxious mechanical and noxious thermal stimuli typical of the post-nerve-injury state (Wang et al. 2001). These studies indicate that while elevated spinal dynorphin is not a factor in the initiation of nerve injury pain, it is essential for the long-term maintenance of abnormal pain after nerve injury.

These studies suggest that abnormally high levels of spinal dynorphin act to maintain, but not to initiate, neuropathic pain. While the exact mechanisms await further study, considerable evidence suggests that elevated levels of spinal dynorphin act through non-opioid mechanisms to enhance the release of excitatory transmitters from primary afferent fibers. Such enhancement of evoked transmitter release may provide a basis by which central changes can enhance the actions of diminished afferent discharge from injured nerves to maintain the neuropathic pain state. Microdialysis studies have demonstrated localized, dose-dependent release of glutamate and aspartate elicited by exogenous dynorphin in the hippocampus and spinal cord (Faden 1992; Skilling et al. 1992). Capsaicin-stimulated release of calcitonin gene-related peptide (CGRP) is potentiated by dynorphin in spinal cord slices in vitro (Claude et al. 1999). Spinal cord tissues obtained from rats with experimental nerve injury demonstrate significantly elevated capsaicin-induced release of CGRP, and this effect was blocked by antiserum to dynorphin; conversely, dynorphin antiserum did not alter capsaicin-induced release of CGRP in spinal cord tissue from sham-operated rats (T.W. Vanderah and F. Porreca, unpublished results). These observations are consistent with previous reports that dynorphin facilitates capsaicin-evoked substance P release from trigeminal nuclear slices, an effect blocked by MK-801 but not by opioid antagonists (Arcaya et al. 1999).

IMPLICATIONS FOR OPIOID EFFICACY

A commonly reported feature of clinical neuropathic pain is its resistance to amelioration by opioids. Increased sensitivity to normally non-noxious mechanical stimulation in animals with experimental nerve injury is completely resistant to spinal morphine, even at doses that are multiples of normally antinociceptive levels in non-injured rats (Bian et al. 1995, 1999; Lee et al. 1995). Additionally, the antinociceptive effect of morphine against acute noxious thermal stimuli applied to the tail is also reduced in rats with injury to spinal nerves that innervate the paw (Ossipov ct al. 1995a). In spite of such lost or reduced spinal efficacy, supraspinal (i.c.v.) morphine measurably suppresses enhanced sensitivity to normally non-noxious mechanical stimulation of the paw in rats with experimental nerve injury. However, the expected synergistic antinociceptive effect of spinal and supraspinal morphine seen in uninjured rats is lost for suppression of responses to both non-noxious mechanical and noxious thermal stimuli in nerve-injured rats (Bian et al. 1995, 1999; Lee et al. 1995). This absence of activity of spinal morphine is probably unrelated to opioid receptor activity because nerve injury is not accompanied by a substantial loss of spinal opioid receptors or of their transduction efficacy (Porreca et al. 1998). Additionally, large-diameter myelinated Aβ afferent fibers, which probably transmit light touch stimuli, do not appear to express opioid receptors (Taddese et al. 1995; Zhang et al. 1998). These findings suggest that the neural changes occurring in the spinal cord effectively inhibit the actions of spinal morphine, resulting in a loss of supraspinal/spinal synergy. The loss of expected site-to-site synergy for systemically given opioids (such as morphine) in the post-nerve-injury state would necessitate higher doses to achieve pain relief. Such loss of synergy may therefore be an important factor contributing to the relative lack of efficacy of systemic opioids in clinical treatment of neuropathic pain.

Manipulations that reduce afferent input are effective in blocking the behavioral manifestations of neuropathic pain and effectively restore the efficacy of opioids in the nerve-injured condition. The application of bupivacaine at the site of spinal nerve injury restored the antinociceptive potency of spinal morphine to suppress the tail-flick response, presumably by reducing afferent tone and thus diminishing the net effect of the facilitated state (Ossipov et al. 1995b). Furthermore, spinal injection of either MK-801 or antiserum to dynorphin restored the antinociceptive potency of spinal morphine and reversed the animals' enhanced sensitivity to normally innocuous mechanical stimulation (Nichols et al. 1997; Bian et al. 1999). Finally, these treatments restore the spinal/supraspinal antinociceptive synergy of morphine (Bian et al. 1999). These observations collectively point to a reduction in afferent input and/or in spinal dynorphin activity as a means of dampening the tonic facilitation initiated by the original insult to the nerve.

CONCLUSION

The data reviewed in this chapter suggest that the processes that initiate neuropathic pain differ from those that are essential to maintaining it. The latter mechanisms are significant because clinical intervention occurs during the maintenance phase. The possibility that spinal plasticity is critical in maintaining neuropathic pain and that these spinal changes may result, in part, from tonic activation of descending facilitation from the brainstem suggests numerous strategies for development of rational therapies for the treatment of neuropathic pain states. The observations presented here raise many questions regarding the mechanisms by which descending facilitation occurs and is sustained. Additionally, the nature of those spinal processes by which the ultimate effects of sustained but diminished degrees of afferent input are potentiated by central plasticity to chronically maintain pain remains to be explored.

REFERENCES

Advokat C. Tolerance to the antinociceptive effect of morphine in spinally transected rats. *Behav Neurosci* 1989; 103:1091–1098.

Al-Chaer ED, Westlund KN, Willis WD. Nucleus gracilis: an integrator for visceral and somatic information. *J Neurophysiol* 1997; 78:521–527.

Arcaya JL, Cano G, Gomez G, Maixner W, Suarez-Roca H. Dynorphin A increases substance P release from trigeminal primary afferent C-fibers. *Eur J Pharmacol* 1999; 366:27–34.

Bakshi R, Faden AI. Competitive and non-competitive NMDA antagonists limit dynorphin A-induced rat hindlimb paralysis. *Brain Res* 1990; 507:1–5.

Bakshi R, Ni RX, Faden AI. *N*-methyl-D-aspartate (NMDA) and opioid receptors mediate dynorphin-induced spinal cord injury: behavioral and histological studies. *Brain Res* 1992; 580:255–264.

Bederson JB, Fields HL, Barbaro NM. Hyperalgesia during naloxone-precipitated withdrawal from morphine is associated with increased on-cell activity in the rostral ventromedial medulla. *Somatosens Mot Res* 1990; 7:185–203.

Bennett GJ, Seltzer Z, Lu GW, Nishikawa N, Dubner R. The cells of origin of the dorsal column postsynaptic projection in the lumbosacral enlargements of cats and monkeys. *Somatosens Mot Res* 1983; 1:131–149.

Bennett GJ, Nishikawa N, Lu GW, Hoffert MJ, Dubner R. The morphology of dorsal column postsynaptic spinomedullary neurons in the cat. *J Comp Neurol* 1984; 224:568–578.

Bian D, Nichols ML, Ossipov MH, Lai J, Porreca F. Characterization of the antiallodynic efficacy of morphine in a model of neuropathic pain in rats. *Neuroreport* 1995; 6:1981–1984.

Bian D, Ossipov MH, Zhong C, Malan TP Jr, Porreca F. Tactile allodynia, but not thermal hyperalgesia, of the hindlimbs is blocked by spinal transection in rats with nerve injury. *Neurosci Lett* 1998; 241:79–82.

Bian D, Ossipov MH, Ibrahim M, et al. Loss of antiallodynic and antinociceptive spinal/supraspinal morphine synergy in nerve-injured rats: restoration by MK-801 or dynorphin antiserum. *Brain Res* 1999; 831:55–63.

Boucher TJ, Okuse K, Bennett DL, et al. Potent analgesic effects of GDNF in neuropathic pain states. *Science* 2000; 290:124–127.

Calejesan AA, Kim SJ, Zhuo M. Descending facilitatory modulation of a behavioral nociceptive response by stimulation in the adult rat anterior cingulate cortex. *Eur J Pain* 2000; 4:83–96.

Caudle RM, Isaac L. A novel interaction between dynorphin(1–13) and an *N*-methyl-D-aspartate site. *Brain Res* 1988; 443:329–332.

Chaplan SR, Bach FW, Pogrel JW, Chung JM, Yaksh TL. Quantitative assessment of tactile allodynia in the rat paw. *J Neurosci Methods* 1994; 53:55–63.

Chaplan SR, Malmberg AB, Yaksh TL. Efficacy of spinal NMDA receptor antagonism in formalin hyperalgesia and nerve injury evoked allodynia in the rat. *J Pharmacol Exp Ther* 1997; 280:829–838.

Chen L, Gu Y, Huang LY. The opioid peptide dynorphin directly blocks NMDA receptor channels in the rat. *J Physiol* 1995; 482:575–581.

Claude P, Gracia N, Wagner L, Hargreaves KM. Effect of dynorphin on ICGRP release from capsaicin-sensitive fibers. *Abstracts: 9th World Congress on Pain.* Seattle: IASP Press, 1999, p. 262.

Craft RM, Carlisi VJ, Mattia A, Herman RM, Porreca F. Behavioral characterization of the excitatory and desensitizing effects of intravesical capsaicin and resiniferatoxin in the rat. *Pain* 1993; 55:205–215.

Devor M. Neuropathic pain and injured nerve: peripheral mechanisms. *Br Med Bull* 1991; 47:619–630.

Devor M. The pathophysiology of damaged peripheral nerves. In: Wall PD, Melzack R (Eds). *Textbook of Pain.* Edinburgh: Churchill Livingstone, 1994, pp 79–100.

Draisci G, Kajander KC, Dubner R, Bennett GJ, Iadarola MJ. Up-regulation of opioid gene expression in spinal cord evoked by experimental nerve injuries and inflammation. *Brain Res* 1991; 560:186–192.

Dubner R, Ruda MA. Activity-dependent neuronal plasticity following tissue injury and inflammation. *Trends Neurosci* 1992; 15:96–103.

England JD, Happel LT, Kline DG, et al. Sodium channel accumulation in humans with painful neuromas. *Neurology* 1996; 47:272–276.

Faden AI. Dynorphin increases extracellular levels of excitatory amino acids in the brain through a non-opioid mechanism. *J Neurosci* 1992; 12:425–429.

Fields HL. Is there a facilitating component to central pain modulation? *Am Pain Soc J* 1992; 1:71–78.

Fields HL, Basbaum AI. Central nervous system mechanisms of pain modulation. In: Wall PD, Melzack R (Eds). *Textbook of Pain.* Edinburgh: Churchill Livingstone, 1999, pp 309–329.

Fields HL, Heinricher MM. Anatomy and physiology of a nociceptive modulatory system. *Philos Trans R Soc Lond B Biol Sci* 1985; 308:361–374.

Fields HL, Rowbotham MC. Multiple mechanisms of neuropathic pain: a clinical perspective. In: Gebhart GF, Hammond DL, Jensen TS (Eds). *Proceedings of the 7th World Congress on Pain*, Progress in Pain Research and Management, Vol. 2. Seattle: IASP Press, 1994, pp 437–454.

Fields HL, Bry J, Hentall I, Zorman G. The activity of neurons in the rostral medulla of the rat during withdrawal from noxious heat. *J Neurosci* 1983; 3:2545–2552.

Fields HL, Heinricher MM, Mason P. Neurotransmitters in nociceptive modulatory circuits. *Annu Rev Neurosci* 1991; 14:219–245.

Fields HL, Malick A, Burstein R. Dorsal horn projection targets of on and off cells in the rostral ventromedial medulla. *J Neurophysiol* 1995; 74:1742–1759.

Fields HL, Rowbotham MC, Devor M. Excitability blockers: anticonvulsants and low concentration local anesthetics in the treatment of chronic pain. In: Dickenson A, Besson JM (Eds). *Handbook of Experimental Pharmacology.* Berlin: Springer Verlag, 1997, pp 93–116.

Gracely RH, Lynch SA, Bennett GJ. Painful neuropathy: altered central processing maintained dynamically by peripheral input. *Pain* 1992; 51:175–194.

Han HC, Lee DH, Chung JM. Characteristics of ectopic discharges in a rat neuropathic pain model. *Pain* 2000; 84:253–261.

Heinricher MM, McGaraughty S. CCK modulates the antinociceptive actions of opioids by an action within the rostral ventromedial medulla: a combined electrophysiological and behavioral study. *Abstracts: 8th World Congress on Pain.* Seattle: IASP Press, 1996, p 472.

Heinricher MM, Roychowdhury SM. Reflex-related activation of putative pain facilitating neurons in rostral ventromedial medulla requires excitatory amino acid transmission. *Neuroscience* 1997; 78:1159–1165.

Heinricher MM, Barbaro NM, Fields HL. Putative nociceptive modulating neurons in the rostral ventromedial medulla of the rat: firing of on- and off-cells is related to nociceptive responsiveness. *Somatosens Mot Res* 1989; 6:427–439.

Heinricher MM, Morgan MM, Fields HL. Direct and indirect actions of morphine on medullary neurons that modulate nociception. *Neuroscience* 1992; 48:533–543.

Houghton AK, Kadura S, Westlund KN. Dorsal column lesions reverse the reduction of homecage activity in rats with pancreatitis. *Neuroreport* 1997; 8:3795–3800.

Kajander KC, Bennett GJ. Onset of a painful peripheral neuropathy in rat: a partial and differential deafferentation and spontaneous discharge in A beta and A delta primary afferent neurons. *J Neurophysiol* 1992; 68:734–744.

Kajander KC, Sahara Y, Iadarola MJ, Bennett GJ. Dynorphin increases in the dorsal spinal cord in rats with a painful peripheral neuropathy. *Peptides* 1990; 11:719–728.

Kajander KC, Wakisaka S, Bennett GJ. Spontaneous discharge originates in the dorsal root ganglion at the onset of a painful peripheral neuropathy in the rat. *Neurosci Lett* 1992; 138:225–228.

Kaplan H, Fields HL. Hyperalgesia during acute opioid abstinence: evidence for a nociceptive facilitating function of the rostral ventromedial medulla. *J Neurosci* 1991; 11:1433–1439.

Kauppila T, Kontinen VK, Pertovaara A. Influence of spinalization on spinal withdrawal reflex responses varies depending on the submodality of the test stimulus and the experimental pathophysiological condition in the rat. *Brain Res* 1998; 797:234–242.

Kim DH, Fields HL, Barbaro NM. Morphine analgesia and acute physical dependence: rapid onset of two opposing, dose-related processes. *Brain Res* 1990; 516:37–40.

Kirk EJ. Impulses in dorsal spinal nerve rootlets in cats and rabbits arising from dorsal root ganglia isolated from the periphery. *J Comp Neurol* 1974; 155:165–175.

Kovelowski CJ, Ossipov MH, Sun H, et al. Supraspinal cholecystokinin may drive tonic descending facilitation mechanisms to maintain neuropathic pain in the rat. *Pain* 2000; 87:265–273.

Lai SL, Gu Y, Huang LY. Dynorphin uses a non-opioid mechanism to potentiate *N*-methyl-D-aspartate currents in single rat periaqueductal gray neurons. *Neurosci Lett* 1998; 247:115–118.

Laughlin TM, Vanderah TW, Lashbrook J, et al. Spinally administered dynorphin A produces long-lasting allodynia: involvement of NMDA but not opioid receptors. *Pain* 1997; 72:253–260.

Lee YW, Chaplan SR, Yaksh TL. Systemic and supraspinal, but not spinal, opiates suppress allodynia in a rat neuropathic pain model. *Neurosci Lett* 1995; 199:111–114.

Lekan HA, Chung K, Yoon YW, Chung JM, Coggeshall RE. Loss of dorsal root ganglion cells concomitant with dorsal root axon sprouting following segmental nerve lesions. *Neuroscience* 1997; 81:527–534.

Liu C, Wall PD, Ben-Dor E, et al. Tactile allodynia in the absence of C-fiber activation: altered firing properties of DRG neurons following spinal nerve injury. *Pain* 2000; 85:503–521.

Liu X, Eschenfelder S, Blenk KH, Jänig W, Häbler H. Spontaneous activity of axotomized afferent neurons after L5 spinal nerve injury in rats. *Pain* 2000; 84:309–318.

Long JB, Rigamonti DD, Oleshansky MA, Wingfield CP, Martinez-Arizala A. Dynorphin A-induced rat spinal cord injury: evidence for excitatory amino acid involvement in a pharmacological model of ischemic spinal cord injury. *J Pharmacol Exp Ther* 1994; 269:358–366.

Ma W, Peschanski M, Ralston HJD. The differential synaptic organization of the spinal and lemniscal projections to the ventrobasal complex of the rat thalamus. Evidence for convergence of the two systems upon single thalamic neurons. *Neuroscience* 1987; 22:925–934.

Malan TP, Ossipov MH, Gardell LR, et al. Extraterritorial neuropathic pain correlates with multisegmental elevation of spinal dynorphin in nerve-injured rats. *Pain* 2000; 86:185–194.

Mansikka H, Pertovaara A. Supraspinal influence on hindlimb withdrawal thresholds and mustard oil-induced secondary allodynia in rats. *Brain Res Bull* 1997; 42:359–365.

McMahon SB, Wall PD. A system of rat spinal cord lamina 1 cells projecting through the contralateral dorsolateral funiculus. *J Comp Neurol* 1983; 214:217–223.

McMahon SB, Wall PD. Descending excitation and inhibition of spinal cord lamina I projection neurons. *J Neurophysiol* 1988; 59:1204–1219.

Merskey H, Bogduk N (Eds). *Classification of Chronic Pain: Descriptions of Chronic Pain Syndromes and Definitions of Pain Terms,* 2nd ed. Seattle: IASP Press, 1994.

Miki K, Iwata K, Tsuboi Y, et al. Responses of dorsal column nuclei neurons in rats with experimental mononeuropathy. *Pain* 1998; 76:407–415.

Miki K, Iwata K, Tsuboi Y, et al. Dorsal column-thalamic pathway is involved in thalamic hyperexcitability following peripheral nerve injury: a lesion study in rats with experimental mononeuropathy. *Pain* 2000; 85:263–271.

Morgan MM, Fields HL. Pronounced changes in the activity of nociceptive modulatory neurons in the rostral ventromedial medulla in response to prolonged thermal noxious stimuli. *J Neurophysiol* 1994; 72:1161–1170.

Nichols ML, Lopez Y, Ossipov MH, Bian D, Porreca F. Enhancement of the antiallodynic and antinociceptive efficacy of spinal morphine by antisera to dynorphin A (1–13) or MK-801 in a nerve-ligation model of peripheral neuropathy. *Pain* 1997; 69:317–322.

Noguchi K, Dubner R, De Leon M, Senba E, Ruda MA. Axotomy induces preprotachykinin gene expression in a subpopulation of dorsal root ganglion neurons. *J Neurosci Res* 1994; 37:596–603.

Ossipov MH, Lopez Y, Nichols ML, Bian D, Porreca F. Inhibition by spinal morphine of the tail-flick response is attenuated in rats with nerve ligation injury. *Neurosci Lett* 1995a; 199:83–86.

Ossipov MH, Lopez Y, Nichols ML, Bian D, Porreca F. The loss of antinociceptive efficacy of spinal morphine in rats with nerve ligation injury is prevented by reducing spinal afferent drive. *Neurosci Lett* 1995b; 199:87–90.

Ossipov MH, Bian D, Malan TP Jr, Lai J, Porreca F. Lack of involvement of capsaicin-sensitive primary afferents in nerve-ligation injury induced tactile allodynia in rats. *Pain* 1999; 79:127–133.

Ossipov MH, Hong Sun T, Malan P Jr, Lai J, Porreca F. Mediation of spinal nerve injury induced tactile allodynia by descending facilitatory pathways in the dorsolateral funiculus in rats. *Neurosci Lett* 2000; 290:129–132.

Payne R. Neuropathic pain syndromes, with special reference to causalgia and reflex sympathetic dystrophy. *Clin J Pain* 1986; 2:59–73.

Pertovaara A. A neuronal correlate of secondary hyperalgesia in the rat spinal dorsal horn is submodality selective and facilitated by supraspinal influence. *Exp Neurol* 1998; 149:193–202.

Pertovaara A, Wei H, Hamalainen MM. Lidocaine in the rostroventromedial medulla and the periaqueductal gray attenuates allodynia in neuropathic rats. *Neurosci Lett* 1996; 218:127–130.

Pohl M, Ballet S, Collin E, et al. Enkephalinergic and dynorphinergic neurons in the spinal cord and dorsal root ganglia of the polyarthritic rat—in vivo release and cDNA hybridization studies. *Brain Res* 1997; 749:18–28.

Porreca F, Tang QB, Bian D, et al. Spinal opioid mu receptor expression in lumbar spinal cord of rats following nerve injury. *Brain Res* 1998; 795:197–203.

Sangameswaran L, Delgado SG, Fish LM, et al. Structure and function of a novel voltage-gated, tetrodotoxin-resistant sodium channel specific to sensory neurons. *J Biol Chem* 1996; 271:5953–5956.

Shir Y, Seltzer Z. A-fibers mediate mechanical hyperesthesia and allodynia and C-fibers mediate thermal hyperalgesia in a new model of causalgiform pain disorders in rats. *Neurosci Lett* 1990; 115:62–67.

Skilling SR, Sun X, Kurtz HJ, Larson AA. Selective potentiation of NMDA-induced activity and release of excitatory amino acids by dynorphin: possible roles in paralysis and neurotoxicity. *Brain Res* 1992; 575:272–278.

Stewart P, Isaac L. A strychnine-sensitive site is involved in dynorphin-induced paralysis and loss of the tail-flick reflex. *Brain Res* 1991; 543:322–326.

Sun H, Ren K, Zhong CM, et al. Nerve-injury induced tactile allodynia is mediated via ascending spinal dorsal column projections. *Pain* 2001; 90:105–111.

Sung B, Na HS, Kim YI, et al. Supraspinal involvement in the production of mechanical allodynia by spinal nerve injury in rats. *Neurosci Lett* 1998; 246:117–119.

Szallasi A, Joo F, Blumberg PM. Duration of desensitization and ultrastructural changes in dorsal root ganglia in rats treated with resiniferatoxin, an ultrapotent capsaicin analog. *Brain Res* 1989; 503:68–72.

Taddese A, Nah SY, McCleskey EW. Selective opioid inhibition of small nociceptive neurons. *Science* 1995; 270:1366–1369.

Tal M, Wall PD, Devor M. Myelinated afferent fiber types that become spontaneously active and mechanosensitive following nerve transection in the rat. *Brain Res* 1999; 824:218–223.

Tang Q, Gandhoke R, Burritt A, et al. High-affinity interaction of (des-Tyrosyl)dynorphin A(2–17) with NMDA receptors. *J Pharmacol Exp Ther* 1999; 291:760–765.

Tang Q, Lynch RM, Porreca F, Lai J. Dynorphin A elicits an increase in intracellular calcium in cultured neurons via a non-opioid, non-NMDA mechanism. *J Neurophysiol* 2000; 83:2610–2615.

Urban MO, Gebhart GF. Characterization of biphasic modulation of spinal nociceptive transmission by neurotensin in the rat rostral ventromedial medulla. *J Neurophysiol* 1997; 78:1550–1562.

Urban MO, Gebhart GF. Supraspinal contributions to hyperalgesia. *Proc Natl Acad Sci USA* 1999; 96:7687–7692.

Urban MO, Zahn PK, Gebhart GF. Descending facilitatory influences from the rostral medial medulla mediate secondary, but not primary hyperalgesia in the rat. *Neuroscience* 1999; 90:349–352.

Vanderah TW, Laughlin T, Lashbrook JM, et al. Single intrathecal injections of dynorphin A or des-Tyr-dynorphins produce long-lasting allodynia in rats: blockade by MK-801 but not naloxone. *Pain* 1996; 68:275–281.

Vanderah TW, Suenaga NM, Ossipov MH, et al. Tonic descending facilitation from the rostral ventromedial medulla mediates opioid-induced abnormal pain and antinociceptive tolerance. *J Neurosci* 2001; 21:279–286.

Wagner R, Deleo JA. Pre-emptive dynorphin and *N*-methyl-D-aspartate glutamate receptor antagonism alters spinal immunocytochemistry but not allodynia following complete peripheral nerve injury. *Neuroscience* 1996; 72:527–534.

Wagner R, DeLeo JA, Coombs DW, Willenbring S, Fromm C. Spinal dynorphin immunoreactivity increases bilaterally in a neuropathic pain model. *Brain Res* 1993; 629:323–326.

Wall PD, Gutnick M. Properties of afferent nerve impulses originating from a neuroma. *Nature* 1974; 248:740–743.

Wall PD, Woolf CJ. The brief and the prolonged facilitatory effects of unmyelinated afferent input on the rat spinal cord are independently influenced by peripheral nerve section. *Neuroscience* 1986; 17:1199–1205.

Wang Z, Gardell LR, Ossipov MH, et al. Pronociceptive actions of dynorphin maintain chronic neuropathic pain. *J Neurosci* 2001; 21:1779–1786.

Wegert S, Ossipov MH, Nichols ML, et al. Differential activities of intrathecal MK-801 or morphine to alter responses to thermal and mechanical stimuli in normal or nerve-injured rats. *Pain* 1997; 71:57–64.

Wiertelak EP, Furness LE, Horan R, et al. Subcutaneous formalin produces centrifugal hyperalgesia at a non-injected site via the NMDA-nitric oxide cascade. *Brain Res* 1994; 649:19–26.

Willis WD. Nociceptive pathways: anatomy and physiology of nociceptive ascending pathways. *Philos Trans R Soc Lond B Biol Sci* 1985; 308:253–270.

Willis WD, Westlund KN. Neuroanatomy of the pain system and of the pathways that modulate pain. *J Clin Neurophysiol* 1997; 14:2–31.

Willis WD, Al-Chaer ED, Quast MJ, Westlund KN. A visceral pain pathway in the dorsal column of the spinal cord. *Proc Natl Acad Sci USA* 1999; 96:7675–7679.

Woolf CJ, Shortland P, Coggeshall RE. Peripheral nerve injury triggers central sprouting of myelinated afferents. *Nature* 1992; 355:75–78.

Xu XJ, Farkas-Szallasi T, Lundberg JM, et al. Effects of the capsaicin analogue resiniferatoxin on spinal nociceptive mechanisms in the rat: behavioral, electrophysiological and in situ hybridization studies. *Brain Res* 1997; 752:52–60.

Zhang X, Bao L, Shi TJ, et al. Down-regulation of mu-opioid receptors in rat and monkey dorsal root ganglion neurons and spinal cord after peripheral axotomy. *Neuroscience* 1998; 82:223–240.

Zhuo M, Gebhart GF. Characterization of descending facilitation and inhibition of spinal nociceptive transmission from the nuclei reticularis gigantocellularis and gigantocellularis pars alpha in the rat. *J Neurophysiol* 1992; 67:1599–1614.

Zhuo M, Gebhart GF. Biphasic modulation of spinal nociceptive transmission from the medullary raphe nuclei in the rat. *J Neurophysiol* 1997; 78:746–758.

Correspondence to: Frank Porreca, PhD, Departments of Pharmacology and Anesthesiology, University of Arizona Health Sciences Center, Tucson, AZ 85724, USA. Tel: 520-626-7421; Fax: 520-626-4182; email: frankp@ u.arizona.edu.

Neuropathic Pain: Pathophysiology and Treatment,
Progress in Pain Research and Management, Vol. 21,
edited by Per T. Hansson, Howard L. Fields, Raymond G.
Hill, and Paolo Marchettini, IASP Press, Seattle, © 2001.

7

The Role of the Sympathetic Nervous System in Neuropathic Pain: Clinical Observations and Animal Models

Wilfrid Jäniga and Ralf Baronb

*Departments of aPhysiology and bNeurology,
University of Kiel, Kiel, Germany*

Interruption of the sympathetic nerve supply to the affected extremity has been used to treat certain pain syndromes for many years. These syndromes include complex regional pain syndromes (CRPS type I, formerly reflex sympathetic dystrophy, and type II, formerly causalgia), post-traumatic neuralgia, phantom limb pain, and to a certain extent acute herpes zoster (Stanton-Hicks et al. 1995; Jänig and Stanton-Hicks 1996; Harden et al. 2001). Patients with CRPS, in particular those with CRPS-I, have pain accompanied by changes that are dependent on the sympathetic nervous system (SNS), such as abnormal regulation of blood flow and sweating; edema of the skin and subcutaneous tissues; and trophic changes of the skin, appendages of skin, and subcutaneous tissues (Blumberg et al. 1994; Blumberg and Jänig 1994; Baron et al. 1996; Jänig and Stanton-Hicks 1996; Baron and Jänig 1998, 2001; Harden et al. 1999; Jänig 1999).

Two therapeutic techniques are commonly used to block sympathetic nerves: (1) injections of a local anesthetic around sympathetic paravertebral ganglia that project to the affected body part (sympathetic ganglion blocks); and (2) regional intravenous (i.v.) application of guanethidine, bretylium, or reserpine (which all deplete norepinephrine in the postganglionic axon) to an isolated extremity blocked with a tourniquet (intravenous regional sympatholysis). However, interventions that block sympathetic activity lack specificity due to inadequate evaluation of the techniques and results of sympathetic blockade and the lack of placebo-controlled studies (see Price et al. 1998).

Neuropathic pain patients can be divided into two groups based on their response to selective sympathetic blockade or antagonism of α-adrenoceptor mechanisms (Arnér 1991; Raja et al. 1991; Price et al. 1998). The pain component that is relieved by specific sympatholytic procedures is considered *sympathetically maintained pain* (SMP). SMP is a general term that includes spontaneous pain and pain evoked by mechanical and thermal stimuli. Thus, SMP is now defined as a *symptom,* not as a clinical entity. The positive effect of a sympathetic blockade is not essential for the diagnosis of a clinical condition such as CRPS. On the other hand, the only way to differentiate between SMP and *sympathetically independent pain* (SIP) is the efficacy of a correctly applied sympatholytic intervention (Stanton-Hicks et al. 1995).

The concept that the (efferent) SNS can contribute to pain is based on longstanding but largely uncontrolled clinical observations (see White and Sweet 1969; Bonica 1990; Blumberg and Jänig 1994; Baron et al. 1996). Systematic studies on patients with CRPS and studies using experimental pain models have established the role of the SNS in generating pain.

HUMAN STUDIES

INFLUENCE OF SYMPATHETIC ACTIVITY AND CATECHOLAMINES ON PRIMARY AFFERENTS AFTER TISSUE INFLAMMATION

Cutaneous application of the algogenic agent capsaicin causes neurogenic inflammation by activating and sensitizing nociceptors. An adrenergic effect on sensitized cutaneous nociceptors was described in this model in human subjects. The heat hyperalgesia that develops after topical application of capsaicin to the skin of human volunteers is enhanced by iontophoresis of norepinephrine (Drummond 1995). Phentolamine, a mixed α_1 and α_2 antagonist, inhibited the norepinephrine-induced pain and mechanical hyperalgesia in capsaicin-sensitized skin (Liu et al. 1996; Kinnman et al. 1997). However, iontophoresis of the nonadrenergic vasoconstrictor agents angiotensin II and vasopressin (Drummond 1998) slightly enhances hyperalgesia in capsaicin-treated skin. Occlusion of blood flow has a similar effect (Drummond et al. 1996). These results suggest that changes in blood flow account for some aspects of the enhanced cutaneous sensibility seen in capsaicin-induced hyperalgesic skin. Modulation of sympathetic cutaneous vasoconstrictor activity in physiological ranges by thermoregulatory stress does not measurably influence capsaicin-induced pain (Baron et al. 1999b). Accordingly, activation of skin sympathetic vasoconstrictor neurons does not change the irritant-induced discharge of single cutaneous C nociceptors in humans (Elam et al. 1996). One controlled study has evaluated the effect of sympathetic blockade on pain after experimental tissue inflammation. Pedersen and colleagues (1997), using a cutaneous heat injury as their pain model, showed that sympathetic blocks with bupivacaine do not alter spontaneous pain and heat hyperalgesia (Raja 1995). In patients with rheumatoid arthritis, however, regional i.v. guanethidine decreases pain and increases pinch strength to elicit pain (Levine et al. 1986a).

INFLUENCE OF SYMPATHETIC ACTIVITY AND CATECHOLAMINES ON PRIMARY AFFERENTS IN PATIENTS WITH NERVE DAMAGE AND CRPS

Clinical studies support the idea that nociceptors develop catecholamine sensitivity after complete or partial nerve lesions. Long after limb amputation, injection of epinephrine around a stump neuroma is intensely painful (Chabal et al. 1992). Recent studies also demonstrate that the perineuromal administration of physiological doses of norepinephrine induces more pain than saline injections (Raja et al. 1998).

Furthermore, intraoperative stimulation of the sympathetic chain increases spontaneous pain in patients with CRPS-II but not in patients with hyperhidrosis (Walker and Nulsen 1948; White and Sweet 1969). In addition, i.v. phentolamine, but not propranolol, relieves SMP (Arnér 1991; Raja et al. 1991). Most researchers agree that pain is relieved by both procedures in patients given both a local anesthetic sympathetic ganglion block and a phentolamine infusion (Raja et al. 1991; Dellemijn et al. 1994).

In CRPS and post-traumatic neuralgias, intracutaneous application of norepinephrine into a symptomatic area rekindles spontaneous pain and dynamic mechanical and cold allodynia that had been relieved by sympathetic blockade, supporting the idea that human nociceptors develop noradrenergic sensitivity after partial nerve lesion (Torebjörk et al. 1995). Furthermore, this group reported that SMP can be maintained for many years (Wahren et al. 1995). Some patients with postherpetic neuralgia experience increased spontaneous pain and mechanical hyperalgesia after intracutaneous injection of epinephrine or phenylephrine (Choi and Rowbotham 1997). A potential criticism of studies in which pain is rekindled with exogenous adrenergic agonists is that the doses of norepinephrine are much higher than are likely to exist in vivo. Therefore, Ali and colleagues (2000) compared the algesic effects of peripheral administration of norepinephrine in physiologically relevant doses in patients with SMP and normal subjects. Intradermal norepinephrine evoked greater pain in the affected regions of patients with SMP than in the contralateral unaffected limb or in control subjects. Most of the patients whose pain increased after injection of norepinephrine

in the affected extremity reported a decrease in pain following systemic administration of phentolamine. These observations suggest that adrenoceptors in
the skin are involved in the mechanisms of SMP.

Patients with CRPS-I and SMP experience more spontaneous pain and
mechanical hyperalgesia when sympathetic cutaneous vasoconstrictor neurons are activated physiologically by cold stress (Fig. 1; R. Baron, unpublished

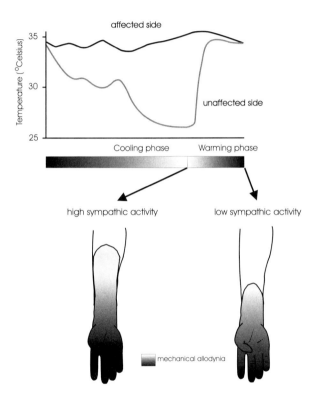

Fig. 1. Influence of cutaneous sympathetic vasoconstrictor activity on pain in patients
with CRPS. Physiological reflex stimuli were applied that activate sympathetic neurons
and lead to norepinephrine release. A thermal suit was supplied by tubes in which
running water at an inflow temperature of 12°C or 50°C was used to cool or warm the
whole body and alter sympathetic activity in cutaneous nerves. Cooling induces a
massive tonic activation of these neurons, whereas warming considerably decreases
their activity. Sympathetic activity to skin thus can be switched on and off in a
controlled manner while pain sensations are measured. High sympathetic activity
during cooling decreases skin temperature due to vasoconstriction (on the unaffected
side). During the experiment the forearm temperature on the affected side was maintained at 35°C by a feedback-controlled heat lamp to exclude temperature effects on the
sensory receptor level. Activation of sympathetic neurons considerably increases the
area of allodynia in patients with SMP, indicating a pathological coupling between
sympathetic and nociceptive neurons in CRPS patients (R. Baron, unpublished observation; see also Wasner et al. 2001).

data). Five patients with CRPS-I who had SMP all experienced greater pain when cold stress was applied to the hand. Sympathetic blocks with local anesthetic increased the skin temperature of the hand to $\geq 35°C$ and significantly decreased spontaneous pain and mechanical allodynia. Results in these patients show a high correlation between pain relief during sympathetic blocks and augmentation of pain during thermoregulatory cold stress. Five patients with CRPS-I who had SIP served as controls; thermoregulatory cold stress did not augment their spontaneous pain or mechanical allodynia, nor did sympathetic blocks bring relief. This experimental study on CRPS patients does not indicate whether the experimentally evoked SMP is generated by direct or indirect coupling between sympathetic and afferent fibers.

Additional lines of evidence support a peripheral α-adrenergic mechanism in SMP. Topical application of the α_2-adrenoceptor agonist clonidine relieves hyperalgesia at the site of application in SMP, but not SIP patients (Davis et al. 1991; Wesselmann et al. 1996). This effect was secondary to a reduction in the release of norepinephrine via activation of the α_2-adrenergic autoreceptor on the sympathetic terminal. Injection of norepinephrine and the α_1-adrenoceptor agonist phenylephrine into the clonidine-treated area produced marked pain and hyperalgesia (Davis et al. 1991). Quantitative autoradiographic studies indicate that the number of α_1-adrenoceptors in hyperalgesic skin of patients with SMP is significantly greater than in the skin of normal subjects (Drummond et al. 1996). Finally, venous α-adrenoceptor responsiveness increases in patients with CRPS-I (Arnold et al. 1993).

INTERPRETATION OF THE CLINICAL AND EXPERIMENTAL DATA OBTAINED IN HUMANS

Although these human studies indicate that the SNS is involved in generating pain, they do not reveal the underlying mechanisms. These clinical observations are interpreted in the following "conventional" way (Fig. 2): Primary afferent nociceptive neurons are excited and possibly sensitized by norepinephrine released by the sympathetic fibers. These nociceptors may have expressed adrenoceptors or their increased excitability may be generated indirectly, via the vascular bed (e.g., change of blood flow) or by other components that are influenced by sympathetic fibers. For example, inflammatory cells in the environment of the nociceptive neurons may influence the excitability of nociceptors. Alternatively, excitability of nociceptors may be modulated directly by molecules released from sympathetic postganglionic neurons (McMahon 1996; Woolf 1996; Jänig and Häbler 2000). Sympathetically maintained spontaneous and evoked activity in nociceptive

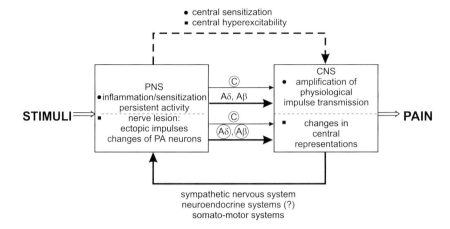

Fig. 2. Generation of peripheral and central hyperexcitability during inflammatory pain and neuropathic pain. The upper, dashed arrow indicates that the central changes result from changes in primary afferent neurons induced by inflammation or persistent stimulation (central sensitization) and from trauma with nerve lesion (central excitability; changes of central representations). The lower, solid arrow indicates efferent feedbacks via the sympathetic nervous system, the somatomotor system, and neuroendocrine systems. Primary afferent nociceptive neurons (in particular those with C fibers) are sensitized during inflammation. The biochemical and physiological changes occurring in these neurons during sensitization are principally reversible. After nerve lesion *all* lesioned primary afferent neurons (unmyelinated as well as myelinated ones) undergo biochemical, physiological, and morphological changes that become irreversible with time. These irreversible changes entail central irreversible changes if primary afferent neurons do not regenerate to their target tissue. The central changes, induced by persistent activity in afferent nociceptive neurons or after nerve lesions, are reflected in the efferent feedback systems. CNS = central nervous system; PNS = peripheral nervous system.

neurons may generate central sensitization and hyperexcitability in dorsal horn neurons and elsewhere. Central sensitization leads to spontaneous pain and pain evoked by stimulation of mechanoreceptors, thermoreceptors, or nociceptors (mechanical and thermal allodynias and hyperalgesias).

   This "conventional" view may be limited. In patients with SMP following nerve lesions (whether induced mechanically, metabolically, or by viral disease), the lesioned primary afferent neurons and corresponding central representations may undergo dramatic biochemical, morphological, and physiological changes. The mechanisms of SMP in these patients could be entirely different from those illustrated in Fig. 2. Sympathetic coupling to afferent neurons with large-diameter axons might be important because activity in these neurons could generate central hyperexcitability and feed into central circuits that have changed as a consequence of the peripheral nerve lesion. However, no experimental evidence supports this idea.

This chapter focuses on mechanisms that depend on activity in sympathetic neurons, based on evidence from clinical observations and experiments in patients. Mechanisms of hyperalgesia that depend on the adrenal medulla or on the innervation by the SNS but not on activity in the sympathetic neurons are discussed elsewhere (Jänig et al. 2000; Jänig and Häbler 2000). This chapter also discusses behavioral and reduced animal models of SMP in vivo and in vitro. Most of these models are based on clinical observations and test various putative contributing mechanisms. This chapter highlights the value of animal models in studying the underlying mechanisms of different components of SMP. However, each animal model has its limitations and must be carefully interpreted within the framework of the experimental setting and its applicability to the clinical situation. Several recent reviews discuss previous results in relation to the clinical background (Jänig 1988; Jänig and Koltzenburg 1991, 1992; Jänig and McLachlan 1994; Jänig and Stanton-Hicks 1996; Jänig et al. 1996; Baron and Jänig 1998; Baron et al. 1999a).

BEHAVIORAL ANIMAL MODELS

Behavioral animal models test the intact organism under controlled conditions. Signs of pain are measured by quantifiable behavioral components such as paw-withdrawal latency to thermal noxious stimulation, frequency and threshold of paw withdrawal to mechanical stimulation with von Frey hairs, and degree of self-mutilation (autotomy). These reactions are interpreted as equivalent to mechanical or thermal hyperalgesia or allodynia or to spontaneous pain in humans. Behavioral models allow researchers to test the degree to which the SNS contributes to these hyperalgesic and allodynic behaviors or to spontaneous pain behavior. Animals are given nerve lesions that are clinically relevant (see Baron et al. 1999a for discussion and references), and behavioral experiments are performed before and after interventions aimed at the sympathetic supply. The strengths of these models include the range of possible experimental manipulations of the SNS and the use of different strains of animals or transgenic animals. Quantitative data obtained in these behavioral experiments guide the design of the reduced animal models discussed below.

Several rat behavioral models for neuropathic pain involving controlled nerve lesions have been used to determine the contribution of the SNS to neuropathic pain. The interventions include surgical or chemical sympathectomy, systemic or local application of adrenoceptor blockers (e.g., phentolamine [α_1, α_2], prazosin [α_1], or yohimbine [α_2]) or of adrenoceptor agonists (e.g., clonidine [α_2]), and intraperitoneal (i.p.) application of guanethidine (which is taken up by the noradrenergic terminals and depletes norepinephrine). In the following text the use of the terms *hyperalgesia* and *allodynia* in the context of animal behavior always refers to hyperalgesic or allodynic behavior, respectively.

AUTOTOMY AFTER LIGATION AND TRANSECTION OF HINDLIMB NERVES

Ligation and transection of the sciatic and saphenous nerves leads to autotomy behavior (self-mutilation; Wall et al. 1979a). This behavior is considered to be an animal model of anesthesia dolorosa (but see Rodin and Kruger 1984; Kauppila 1998). Repeated i.p. application of guanethidine (60 mg/kg) for several days prevents or significantly reduces autotomy (Wall et al. 1979b). Coderre and coworkers (1984, 1986) confirmed these results by showing in rats that guanethidine significantly reduced autotomy when injected subcutaneously at doses of 30 mg/kg repeatedly over 4 days before ligation and section of the sciatic and saphenous nerves. Repeated subcutaneous injections of norepinephrine (1 mg/kg, three once-daily injections starting the day of nerve lesion) plus pargyline (a monoamine oxidase inhibitor, five once-daily injections starting 2 days before the nerve lesion) significantly enhanced the autotomy behavior (Coderre and Melzack 1986, Coderre et al. 1986).

These changes in self-mutilation behavior were interpreted to mean that activity in sympathetic neurons maintains ectopic activity in lesioned afferents, which in turn triggers the autotomy behavior. However, the investigators did not test whether *surgical* sympathectomy, either prior to or after the peripheral nerve lesion, would prevent or alleviate autotomy. Furthermore, the interpretation of the results fully depends on the application of pharmacological substances in high doses. Finally, there is no indication that spontaneous ectopic activity in lesioned afferent neurons is maintained by activity in sympathetic neurons.

PARTIAL LESION OF THE SCIATIC NERVE

Partial ligation of one-third to one-half of the sciatic nerve leads to signs of spontaneous pain, thermal hyperalgesia, mechanical allodynia, and mechanical hyperalgesia (Seltzer et al. 1990). Chemical sympatholysis with guanethidine, injected i.p. repeatedly over several days prior to nerve injury, prevented thermal hyperalgesia but had little effect on mechanical hyperalgesia (Shir and Seltzer 1991). When performed months after nerve lesion, sympatholysis by guanethidine alleviated all sensory disorders (Shir and Seltzer 1991). Similarly, Tracey et al. (1995a) showed that norepinephrine injected locally into the affected paw exacerbated, while both the α_2-adrenoceptor antagonist yohimbine and chemical sympathectomy significantly relieved mechanical and thermal hyperalgesic behavior. Local injection of indomethacin also eliminated hyperalgesia, so the authors concluded that prostaglandins might be involved, as suggested by Levine et al. (1986b). Based on behavioral testing (mechanical hyperalgesia) in an acute inflammatory model (repetitive treatment of the hairy skin of the rat hindpaw with chloroform) and pharmacological interventions, Levine et al. (1986b) proposed that norepinephrine released by sympathetic fibers acts on α_2-adrenoceptors in the varicosities of the sympathetic terminals. The authors believed that this mechanism leads to release of a prostaglandin that sensitizes the nociceptors for mechanical stimulation. However, the partial nerve lesion model of Tracey et al. (1995a) did not show that thermal and mechanical hyperalgesia were enhanced by the α_2-adrenoceptor agonist clonidine. Furthermore, the model of Levine et al. (1986b) and the partial nerve lesion model are probably fundamentally different, the former representing an inflammatory pain and the latter a neuropathic pain.

Finally, neuropeptide Y (NPY) acting via peripheral Y2 receptors also seemed to be involved in the generation of hyperalgesia in the partial sciatic nerve lesion model (Tracey et al. 1995b). However, the effects of surgical sympathectomy performed 1 week after partial sciatic nerve lesion on mechanical and cold allodynia and ongoing pain were not significant (Kim et al. 1997). Evaluation of these results depends heavily on the interpretation of the pharmacological interventions.

CHRONIC CONSTRICTION INJURY OF THE SCIATIC NERVE

Chronic constriction injury of the sciatic nerve generates mechanical and thermal hyperalgesic behavior (Bennett and Xie 1988). Guilbaud and collaborators (Neil et al. 1991a,b; Desmeules et al. 1995) reported that both surgical sympathectomy and depletion of sympathetic transmitters by guanethidine reduce thermal hyperalgesia but have little effect on mechanical hyperalgesia. Self-mutilating behavior and spontaneous pain behavior were not changed after guanethidine or surgical sympathectomy, respectively. However, Kim et al. (1997) found only a slight, statistically nonsignificant reduction of mechanical and cold allodynia after surgical sympathectomy.

CRYOLYSIS OF THE SCIATIC NERVE

Rats with cryoneurolysis of the sciatic nerve also develop signs of mechanical allodynia but display no thermal hyperalgesic behavior. Surgical sympathectomy performed prior to or after the cryoneurolysis did not influence the development or maintenance of the mechanical allodynic behavior (Willenbring et al. 1995).

SPINAL NERVE LESION

Ligation and transection of the spinal nerves L5 and L6 or only the spinal nerve L5 is followed by mechanical hyperalgesia and allodynia and thermal hyperalgesia (Kim and Chung 1992; Choi et al. 1994; Blenk et al. 1997). Chung and collaborators, who invented this model, found that these pain behaviors were permanently reversed by surgical lumbar sympathectomy (Kim and Chung 1991; Kim et al. 1993, 1997; Choi et al. 1994; Kinnman and Levine 1995). Pain behaviors were also prevented by surgical sympathectomy prior to spinal nerve lesion (Kim et al. 1993) and were temporarily reversed by i.p. injection of phentolamine (to block α-adrenoceptors) or guanethidine (to prevent release of norepinephrine) (Kim et al. 1993). These findings suggest that a coupling between the SNS and afferent neurons is critical for both the development and maintenance of the behavioral changes. Thus, the spinal nerve ligation (SNL) model appeared to be a promising behavioral animal model for human SMP in neuropathic conditions. However, considerable differences exist between rat strains and substrains in the development of signs of mechanical allodynia and heat hyperalgesia and in the dependence of mechanical allodynic behavior on adrenoceptors in animals with spinal nerve lesion (Yoon et al. 1999). For example, mechanical allodynic behavior after spinal nerve lesion was temporarily abolished in Lewis rats by i.p. phentolamine (≤ 2 mg/kg), while the same intervention had little or no effect in Fischer, Sprague-Dawley, and Wistar rats (Lee et al. 1997). Surgical sympathectomy completely abolished mechanical allodynic behavior in Sprague-Dawley rats with spinal nerve lesion (Kim et al. 1993).

The effect of surgical sympathectomy (performed prior to or after spinal nerve lesion) on the mechanical allodynic and hyperalgesic behavior of nerve-lesioned rats could not be reproduced by two laboratories using two different strains of rat (Sprague-Dawley and Wistar) and two different testing procedures, measuring frequency and threshold of paw withdrawal with von Frey hairs of different strengths (Ringkamp et al. 1999). The results obtained by these two groups were completely opposite to those obtained by Chung and coworkers. Finally, Eschenfelder et al. (2000) demonstrated that the mechanical allodynic/hyperalgesic behavior that develops in rats after lesion of the spinal nerve L5 does *not disappear* after transection of the dorsal root L5. Moreover, transection of the dorsal root L5 alone was followed by mechanical allodynic/hyperalgesic behavior, regardless of whether local anesthetics were used to block conduction in that dorsal root to prevent ectopic impulse generation at the site of the lesion. Similar results were described by Colburn et al. (1999) and Li et al. (2000). These results are also completely at variance with those published by Chung and coworkers (Sheen and Chung 1993; Na et al. 1995; Yoon et al. 1996) and Kinnman and Levine (1995) and conflict with the general hypothesis underlying the nerve lesion models (see Fig. 2).

CONCLUSIONS FROM BEHAVIORAL ANIMAL MODELS

The controversial results of the rat behavioral models of nerve injury provide conflicting evidence on the role of the SNS in generating pain behavior. These controversies indicate that behavioral animal models must be designed with the utmost care. Small changes in the experimental procedures may create major behavioral changes. Behavioral testing should be performed in a blinded fashion if possible, and the models must be designed in close association with the clinical situation to be certain to test what is intended to be tested. The results of systemic pharmacological interventions (e.g., application of adrenoceptor agonists and antagonists, guanethidine, and chemical sympathectomy with 6-hydroxy-dopamine) do not necessarily allow functional interpretations, partly because of the widespread systemic effects of these agents. Finally, the controversial results obtained from the animal behavior models may argue that the models do not reflect SMP as defined clinically.

Apparently the situation of the behavioral animal models is comparable to the clinical situation because not only is it difficult to determine whether a particular patient has SMP, but patients with apparently identical clinical findings may or may not have SMP. Furthermore, there may be different types of SMP, most likely with different underlying mechanisms. For example, the mechanisms of SMP in patients with CRPS-II, which the behavioral animal models mentioned above are supposed to represent, most likely differ from those in patients with CRPS-I. Finally, only a small percentage (about 5% or less) of patients with traumatic nerve injury (e.g., of the median or tibial nerve) develop neuropathic pain, and only a fraction of these patients have evidence for a sympathetically maintained component to their pain.

This controversial situation does not mean that behavioral animal models are useless and cannot simulate the clinical situation. On the contrary, there are good reasons to assume that we are dependent on the design of these animal models if we want to discover the mechanisms behind the different types of pathological pain in which the SNS is involved. However, the same behavioral model cannot be expected to represent SMP in different groups of patients (e.g., those with CRPS-I or CRPS-II).

REDUCED ANIMAL MODELS IN VIVO

Reduced animal models in vivo use neurophysiological recordings from afferent neurons, controlled stimulation of the sympathetic supply, and application of pharmacological agents such as adrenoceptor agonists and antagonists to study sympathetic-primary afferent coupling. This phenomenon may follow various types of clinically relevant nerve lesions as well as traumas without significant nerve lesion. These reduced models allow changes in ongoing and reflex-evoked efferent activity in the sympathetic neurons to be measured in parallel with the effector responses such as blood flow and sweating. Furthermore, abnormal activity after sympathetic-afferent coupling can be investigated together with its consequences for central information processing (e.g., in dorsal horn neurons). Results from morphological investigations can be correlated with functional and behavioral data to reveal which structural changes are relevant in various forms of SMP.

Following peripheral nerve injury, sympathetic noradrenergic neurons may influence afferent neurons in several ways. Experiments in reduced animal models of nerve injury in vivo have shown that sympathetic-primary afferent coupling may occur at or close to the site of nerve lesion or else remote from the lesion site.

SYMPATHETIC-AFFERENT COUPLING IN A NEUROMA FOLLOWING NERVE LESION OR LIGATION

Coupling between sympathetic fibers and afferent terminals is rare in neuromas after nerve lesion or ligation, particularly in old neuromas. It may occur in myelinated as well as unmyelinated nerve fibers and is mediated by norepinephrine and by α-adrenoceptors. Electrical stimulation of the sympathetic neurons can only elicit afferent discharges at frequencies of ≥10 Hz (Devor and Jänig 1981; Blumberg and Jänig 1984); such frequencies never occur in sympathetic neurons in vivo. There is no evidence that ongoing activity in neuroma fibers is dependent on sympathetic activity. These data are compatible with clinical experience showing that neuroma pain is not dependent on sympathetic activity and support histological observations that catecholamine-containing axon profiles are rare within the neuroma many weeks after nerve lesion and ligation (E.M. McLachlan, personal communication; see also Goldstein et al. 1988; for general discussion see Jänig 1988).

SYMPATHETIC-AFFERENT COUPLING AFTER REGENERATION OF AFFERENT AND SYMPATHETIC FIBERS TO THE TARGET TISSUE

Norepinephrine- and α-adrenoceptor-mediated coupling has been reported in unmyelinated afferent fibers that were allowed to regenerate to the target tissue. Strong afferent excitation was generated by electrical stimulation of the sympathetic neurons at frequencies of ≥0.5 Hz more than 1 year after cross-union of the proximal stump of the sural nerve to the distal stump of the tibial nerve (Häbler et al. 1987). The excitation was not mediated by changes of blood flow. The afferent nerve fibers had some spontaneous activity. Reflex activation of the sympathetic neurons also generated some afferent impulses. The sympathetically induced discharges could be mimicked by epinephrine and norepinephrine applied systemically and were blocked by the α-adrenoceptor antagonist phentolamine. The functional class of the affected primary afferent fibers was not determined. However, these fibers were unmyelinated and therefore most likely nociceptive. This is still the *only* experimental study to illustrate that activity in sympathetic neurons at *physiological frequencies* (Jänig 1985, 1995; Häbler et al. 1994) can elicit impulses in primary afferent nerve fibers.

COUPLING BETWEEN UNLESIONED POSTGANGLIONIC AND AFFERENT NERVE TERMINALS AFTER PARTIAL NERVE LESION

C-fiber polymodal nociceptors may develop sensitivity to sympathetic nerve stimulation and to norepinephrine following partial nerve injury. Sympathetic stimulation excites polymodal nociceptors and sensitizes them to heat stimuli. Both types of sensitivity develop 4 to 10 days after partial nerve lesion, persist for at least 150 days, and are preferentially mediated by $α_2$-adrenoceptors (Sato and Perl 1991; Perl 1994; O'Halloran and Perl 1997; Birder and Perl 1999). Again, the sympathetic-afferent coupling that activates and sensitizes nociceptors requires electrical stimulation of sympathetic neurons at frequencies that do not occur under physiological conditions (Jänig 1985, 1995; Häbler et al. 1994). O'Halloran and Perl (1997) proposed that circulating epinephrine could act via an α-adrenoceptor subtype. However, this interesting proposal remains unproven because the epinephrine concentrations used by O'Halloran and Perl to excite the nociceptive afferents in this study (50 ng/0.2 mL injected intra-arterially) were about 100 to 1000 times higher than normal circulating epinephrine concentrations in the plasma of rats, which is in the range of 0.15 ng/mL under resting conditions to about 2 ng/mL under immobilization stress (Kvetnansky et al. 1998).

SYMPATHETIC-AFFERENT COUPLING IN THE NERVE PROXIMAL TO THE NERVE LESION

A nerve lesion is followed by dramatic changes in the entire nerve proximal to the lesion. Many neurons with unmyelinated axons die with time after nerve lesion (Jänig and McLachlan 1984; Jänig 1988). Peptidergic and nonpeptidergic afferent and postganglionic fibers start to sprout retro- and anterogradely, endoneural blood vessels become innervated, peptide content of the afferent neurons changes quantitatively and qualitatively, and norepinephrine levels decrease in the postganglionic neurons. The nerve proximal to the lesion undergoes a continuous reorganization, showing many signs of sterile inflammation (Barrett and McLachlan 1999). These changes raise the question of whether sympathetic-afferent coupling occurs in the nerve proximal to the lesion and if so, whether it is mediated directly by norepinephrine, indirectly via the vascular bed, or by a combination of mechanisms.

SYMPATHETIC COUPLING AND SPROUTING OF SYMPATHETIC FIBERS IN THE DRG AFTER PERIPHERAL NERVE LESION

Following transection and ligation of a peripheral nerve (e.g., the sciatic nerve or a spinal nerve in rats), perivascular catecholamine-containing axons start to invade the dorsal root ganglia (DRG) containing somata with lesioned axons. This novel sprouting in the DRG increases with time. Depending on the distance between the lesion site and the DRG, within days to many weeks after the nerve lesion some somata are partially or almost completely surrounded by varicose catecholaminergic terminals. These terminals preferentially surround large-diameter neurons (McLachlan et al. 1993; Chung et al. 1996). Sprouting of sympathetic fibers in the DRG may be related to cytokine-induced production of neurotrophins. The low-affinity neurotrophin receptor p75 is expressed by satellite cells preferentially surrounding the large DRG cells. The p75 receptor may then display the released neurotrophins as a trophic gradient and may initiate sprouting of postganglionic axons around these DRG cells (Zhou et al. 1996; Ramer et al. 1999).

Electrical stimulation of the sympathetic neurons innervating the DRG that contain cell somata of axotomized afferents can excite or depress some primary afferent neurons via coupling in the DRG. In recent studies, spontaneously active neurons with myelinated axons and a few spontaneously active DRG cells with unmyelinated fibers were influenced. However, most cells with unmyelinated fibers were *inhibited* (Devor et al. 1994; Michaelis et al. 1996). The type of adrenoceptor mediating these effects was preferentially α_2 (Chen et al., 1996). This finding corresponds to the increased expression of α_2-adrenoceptors in axotomized small-diameter DRG cells (Birder and Perl 1999; Shi et al. 2000). However, similar experiments on rats with spinal nerve lesion reported a low incidence of spontaneously active afferent neurons that were excited by stimulation of the sympathetic chain, even when a high frequency was used (Häbler et al. 2000).

Serious caveats remain as to whether these exciting morphological and neurophysiological findings can account for sympathetic-afferent coupling in the generation of pain in patients with nerve lesions or in the generation of hyperalgesic and allodynic behavior in animals with nerve lesions. Several arguments must be considered.

First, catecholaminergic baskets appear predominantly around large DRG cells and are rare around small DRG cells (McLachlan et al. 1993). After sciatic nerve lesion in rats, catecholaminergic baskets appear at ≥ 4 weeks and increase in number up to 250 days post-lesion (E.M. McLachlan, unpublished observation). In the chronic constriction injury and partial sciatic nerve injury models, baskets form even later (≤ 20 weeks) (Lee et al. 1998). However, excitation of axotomized afferent neurons via their cell bodies following sympathetic stimulation is most prominent shortly after sciatic nerve lesion when the baskets are almost absent. Later on, when the baskets are present, depression of activity is dominant (Devor et al. 1994; Michaelis et al. 1996).

Second, the vast majority of axotomized C-fiber DRG neurons and most axotomized A-fiber DRG neurons are not influenced by sympathetic stimulation. The sympathetic supply had to be stimulated at $\geq 5–10$ Hz to generate responses in the axotomized afferent neurons. Discharge frequencies of $\geq 5–10$ Hz rarely occur in sympathetic neurons under physiological conditions (Jänig 1985, 1995; Häbler et al. 1994).

Third, the rate of ectopic spontaneous activity in DRG neurons 15–45 days after spinal nerve lesion is not significantly different between sympathectomized animals and those with intact sympathetic supply (Liu et al. 2000). There is little evidence that ongoing ectopic activity in lesioned afferent nerve fibers is dependent on sympathetic activity. In contrast, Lee et al. (1999) found that α_1-adrenoceptor antagonists temporarily reduced ongoing discharges in lesioned afferent A-fiber neurons recorded in vivo after spinal nerve lesion in Lewis rats. This result suggests a causative role of sympathetic neurons in generating ectopic activity.

Fourth, the degree of activation of axotomized DRG neurons by sympathetic stimulation is highly correlated with the decrease of blood flow through the DRG. The incidence of excitatory responses in axotomized DRG cells induced by sympathetic stimulation significantly increased and the effective stimulation frequency necessary to excite the afferent cells significantly decreased when the vascular bed in the DRG was constricted. These experiments favor the idea that sympathetically induced discharges in axotomized DRG cells occur mainly when perfusion of the DRG is impaired. The decrease in blood flow might be related to the perivascular sprouting of postganglionic nerve fibers (Häbler et al. 2000).

Fifth, sympathetic sprouting in the DRG was not correlated with whether or not neuropathic pain behavior was found to be sympathetically dependent or independent in rats after sacral spinal nerve lesions (Kim et al. 1998, 1999).

Finally, ectopic spontaneous activity generated in the DRG after peripheral nerve lesion appears in axotomized and also in intact muscle afferent neurons with myelinated axons of low and medium conduction velocity and not in cutaneous afferent neurons. About 20% of the myelinated muscle afferent neurons exhibit spontaneous activity (Michaelis et al. 2000). Because sympathetic stimulation largely influences spontaneously active DRG cells after nerve lesion, we conclude that only muscle afferent neurons are affected by sympathetic stimulation via the DRG. The percentage of affected DRG cells is low, approximately in the range of 1–2% of all DRG cells, assuming that cutaneous afferents are 2–3 times more common than deep somatic afferents (see Baron et al. 1988).

REDUCED ANIMAL MODELS IN VITRO

Reduced in vitro models use isolated tissues and organs from animals that have undergone controlled nerve lesions, including preparations of skin and nerve tissue, DRG cells with attached nerves, isolated nerves with a nerve-end neuroma or neuroma-in-continuity, and isolated DRG cells. These preparations contribute significantly to the study of mechanisms of sympathetic-afferent coupling at the cellular and subcellular level, allowing researchers to investigate changes in adrenoreceptor expression and altered coupling to ionic channels, which could enhance excitability (e.g., by generating ectopic impulse activity in primary afferent neurons). Such studies may lead to the development of new pharmacological tools and therapeutics. Limitations of this approach include possible alterations of the physiology of isolated tissues and neurons compared to their behavior in situ because the expression of receptors and ionic channels may change rapidly. Data obtained in these preparations must be interpreted cautiously and within the context of results obtained from reduced animal models in vivo, from behavioral animal models, and from the clinical situation in humans.

In vitro experiments have shown that lesioned afferents after chronic constriction or L5 spinal nerve injury and intact afferents after intrathecal NGF treatment have excitatory responses to norepinephrine (Petersen et al. 1996; Zhang et al. 1997; Jones et al. 1999) or epinephrine (Lee et al. 1999). However, the doses used were relatively high and in similar in vitro experiments, small depolarizations of both intact and lesioned somata in response to norepinephrine could not be blocked by adrenoceptor antagonists (Lopez de Armentia et al. 1999), indicating that the observed effects may have been nonspecific. In monkeys, in an in vitro skin-nerve preparation, uninjured C-fiber nociceptors after partial denervation of the skin resulting from an L6 spinal nerve lesion acquired spontaneous activity displayed a higher incidence of responses to both α_1- and α_2-adrenergic agonists as compared to controls (Ali et al. 1999).

CONCLUSIONS FROM IN VIVO AND IN VITRO EXPERIMENTS

The reduced animal models, both in vivo and in vitro, show that sympathetic-afferent coupling can occur under pathophysiological conditions, involving expression of functional adrenoceptors by the lesioned afferent neurons and plastic changes of both sympathetic and afferent neurons. However, the data from these models are inconsistent with observations of SMP in patients. The experimental interventions used in the animal models (e.g., frequency of stimulation of sympathetic neurons, concentrations of applied adrenoceptor agonists) seem out of proportion to biological events. Therefore, the experimental data must be considered with the utmost caution.

SYNOPSIS

Despite the considerable research efforts reviewed above, the role of the SNS in the generation of pain is still unclear. The clinical characteristics of CRPS-I are distinct from those of CRPS-II (Stanton-Hicks et al. 1995; Jänig and Stanton-Hicks 1996; Baron and Jänig 1998; Harden et al. 2001): (a) they may develop after trauma with minimal or undetectable nerve lesion; (b) the trauma may be remote from the affected extremity (e.g., central trauma, visceral trauma); (c) ongoing pain, hyperalgesia, and allodynia are mostly localized in deep somatic tissues.

Patients with both CRPS-I and CRPS-II may have pain associated with swelling of the extremity and abnormal regulation of blood flow and sweating generated by the SNS. However, these characteristics are probably more prominent in patients with CRPS-I. Although patients with either CRPS-I or CRPS-II may have SMP, the underlying pathophysiology may differ in the two groups. While there is partial overlap in the clinical phenomenology of patients with CRPS-I and CRPS-II, we feel there is merit in categorizing CRPS-II, but not necessarily CRPS-I, as a form of neuropathic pain (see Jänig 2001).

The available human models and behavioral and reduced animal models may be representative of SMP in patients with CRPS-II and other neuropathic pain syndromes, but not in CRPS-I patients. The strengths and limitations of the different classes of models are as follows.

Human models. Human models provide access to the subjective experience of experimental subjects. Spontaneous and evoked pain can be measured quantitatively using psychophysical scales; conclusions are drawn from the correlation between the psychophysical data and the experimental interventions. The obvious advantages of human experimental models are that they can provide information on the human experience of pain and can help bridge the gap between experimental animal models and the clinical situation. The human models are limited by the restrictions on invasive surgical and pharmacological interventions so that it is difficult to test specific pathophysiological mechanisms. Human models clearly show that the SNS is involved in pain and most likely produces associated tissue changes in patients with CRPS-I and CRPS-II.

Behavioral animal models. Behavioral models allow researchers to test the degree of SNS involvement in the animals' hyperalgesic and allodynic behaviors. Following nerve lesions, which attempt to model specific clinical phenomena, behavioral experiments are performed before and after interventions designed to alter the sympathetic supply. These models have provided conflicting evidence regarding the role of the SNS in nerve injury pain. The behavioral animal models for SMP and associated changes in patients with CRPS-I are quite limited.

Reduced animal models in vivo. In these functional animal models, changes of ongoing and reflex activity in the sympathetic neurons generated by controlled nerve lesions can be correlated with the effector responses. Furthermore, researchers can investigate the consequences of abnormal activity following sympathetic-afferent coupling (e.g., information processing in the dorsal horn). Results from morphological investigations (using immunohistochemical, electron-microscopic, and other techniques) can be

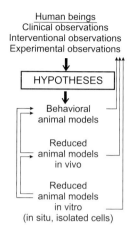

Fig. 3. Hierarchy of human and animal models and clinical investigations in experimental research on the role of the sympathetic nervous system in pain. This hierarchy consists of different levels that interact reciprocally with each other. The scientific questions to be asked are formulated based on the clinical observations. The human and the behavioral animal models mostly focus on one component (e.g., SMP, autonomic abnormalities, motor abnormalities, or edema in CRPS-I or -II). Experimental behavioral animal models and experimental human models are the basis for the formulation of questions for the more reduced animal models. These reduced models focus on one component (e.g., sympathetic-afferent coupling in the periphery or in the dorsal root ganglion). Thus the results obtained in the behavioral models are anchored in the clinical observations, the results obtained on the reduced animal models in vivo are based on the behavioral animal models and the human experimental models, and the reduced animal models in vitro are mainly based on the animal models in vivo. Research performed on the various animal models affects the clinical research performed on patients with SMP. This interactive research strategy applies to most experimental research that aims to elucidate the pathophysiological processes underlying diseases.

correlated with the functional data to suggest which structural changes are relevant in various forms of SMP. Some of these approaches, using reduced animal models in vivo, appear to be relevant to SMP in CRPS-II, but not in CRPS-I.

Reduced animal models in vitro. Because the tissue for in vitro experiments is subjected to significant surgical manipulation and rapid changes in the expression of receptors and ionic channels may result from the experimental preparation, the longer-term abnormalities observed must be interpreted with caution. Data obtained in these preparations must be correlated closely with results obtained from reduced animal models in vivo and data obtained from experiments on humans to determine their relevance to clinical SMP.

In fact, many of the observations made in these animal models do not match those in patients with SMP. Therefore, future research using animal models must be better integrated with observations on human patients. Furthermore, design of behavioral and reduced animal models must be more closely integrated to assure a continuous interaction among the different models (Fig. 3). Only an integrated approach has any chance of uncovering the pathophysiology and improving treatment.

ACKNOWLEDGMENT

Supported by the German Research Foundation and the Sander Foundation.

REFERENCES

Ali Z, Ringkamp M, Hartke TV, et al. Uninjured C-fiber nociceptors develop spontaneous activity and α-adrenergic sensitivity following L_6 spinal nerve ligation in monkey. *J Neurophysiol* 1999; 81:455–466.

Ali Z, Raja SN, Wesselmann U, et al. Intradermal injection of norepinephrine evokes pain in patients with sympathetically maintained pain. *Pain* 2000; 88:161–168.

Arnér S. Intravenous phentolamine test: diagnostic and prognostic use in reflex sympathetic dystrophy. *Pain* 1991; 46:17–22.

Arnold JM, Teasell RW, MacLeod AP, et al. Increased venous alpha-adrenoceptor responsiveness in patients with reflex sympathetic dystrophy. *Ann Intern Med* 1993; 118:619–621.

Baron R, Jänig W. Schmerzsyndrome mit kausaler Beteiligung des Sympathikus. *Anaesthesist* 1998; 47:4–23.

Baron R, Jänig W. Neuropathische Schmerzen. In: Zenz M, Jurna I (Eds). *Lehrbuch der Schmerztherapie*. Stuttgart: Wissenschaftliche Verlagsgesellschaft, 2001, pp 65–87.

Baron R, Jänig W, Kollmann W. Sympathetic and afferent somata projecting in hindlimb nerves and the anatomical organization of the lumbar sympathetic nervous system of the rat. *J Comp Neurol* 1988; 275:460–468.

Baron R, Blumberg H, Jänig W. Clinical characteristics of patients with CRPS type I and type II in Germany with special emphasis on vasomotor function. In: Jänig W, Stanton-Hicks M (Eds). *Reflex Sympathetic Dystrophy: A Reappraisal*, Progress in Pain Research and Management, Vol. 6. Seattle: IASP Press, 1996, pp 25–48.

Baron R, Levine JD, Fields HL. Causalgia and reflex sympathetic dystrophy: does the sympathetic nervous system contribute to the generation of pain? *Muscle Nerve* 1999a; 22:678–695.

Baron R, Wasner GL, Borgstedt R, et al. Effect of sympathetic activity on capsaicin evoked spontaneous pain, hyperalgesia and vasodilatation. *Neurology* 1999b; 23:923–932.

Barrett LG, McLachlan EM. Long-term changes in peripheral nerve trunks following nerve ligation in rats. *Proc Aust Neurosci Soc* 1999; 10:116.

Bennett GJ, Xie YK. A peripheral mononeuropathy in rat that produces disorders of pain sensation like those seen in man. *Pain* 1988; 33:87–107.

Birder LA, Perl ER. Expression of $α_2$-adrenergic receptors in rat primary afferent neurones after peripheral nerve injury or inflammation. *J Physiol* 1999; 515:533–542.

Blenk K-H, Häbler H-J, Jänig W. Neomycin and gadolinium applied to an L5 spinal nerve lesion prevent mechanical allodynia-like behaviour in rats. *Pain* 1997; 70:155–165.

Blumberg H, Jänig W. Discharge pattern of afferent fibers from a neuroma. *Pain* 1984; 20:335–353.

Blumberg H, Jänig W. Clinical manifestations of reflex sympathetic dystrophy and sympathetically maintained pain. In: Wall PD, Melzack R (Eds). *Textbook of Pain,* 3rd ed. Edinburgh: Churchill Livingstone, 1994, pp 685–697.

Blumberg H, Hoffmann U, Mohadjer M, Scheremet R. Clinical phenomenology and mechanisms of reflex sympathetic dystrophy: emphasis on edema. In: Gebhart GF, Hammond DL, Jensen TS (Eds). *Proceedings of the 7th World Congress on Pain,* Progress in Pain Research and Management, Vol. 2. Seattle: IASP Press, 1994, pp 455–481.

Bonica JJ. Causalgia and other reflex sympathetic dystrophies. In: Bonica JJ (Ed). *The Management of Pain.* Philadelphia: Lea and Febiger, 1990, pp 220–243.

Chabal C, Jacobson L, Russell LC, Burchiel KJ. Pain response to perineuromal injection of normal saline, epinephrine, and lidocaine in humans. *Pain* 1992; 49:9–12.

Chen Y, Michaelis M, Jänig W, Devor M. Adrenoceptor subtype mediating sympathetic-sensory coupling in injured sensory neurons. *J Neurophysiol* 1996; 76:3721–3730.

Choi B, Rowbotham MC. Effect of adrenergic receptor activation on post-herpetic neuralgia pain and sensory disturbances. *Pain* 1997; 69:55–63.

Choi Y, Yoon YW, Na HS, Kim SH, Chung JM. Behavioral signs of ongoing pain and cold allodynia in a rat model of neuropathic pain. *Pain* 1994; 59:369–376.

Chung K, Lee BH, Yoon YW, Chung JM. Sympathetic sprouting in the dorsal root ganglia of the injured peripheral nerve in a rat neuropathic pain model. *J Comp Neurol* 1996; 376:241–252.

Coderre TJ, Melzack R. Procedures which increase acute pain sensitivity also increase autotomy. *Exp Neurol* 1986; 92:713–722.

Coderre TJ, Abbott FV, Melzack R. Effect of peripheral antisympathetic treatments in the tail-flick, formalin and autotomy tests. *Pain* 1984; 18:13–23.

Coderre TJ, Grimes RW, Melzack R. Deafferentation and chronic pain in animals: an evaluation of evidence suggesting autotomy is related to pain. *Pain* 1986; 26:61–84.

Colburn RW, Rickman AJ, DeLeo JA. The effect of site and type of nerve injury on spinal glial activation and neuropathic pain behavior. *Exp Neurol* 1999; 157:289–304.

Davis KD, Treede RD, Raja SN, Meyer RA, Campbell JN. Topical application of clonidine relieves hyperalgesia in patients with sympathetically maintained pain. *Pain* 1991; 47:309–317.

Dellemijn PL, Fields HL, Allen RR, McKay WR, Rowbotham MC. The interpretation of pain relief and sensory changes following sympathetic blockade. *Brain* 1994; 117:1475–1487.

Desmeules JA, Kayser V, Weil-Fuggaza J, Bertrand A, Guilbaud G. Influence of the sympathetic nervous system in the development of abnormal pain-related behaviours in a rat model of neuropathic pain. *Neuroscience* 1995; 67:941–951.

Devor M, Jänig W. Activation of myelinated afferents ending in a neuroma by stimulation of the sympathetic supply in the rat. *Neurosci Lett* 1981; 24:43–47.

Devor M, Jänig W, Michaelis M. Modulation of activity in dorsal root ganglion (DRG) neurons by sympathetic activation in nerve-injured rats. *J Neurophysiol* 1994; 71:38–47.

Drummond PD. Noradrenaline increases hyperalgesia to heat in skin sensitized by capsaicin. *Pain* 1995; 60:311–315.

Drummond PD. The effect of noradrenaline, angiotensin II and vasopressin on blood flow and sensitivity to heat in capsaicin-treated skin. *Clin Auton Res* 1998; 8:87–93.

Drummond PD, Skipworth S, Finch PM. Alpha 1-adrenoceptors in normal and hyperalgesic human skin. *Clin Sci (Colch)* 1996; 91:73–77.

Elam M, Skarphedinsson JO, Olhausson B, Wallin BG. No apparent sympathetic modulation of single C-fiber afferent transmission in human volunteers. In: *Abstracts: 8th World Congress on Pain.* Seattle: IASP Press, 1996, pp 398.

Eschenfelder S, Häbler H-J, Jänig W. Dorsal root section elicits signs of neuropathic pain rather than reversing them in rats with L5 spinal nerve injury. *Pain* 2000; 87:213–219.

Goldstein RS, Raber P, Govrin-Lippmann R, Devor M. Contrasting time course of catechola- mine accumulation and of spontaneous discharge in experimental neuromas in the rat. *Neurosci Lett* 1988; 94:58–63.

Häbler H-J, Jänig W, Koltzenburg M. Activation of unmyelinated afferents in chronically lesioned nerves by adrenaline and excitation of sympathetic efferents in the cat. *Neurosci Lett* 1987; 82:35–40.

Häbler H-J, Jänig W, Krummel M, Peters OA. Reflex patterns in postganglionic neurons supplying skin and skeletal muscle of the rat hindlimb. *J Neurophysiol* 1994; 72:2222–2236.

Häbler H-J, Eschenfelder S, Liu X-G, Jänig W. Sympathetic-sensory coupling after L5 spinal nerve lesion in the rat and its relation to changes in dorsal root ganglion blood flow. *Pain* 2000; 87:335–345.

Harden RN, Bruehl S, Galer BS, et al. Complex regional pain syndrome: are the IASP diagnostic criteria valid and sufficiently comprehensive? *Pain* 1999; 83:211–219.

Harden RN, Baron R, Jänig W (Eds). *Complex Regional Pain Syndrome,* Progress in Pain Research and Management, Vol. 22. Seattle: IASP Press, 2001, in press.

Jänig W. Organization of the lumbar sympathetic outflow to skeletal muscle and skin of the cat hindlimb and tail. *Rev Physiol Biochem Pharmacol* 1985; 102:119–213.

Jänig W. Pathophysiology of nerve following mechanical injury. In: Dubner R, Gebhart GF, Bond MR (Eds). *Pain Research and Clinical Management,* Vol. 3. Amsterdam: Elsevier Science, 1988, pp 89–108.

Jänig W. Ganglionic transmission *in vivo.* In: McLachlan ME (Ed). *Autonomic Ganglia,* The Autonomic Nervous System, Vol. 5. Chur, Switzerland: Harwood Academic, 1995, pp 349– 395.

Jänig W. Pain and the sympathetic nervous system: pathophysiological mechanisms. In: Mathias CJ, Bannister R (Eds). *Autonomic Failure,* 4th. ed. Oxford: Oxford University Press, 1999, pp 99–108.

Jänig W. CRPS-I and CRPS-II: A strategic view. In: Harden RN, Baron R, Jänig W (Eds). *Complex Regional Pain Syndrome,* Progress in Pain Research and Management, Vol. 22. Seattle: IASP Press, 2001, in press.

Jänig W, Häbler H-J. Sympathetic nervous system: contribution to chronic pain. In: Sandkühler J, Bromm B, Gebhart GF (Eds). Nervous System Plasticity and Chronic Pain. *Progr Brain Res* 2000; 129:453–470.

Jänig W, Koltzenburg M. What is the interaction between the sympathetic terminal and the primary afferent fiber? In: Basbaum AI, Besson J-M (Eds). *Towards a New Pharmacotherapy of Pain,* Dahlem Workshop Reports. Chichester: John Wiley & Sons, 1991, pp 331–352.

Jänig W, Koltzenburg M. Possible ways of sympathetic afferent interaction. In: Jänig W, Schmidt RF (Eds). *Reflex Sympathetic Dystrophy: Pathophysiological Mechanisms and Clinical Implications.* New York: VCH Verlagsgesellschaft, 1992, pp 213–243.

Jänig W, McLachlan EM. On the fate of sympathetic and sensory neurons projecting into a neuroma of the superficial peroneal nerve in the cat. *J Comp Neurol* 1984; 225:302–311.

Jänig W, McLachlan EM. The role of modifications in noradrenergic peripheral pathways after nerve lesions in the generation of pain. In: Fields HL, Liebeskind JC (Eds). *Pharmacologi- cal Approaches to the Treatment of Pain: New Concepts and Critical Issues,* Progress in Pain Research and Management, Vol. 1. Seattle: IASP Press, 1994, pp 101–128.

Jänig W, Stanton-Hicks M (Eds). *Reflex Sympathetic Dystrophy: A Reappraisal,* Progress in Pain Research and Management, Vol. 6. Seattle: IASP Press, 1996.

Jänig W, Levine JD, Michaelis M. Interaction of sympathetic and primary afferent neurons following nerve injury and tissue trauma. In: Kumazawa T, Kruger L, Mizumura K (Eds). The Polymodal Receptor—a Gateway to Pathological Pain. *Progr Brain Res* 1996; 112:161– 184.

Jänig W, Khasar SG, Levine JD, Miao FJ-P. The role of vagal visceral afferents in the control of nociception. In: Mayer EA, Saper CB (Eds). The biological basis for mind body interaction. *Prog Brain Res* 2000; 122:271–285.

Jones MG, Munson JB, Thompson SWN. A role for nerve growth factor in sympathetic sprouting in rat dorsal root ganglia. *Pain* 1999; 79:21–29.

Kauppila T. Correlation between autotomy-behavior and current theories of neuropathic pain. *Neurosci Beh Rev* 1998; 23:111–129.

Kim SH, Chung JM. Sympathectomy alleviates mechanical allodynia in an experimental animal model for neuropathy in the rat. *Neurosci Lett* 1991; 134:131–134.

Kim SH, Chung JM. An experimental model for peripheral neuropathy produced by segmental spinal nerve ligation in the rat. *Pain* 1992; 50:355–363.

Kim SH, Na HS, Sheen K, Chung JM. Effects of sympathectomy on a rat model of peripheral neuropathy. *Pain* 1993; 55:85–93.

Kim KJ, Yoon YW, Chung JM. Comparison of three rodent neuropathic pain models. *Exp Brain Res* 1997; 113:200–206.

Kim HJ, Na HS, Sung B, Hong SK. Amount of sympathetic sprouting in the dorsal root ganglia is not correlated to the level of sympathetic dependence of neuropathic pain in a rat model. *Neurosci Lett* 1998; 245:21–24.

Kim HJ, Na HS, Sung B, et al. Is sympathetic sprouting in the dorsal root ganglia responsible for the production of neuropathic pain in a rat model? *Neurosci Lett* 1999; 269:103–106.

Kinnman E, Levine JD. Sensory and sympathetic contributions to nerve injury-induced sensory abnormalities in the rat. *Neuroscience* 1995; 64:751–767.

Kinnman E, Nygards EB, Hansson P. Peripheral alpha-adrenoreceptors are involved in the development of capsaicin induced ongoing and stimulus evoked pain in humans. *Pain* 1997; 69:79–85.

Kvetnansky R, Pacak K, Sabban EL, Kopin IJ, Goldstein DS. Stressor specificity of peripheral catecholaminergic activation. *Adv Pharmacol* 1998; 42:556–560.

Lee BH, Yoon YW, Chung K, Chung JM. Comparison of sympathetic sprouting in sensory ganglia in three animal models of neuropathic pain. *Exp Brain Res* 1998; 120:432–438.

Lee DH, Chung K, Chung JM. Strain differences in adrenergic sensitivity of neuropathic pain behaviors in an experimental rat model. *Neuroreport* 1997; 8:3453–3456.

Lee DH, Liu X, Kim HAT, Chung K, Chung JM. Receptor subtype mediating the adrenergic sensitivity of pain behavior and ectopic discharges in neuropathic Lewis rats. *J Neurophysiol* 1999; 81:2226–2233.

Levine JD, Fye K, Heller P, Basbaum AI, Whiting-O'Keefe Q. Clinical response to regional intravenous guanethidine in patients with rheumatoid arthritis. *J Rheumatol* 1986a; 13:1040–1043.

Levine JD, Taiwo YO, Collins SD, Tam JK. Noradrenaline hyperalgesia is mediated through interaction with sympathetic postganglionic neurone terminals rather than activation of primary afferent nociceptors. *Nature* 1986b; 323:158–160.

Li Y, Dorsi MJ, Meyer RA, Belzberg AJ. Mechanical hyperalgesia after an L5 spinal nerve lesion is not dependent on input from injured nerve fibers. *Pain* 2000; 85:493–502.

Liu M, Max MB, Parada S, Rowan JS, Bennett GJ. The sympathetic nervous system contributes to capsaicin-evoked mechanical allodynia but not pinprick hyperalgesia in humans. *J Neurosci* 1996; 16:7331–7335.

Liu X-G, Eschenfelder S, Blenk K-H, Jänig W, Häbler H-J. Spontaneous activity of axotomized afferent neurons after L5 spinal nerve injury in the rat. *Pain* 2000; 84:309–318.

Lopez de Armentia M, Stebbing M, Hodges PW. Noradrenaline produces non-specific effects in axotomized neurons in DRG isolated in vitro. *Soc Neurosci Abstracts* 1999; 25:770.4.

McLachlan EM, Jänig W, Devor M, Michaelis M. Peripheral nerve injury triggers noradrenergic sprouting within dorsal root ganglia. *Nature* 1993; 363:543–546.

Michaelis M, Devor M, Jänig W. Sympathetic modulation of activity in dorsal root ganglion neurons changes over time following peripheral nerve injury. *J Neurophysiol* 1996; 76:753–763.

Michaelis M, Liu XG, Jänig W. Axotomized and intact muscle afferents but no skin afferents develop ongoing discharges of dorsal root ganglion origin after peripheral nerve lesion. *J Neurosci* 2000; 20:2742–2748.

McMahon SB. NGF as a mediator of inflammatory pain. *Phil Trans R Soc Lond B Biol Sci* 1996; 351:431–440.

Na HS, Kim YI, Ko KH, Hong SK. The role of signals from dorsal root ganglion in neuropathic pains induced by nerve injury. *Soc Neurosci Abstracts* 1995; 21:896.

Neil A, Attal N, Guilbaud G. Effects of guanethidine on sensitization to natural stimuli and self-mutilating behaviour in rats with a peripheral neuropathy. *Brain Res* 1991a; 565:237–246.

Neil A, Attal N, Guilbaud G. Effects of adrenergic depletion with guanethidine before and after the induction of a peripheral neuropathy on subsequent mechanical, heat and cold sensitivities in rats. In: Bond MR, Charlton JE, Woolf CJ (Eds). *Proceedings of the VIth World Congress on Pain.* Amsterdam: Elsevier, 1991b, pp 383–388.

O'Halloran KD, Perl ER. Effects of partial nerve injury on the responses of C-fiber polymodal nociceptors to adrenergic agonists. *Brain Res* 1997; 759:233–240.

Pedersen JL, Rung GW, Kehlet H. Effect of sympathetic nerve block on acute inflammatory pain and hyperalgesia. *Anesthesiology* 1997; 86:293–301.

Perl ER. A reevaluation of mechanisms leading to sympathetically related pain. In: Fields HL, Liebeskind JC (Eds). *Pharmacological Approaches to the Treatment of Chronic Pain: New Concepts and Critical Issues,* Progress in Pain Research and Management, Vol. 1. Seattle: IASP Press, 1994, pp 129–150.

Petersen M, Zhang J, Zhang JM, LaMotte RH. Abnormal spontaneous activity and responses to norepinephrine in dissociated dorsal root ganglion cells after chronic nerve constriction. *Pain* 1996; 67:391–397.

Price DD, Long S, Wilsey B, Rafii A. Analysis of peak magnitude and duration of analgesia produced by local anesthetics injected into sympathetic ganglia of complex regional pain syndrome patients. *Clin J Pain* 1998; 14:216–226.

Raja SN. Role of the sympathetic nervous system in acute pain and inflammation. *Ann Med* 1995; 27:241–246.

Raja SN, Treede RD, Davis KD, Campbell JN. Systemic alpha-adrenergic blockade with phentolamine: a diagnostic test for sympathetically maintained pain. *Anesthesiology* 1991; 74:691–698.

Raja SN, Abatzis V, Frank SM. Role of a-adrenoceptors in neuroma pain in amputees. *Anesthesiology* 1998; 89:A1083.

Ramer MS, Thompson SWN, McMahon SB. Causes and consequences of sympathetic basket formation in dorsal root ganglia. *Pain* 1999; (Suppl 6):S111–S120.

Ringkamp M, Eschenfelder S, Grethel EJ, et al. Lumbar sympathectomy failed to reverse mechanical allodynia- and hyperalgesia-like behavior in rats with L5 spinal nerve injury. *Pain* 1999; 79:142–153.

Rodin BE, Kruger L. Deafferentation in animals as a model for the study of pain: an alternative hypothesis. *Brain Res* 1984; 319:213–228.

Sato J, Perl ER. Adrenergic excitation of cutaneous pain receptors induced by peripheral nerve injury. *Science* 1991; 251:1608–1610.

Seltzer Z, Dubner R, Shir Y. A novel behavioral model of neuropathic pain disorders produced in rats by partial sciatic nerve injury. *Pain* 1990; 43:205–218.

Sheen K, Chung JM. Signs of neuropathic pain depends on signals from injured nerve fibers in a rat model. *Brain Res* 1993; 610:62–68.

Shi TJS, Winzer-Serhan U, Leslie F, Hökfelt T. Distribution and regulation of α_2-adrenoceptors in rat dorsal root ganglia. *Pain* 2000; 84:319–330.

Shir Y, Seltzer Z. Effects of sympathectomy in a model of causalgiform pain produced by partial sciatic nerve injury in rats. *Pain* 1991; 45:309–320.

Stanton-Hicks M, Jänig W, Hassenbusch S, et al. Reflex sympathetic dystrophy: changing concepts and taxonomy. *Pain* 1995; 63:127–133.

Torebjörk E, Wahren LK, Wallin BG, Hallin R, Koltzenburg M. Noradrenaline-evoked pain in neuralgia. *Pain* 1995; 63:11–20.

Tracey DJ, Cunningham JE, Romm MA. Peripheral hyperalgesia in experimental neuropathy: mediation by alpha 2-adrenoreceptors on post-ganglionic sympathetic terminals. *Pain* 1995a; 60:317–327.

Tracey DJ, Romm MA, Yao NN. Peripheral hyperalgesia in experimental neuropathy: exacerbation by neuropeptide Y. *Brain Res* 1995b; 669:245–254.

Wahren LK, Gordh T Jr, Torebjörk E. Effects of regional intravenous guanethidine in patients with neuralgia in the hand; a follow-up study over a decade. *Pain* 1995; 62:379–385.

Walker AE, Nulsen F. Electrical stimulation of the upper thoracic portion of the sympathetic chain in man. *Arch Neurol Psychiatry* 1948; 5559–5560.

Wall PD, Devor M, Inbal R, et al. Autotomy following peripheral nerve lesions: experimental anaesthesia dolorosa. *Pain* 1979a; 7:103–113.

Wall PD, Scadding JW, Tomkiewicz MM. The production and prevention of experimental anaesthesia dolorosa. *Pain* 1979b; 6:175–182.

Wasner G, Schattschneider J, Heckmann K, Maier C, Baron R. Vascular abnormalities in reflex sympathetic dystrophy (CRPS I)—mechanisms and diagnostic value. *Brain* 2001; 124:587–599.

Wesselmann UI, Ali Z, Meyer RA, Raja SN. Topical clonidine attenuates ongoing pain and hyperalgesia in patients with sympathetically maintained pain (SMP). *Soc Neurosci Abstracts* 1996; 22:1803.

White JC, Sweet WH. *Pain and the Neurosurgeon: A Forty Year Experience*. Springfield, IL: Charles C. Thomas, 1969.

Willenbring S, Beauprie IG, DeLeo JA. Sciatic cryoneurolysis in rats: a model of sympathetically independent pain. Part 1: Effects of sympathectomy. *Anesth Analg* 1995; 81:544–548.

Woolf CJ. Phenotypic modification of primary sensory neurons: the role of nerve growth factor in the production of persistent pain. *Philos Trans R Soc Lond B Biol Sci* 1996; 351:441–448.

Yoon YW, Na HS, Chung JM. Contributions of injured and intact afferents to neuropathic pain in an experimental rat model. *Pain* 1996; 64:27–36.

Yoon YW, Lee DH, Lee, BH, Chung JM. Different strains and substrains of rat show different levels of neuropathic pain behaviors. *Exp Brain Res* 1999; 129:167–171.

Zhang JM, Song XJ, LaMotte RH. An in vitro study of ectopic discharge generation and adrenergic sensitivity in the intact nerve-injured rat dorsal root ganglion. *Pain* 1997; 72:51–57.

Zhou XF, Rush RA, McLachlan EM. Differential expression of the p75 nerve growth factor receptor in glia and neurons of the dorsal root ganglia after peripheral nerve transection. *J Neurosci* 1996; 16:2901–2911.

Correspondence to: Wilfrid Jänig, Dr med, Physiologisches Institut, Christian-Albrechts-Universität zu Kiel, Olshausenstr. 40, 24098 Kiel, Germany. Tel: 431/8802036; Fax: 431/8805256; email: w.janig@physiologie.uni-kiel.de.

Neuropathic Pain: Pathophysiology and Treatment,
Progress in Pain Research and Management, Vol. 21,
edited by Per T. Hansson, Howard L. Fields, Raymond G.
Hill, and Paolo Marchettini, IASP Press, Seattle, © 2001.

8

Postherpetic Neuralgia—A Model for Neuropathic Pain?

Turo J. Nurmikko

*Pain Research Institute, Department of Neurological Science,
University of Liverpool, Liverpool, United Kingdom*

Each year 2 out of 1000 people in the United States, mainly over 50 years of age, develop herpes zoster (HZ) (Donohue et al. 1995). Most patients must cope with a segmental rash, pain and allodynia for a few weeks, will be diagnosed by primary care physicians, and will receive antivirals and analgesics. Almost all will be reassured of the inherently good prognosis of the condition. A small percentage will develop postherpetic neuralgia (PHN). In this group pain will continue long after the rash has resolved, causing a great deal of suffering and disability.

Compared with other chronic pain conditions (such as low back pain, fibromyalgia, and migraine), PHN is relatively uncommon. Its true prevalence is not known, not only because epidemiological data are scarce, but also because of a lack of consensus on the definition of PHN. It is commonly considered to have developed if pain persists beyond a certain defined period after the cutaneous eruption (or its resolution). The transition from HZ to PHN is deemed by different investigators to occur immediately after the rash, or at 1 month, 3 months, or 6 months after crusting of the skin lesions (Dworkin and Portenoy 1996). Some advocate use of the term *zoster-associated pain* (ZAP), defined as pain occurring any time from the onset of rash until a predefined minimum level of pain (or total resolution of pain) has been reached (Dworkin and Portenoy 1996).

The practice of time-linked diagnostic definition has its weaknesses. Notably, any evaluation of a patient with long-lasting pain after HZ will raise the question of whether at a given time point the pain is just tailing off or whether a chronic condition has become established. Prevalence estimates will be profoundly affected by the timing criteria because of the tendency of the condition to spontaneously improve over time, especially in the first 6 months. Studies on the pathophysiology of PHN may also be influenced by the decision of the investigator to focus either on more recent or truly chronic cases.

Recent and past epidemiological data on the incidence of HZ and cohort studies on its natural course allow rough estimates of the overall burden of prolonged postzoster pain in Western countries. While acute zoster is frequently, though not exclusively painful, pain rapidly decreases as recovery takes place. The classic prospective study by Hope-Simpson of all 321 HZ cases seen in one general practice in Cirencester, England between 1947 and 1972 demonstrated that 10% of patients had pain at 3 months and 4% at 12 months. Two recent prospective studies obtained similar results (Haanpää et al. 1999; Helgason et al. 2000). Those over 60 years of age are at risk for prolonged pain (Fig. 1). These figures are at conflict with much higher percentages frequently quoted in the literature (Burgoon et al. 1957; de Moragas and Kierland 1957); however, the latter are based on reports of hospital admissions of patients and therefore are not representative of the general population. These studies suggest that those who still have significant pain at 12 months are at considerable risk of continuing to suffer from PHN for several years (Watson et al. 1991b; Helgason et al. 2000).

Every year approximately 600,000 Americans will suffer an attack of HZ, and some 8% (48,000) will have pain at 1 month (Choo et al. 1997). If other existing data on the natural course of HZ in the general population are reliable, 20,000 to 32,000 of these patients still will have some pain left

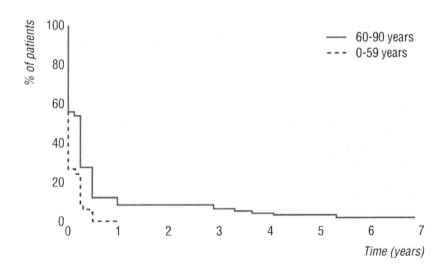

Fig. 1. Kaplan-Meier plot of duration of postzoster pain in two age groups. From Helgason et al. (2000), with permission.

after 12 months (Hope-Simpson 1975; Haanpää et al. 2000; Helgason et al. 2000). However, fewer than half will rate their pain as moderate or severe (Helgason et al. 2000). Many of these patients will go on to develop chronic PHN, which may take years to resolve or could last a lifetime. The relative contribution of the newly acquired and chronic PHN on the overall prevalence of the condition has not been calculated but is likely to be considerable. In a recent survey of 1079 elderly patients with a median age of 80 years for lifetime prevalence of PHN, 11 (1%) complained of postzoster pain that had lasted more than 12 months (Bowsher 1999) (The figure may turn out to be higher, as some patients with ongoing pain were interviewed within 12 months of the onset of shingles.) Assuming that the study population was representative of the elderly British population at the time, these numbers translate to a population of almost 100,000 citizens over 65 with chronic PHN in the United Kingdom. The equivalent in the United States would be on the order of 500,000. Because this retrospective study was part of a survey on the prevalence of psychiatric illness, and because no attempt was made to estimate the intensity of or disability caused by the pain, we must view these figures with caution. However, the study does give a rough estimate of the magnitude of the problem, and prevalence may be on the increase as people are living longer and the incidence of herpes zoster is increasing (Donahue et al. 1995).

In addition to the group of patients with chronic PHN of more than 1 year's duration, there is at any given time a steadily changing group of patients with protracted pain following shingles (1, 3, or 6 months, depending on the definition) who may recover within a year of contracting HZ. In the absence of prospective studies it would be bold to suggest that these two groups share the same pathophysiological mechanisms for their pain, or that their responses to various treatments would be identical. In this chapter I will discuss some controversies that have emerged in relation to the pathophysiology of PHN.

MECHANISMS OF NERVE DAMAGE IN SHINGLES

HZ results from activation of the varicella-zoster virus (VZV), which has remained latent in the dorsal root ganglion (DRG) since the first infection (usually chickenpox). During latency the virus persists in a noninfectious form in several ganglia and is predominantly found in neurons (Kennedy et al. 2000). The molecular mechanisms of how latency is established and maintained for years and decades are incompletely understood, but a precise interaction seems to take place between the host immune response and several VZV-encoded transcripts and proteins (genes 4, 21, 29, 62, and 63).

Reactivation is associated with a decline in cell-mediated immunity, but the role of other factors and the precise mechanisms underlying the transition from latency to active viral replication are unknown (Gilden et al. 2000). During recrudescence the virus replicates in the ganglionic nerve cells, which start infecting neighboring cells. As a result, a local ganglionitis develops, followed by transmission of the infection down the nerve to the skin. How the virus is transported in the affected axons is not known. The infection also spreads centrally, leading to inflammation of the leptomeninges and the ipsilateral posterior and anterior horns of the spinal cord, and to vacuolization of the posterior columns. Occasional observations of inflammatory changes in the contralateral spinal ganglia come from human postmortem studies (Watson et al. 1991a).

Recent studies suggest that extension of the viral inflammation into the central nervous system (CNS) during HZ is common, though usually subclinical. Of 46 patients with uncomplicated HZ of fewer than 18 days' duration, abnormalities of the cerebrospinal fluid suggestive of VZV infection were found in 61% (Haanpää et al. 1998). In a subgroup of 16 patients with cranial or cervical HZ, MRI revealed inflammatory changes in 9 patients. Another study of 40 patients given HZ electromyographic tests suggested motor involvement in 21 (53%); in many cases this change was bilateral, indicating transmission of the virus-induced inflammation across the spinal cord (Haanpää et al. 1997).

Histopathological studies of acute and subacute HZ show evidence of neuronal loss and inflammatory infiltrates in ganglia, nerves, and nerve roots. In some cases the affected ganglia are extensively necrotic. Most changes in the peripheral nerve appear to result from Wallerian degeneration occurring in both large- and small-diameter fibers (Denny-Brown et al. 1944). Inflammatory changes are then slowly replaced by fibrous tissue. These changes have been described following shingles in those with and without PHN (Zacks et al. 1964; Watson et al. 1991a).

From the relatively few histopathological studies on HZ and PHN published to date, degenerative changes affecting the nerve seem to be a uniform consequence; however, the meager data seem to involve patients predominantly with severe infections. Surprisingly, reports of involvement of the ganglia, nerve roots, and CNS vary greatly. Thus, Watson and colleagues (1991a, 2000) found major dorsal horn atrophy in four cases of thoracic PHN but no changes in one further case of trigeminal PHN. They found no atrophy in two patients with a history of shingles but without subsequent PHN; however, one of these patients showed evidence of post-inflammatory swelling of the dorsal horn (Watson et al. 1991a). Watson et al. (1991a) and Zacks et al. (1964) have described degenerative changes in the spinal and trigeminal ganglia to varying degrees without any correlation with PHN pain. It is therefore difficult to associate these findings with any pain mechanism, and the sensory data provided are too limited to draw conclusions about the pathophysiology of pain and/or allodynia.

Furthermore, increasing evidence indicates that abnormalities are not confined to the affected side only. Watson et al. (2000) showed in their case study that the nonaffected ophthalmic branch of the trigeminal nerve had undergone major degenerative changes as well. Oaklander et al. (1998) showed a relative reduction in the density of epidermal nerve fibers obtained by skin punch biopsy and stained with the pan-neuronal marker PGP9.5. This finding is not surprising in light of electromyographic evidence of contralateral nerve root involvement in the acute stages, findings at autopsy of inflammatory cells in the contralateral ganglia, and evidence of VZV latency in the contralateral ganglia in the experimental VZV model.

ANIMAL STUDIES

The varicella-zoster virus has a very narrow host range, and natural infections occur only in humans and primates. In recent years several groups have reported success in establishing a latent infection in rat dorsal ganglia by subcutaneous inoculation of the foot pad or paraspinal skin with infected cells or with cell-free virus preparations (Sadzot-Delvaux et al. 1995; Annunziato et al. 1998; Fleetwood-Walker et al. 1999). One group found evidence of VZV DNA in the contralateral DRG as well, although the mechanism of the migration of the virus remained uncertain (Annunziato et al. 1998). None of the animals showed signs of infection, nor did they show any of the characteristic behavioral signs associated with rodent models of neuropathic pain (e.g., guarding, grooming, and abnormal posture).

However, when graded innocuous and noxious mechanical and thermal stimuli were applied to the inoculated foot pad of the rat, the investigators noted a significant reduction in the thresholds for the limb-withdrawal reflex (Fleetwood-Walker et al. 1999). Histopathological analyses of the corresponding DRG showed expression of the VZV-specific protein IE 63, but no evidence of inflammation or cell death. The authors suggested that VZV latency alone is capable of establishing this heightened sensitivity to mechanical and thermal stimuli. Using an in vitro model for latent VZV infection, another group recently reported development of norepinephrine sensitivity in small capsaicin-sensitive neurons; further analyses showed that this was due to upregulation of expression of α_1-adrenergic receptors in these fibers (Kress and Fickenscher 2001).

The experimental models described are not representative of the full-blown human form of HZ and PHN, but these important observations suggest that at some level of latent infection, VZV may be capable of inducing abnormalities in afferent function. It is generally accepted that subclinical reactivations may occur during latency, which suggests that the host's immune response and the existing viral burden are not in harmonious balance (Sadzot-Delvaux et al. 1998). The transition of the latent virus from a quiescent state into a progressive state of replication is not an explosive all-or-nothing phenomenon, but rather a shift in balance in the complex interactions between the virus and the host factors curtailing its activation. If so, the unusually long episodes of neuralgia preceding the rash by months (Haanpää et al. 1999) could represent a form of neuritis, which is partially contained by the host's defenses until they are finally overwhelmed by the viral burden. Similarly, the virus may not have been completely defeated by the time the skin has healed. Post mortem studies have shown evidence of inflammation in the DRG months after the rash has resolved (Watson et al. 1991b). One laboratory has reported detection of VZV DNA in mononuclear cells of some patients with PHN (Vafai et al. 1998). Further studies are needed to evaluate whether, following shingles, VZV persists in ganglia at a greater level than during latency and whether this correlates with the duration or intensity of pain.

CLINICAL FEATURES OF HZ AND PHN

With few exceptions (Lampl et al. 1998; Schott 1998; Haanpää et al. 1999), pain associated with HZ infection starts before or at the time of the cutaneous eruption and runs a variable course until it is resolved or becomes permanent. On some occasions pain may appear many years after the initial episode, usually provoked by a local injury (Schott 1998). Some 40% of patients pain experience preherpetic neuralgia (Haanpää et al. 1999).

The quality of pain in both acute HZ and PHN can be variable. In both conditions, either spontaneous pain or evoked pain may dominate the picture. Though several investigators have pointed out features that distinguish the two conditions, the similarities are undeniable, and would be practically impossible to separate the two conditions by pain description or clinical examination, if it were not for the presence of rash. Using the McGill Pain Questionnaire, Bhala et al. (1988) noted some differences in choice of somatic and evaluative words between patients with HZ and PHN. However, among the 10 most commonly chosen words, 6 featured in both groups and in the rest the difference was in nuances rather than quality (e.g., as opposed to the descriptor "hot" in shingles, the term "burning" was preferred in PHN, and the words "stabbing" and "shooting" entered the top 10 in the HZ group compared to "shooting" alone in PHN).

Similarly, evoked pain is a common feature in HZ and PHN. In Table I, observations from several studies are presented as percentages of patients displaying one or several types of allodynia or hyperalgesia. While no direct comparisons have been made, the results suggest that heat hyperalgesia is as prevalent in HZ as in PHN, and that mechanical allodynia is only marginally more common in PHN, although this may be due to patient selection bias. The difference in the prevalence of evoked pain between HZ and PHN is modest, suggesting that whatever neural aberrations underlie these pains, they are unlikely to be unique to HZ or PHN. Any difference in the intensity of allodynia and hyperalgesia between HZ and PHN appears not to have been determined.

Several subtypes of mechanical allodynia are seen in HZ and PHN (Table I, Fig. 2) and may coexist in a given patient, as shown by Venn's diagram from the study of Pappagallo et al. (2000) (Fig. 2). It seems important to be able to delineate the mechanisms of each type of pain and apply treatments accordingly. At the present stage, truly comprehensive pathophysiological studies in either HZ and PHN are few, and no study has been able to link a pain subtype with a unique mechanism for which a preferred treatment is available.

Table I
Percentages of acute herpes zoster and postherpetic neuralgia patients
with one or several types of allodynia or hyperalgesia

	Acute Herpes Zoster		Postherpetic Neuralgia		
	Haanpää et al. 1999 ($n = 113$)	Nurmikko et al. 1991 ($n = 31$)	Nurmikko and Bowsher 1990 ($n = 42$)	Pappagallo et al. 2000 ($n = 63$)	Rowbotham and Fields 1996 ($n = 35$)
Mechanical Allodynia	*45*	*55*	*87*	*78*	*100**
Dynamic	32	55	87	60	100
Static	31	ND	ND	52	ND
Punctate	ND	ND	ND	37	ND
Skin stretch	17	ND	17	ND	ND
Thermal Hyperalgesia			*40*		
Heat	11	25	8	29	34
Cold	ND	ND	10	17	ND

Abbreviation: ND = not determined.
* Patients were chosen on the basis of allodynia.

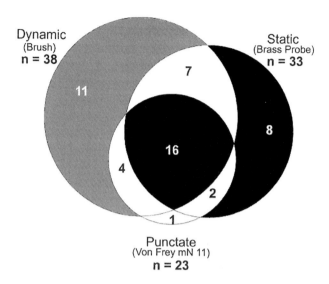

Fig. 2. Venn diagram indicating the relative proportion of 63 patients with PHN and mechanical allodynia; 49% of patients had at least one type of allodynia. From Pappagallo et al. (2000), with permission.

PATHOPHYSIOLOGICAL STUDIES OF POSTHERPETIC NEURALGIA

Several lines of investigations have looked into the mechanisms of PHN. Investigations have tended to be hypothesis-testing rather than hypothesis-generating. Implicit in this line of approach is the assumption of the relative homogeneity and stability of PHN as a clinical syndrome. As will be discussed below, this may not be the case. The investigations to date have been conducted in a relatively small group of patients with PHN, usually presenting with a wide distribution of duration and intensity of pain. Baron and Saguer (1993) and Rowbotham and Fields (1996) were selective in enrolling only patients with cutaneous allodynia, but most studies used no particular restrictions in the selection process. Methods used to date have included psychophysical tests (Rowbotham and Fields 1996), selective neural blockade (Nurmikko et al. 1991), chemical pain induction (Baron and Saguer 1993; Choi and Rowbotham 1997; Petersen et al. 2000), and evaluation of treatment (Rowbotham et al. 1995, 1996a).

The results of these studies are so diverse that it is now clear that no single pathology can possibly explain the whole spectrum of pain-generating mechanisms in PHN. Moreover, the existing evidence points to a significant contribution to the pathology from both the peripheral and central nervous systems. The relative weight of each contribution varies among individual patients and may be more decisive in terms of prognosis and treatment effectiveness than age, comorbidity, or drug dosage. Below, we briefly discuss the various hypotheses of PHN. Many of the comments may also apply to HZ, but the current level of understanding of pain mechanisms in the latter condition precludes any firm conclusions.

EVIDENCE SUGGESTING A PERIPHERAL MECHANISM

Groupwise analyses in PHN and HZ have shown impaired sensation of all modalities in the affected skin, but frequent observations indicate that the degree of sensory loss varies greatly (Rowbotham and Fields 1989; Nurmikko and Bowsher 1990; Haanpää et al. 1999; Zaal et al. 2000). In their 1989 paper, Rowbotham and Fields comment on the fact that some patients had minimal or no sensory loss in the affected skin while in others the skin appeared almost insensate. Similarly, when analyzing a group of 42 patients with chronic PHN, Nurmikko and Bowsher (1990) found elevations of all sensory thresholds in the affected dermatome when compared to the contralateral homologous site. Yet when the abnormality of the sensory loss was estimated against an "asymmetry index" derived from healthy age-matched controls, threshold elevation fell outside the normal range in 27–78% of patients, depending on the sensory modality subtype (Nurmikko and Bowsher 1990). For example, touch was within normal limits in 22% and heat pain in 40% of cases. In acute HZ, elevated thresholds for warmth were reported in 22%, for cold in 20%, and for touch in 25% of the patients tested (Haanpää et al. 2000). According to this study, these changes did not correlate with either pain or allodynia and tended to normalize quickly in a matter of months. Another group, however, reported major sensory impairment 2 months after the cutaneous eruption in 20% of cases and concluded that it was associated with increased levels of spontaneous pain (Zaal et al. 2000).

Despite these variable results, clear evidence shows that some patients with HZ and PHN have little if any sensory loss. To explore this phenomenon further, Rowbotham and Fields (1996) established a pattern of cutaneous sensory change in the most painful area of the patients with PHN, all of whom had dynamic mechanical allodynia. They found an inverse correlation between pain and thermal sensory deficit. Those who were hyperalgesic to heat showed higher ratings for spontaneous pain (Fig. 3a) and for allodynia. This finding was interpreted as representing sensitization of nociceptors (and/or central sensitization) as the pain-maintaining mechanism.

Similar results were obtained by Pappagallo et al. (2000), who performed an almost identical analysis in their 63 patients with PHN. The difference is

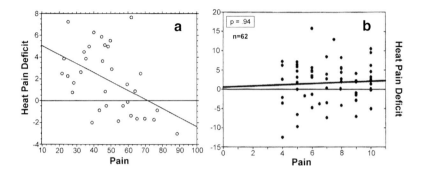

Fig. 3. Scatter plots (with slight modifications) from two studies evaluating the relationship between heat pain deficit (expressed in degrees Celsius) and ongoing pain (measured on a visual analogue scale of 0–100 [a] and 0–10 [b]). Heat pain deficit denotes heat pain threshold measured on the affected side minus the same threshold on the contralateral unaffected side. Negative values indicate heat hyperalgesia, and positive values denote heat hypoesthesia. Rowbotham and Fields (Fig. 3a) found that heat pain deficit, when plotted against PHN pain scores, correlated inversely with ongoing pain ($r^2 = 0.24$, $P < 0.003$), whereas Pappagallo et al. (Fig. 3b) did not. Note the different scales used for heat pain deficit and pain. From Rowbotham and Fields (1996) and Pappagallo et al. (2000), with permission.

that they were unable to find a correlation between pain and heat pain thresholds (Fig. 3b). However, as they pointed out, approximately one-fourth of their patients had hyperalgesia to heat, and would qualify for the sensitized nociceptor group that formed one-third of Rowbotham and Fields' study population. Importantly, Fig. 3a,b shows the wide scatter of values, with several patients in both studies showing both intense pain and hypoalgesia, rather than hyperalgesia, to heat.

The role of the peripheral afferent dysfunction in PHN has been further evaluated by infiltrating the skin with a variety of pharmacological agents. In a double-blind study in 15 patients with chronic PHN of the allodynic subtype, a cutaneous injection of an adrenergic agonist (epinephrine or phenylephrine) intensified ongoing pain and mechanical allodynia, whereas saline did not (Choi and Rowbotham 1997). Detailed analysis of their data shows that this aggravation of symptoms occurred to any significant degree in only five subjects. However, it is reasonable to assume that these patients had developed noradrenergic sensitivity induced by the viral invasion and subsequent nerve damage. This upregulation of adrenergic receptors is thought to explain the occasional success from sympathetic blockade, especially in HZ and early PHN. In chronic cases sympathetic blockade is almost always ineffective (Nurmikko et al. 1991).

Another study by the same group analyzed the effect of stimulating capsaicin-sensitive nerve fibers in 17 patients with PHN and mechanical dynamic allodynia (Petersen et al. 2000). Topical capsaicin was applied to the affected skin and to the contralateral mirror image site. Eleven of these patients experienced a pronounced increase in their ongoing pain or showed expansion of the allodynic area. In the other patients, the response to local application of capsaicin did not differ between the affected and healthy skin. Interestingly, the expansion of allodynia in three patients extended well into the previously nonpainful skin, in which sensory thresholds and intraepidermal nerve fiber density were determined by skin punch biopsy to be normal.

In comparison with the 6 nonresponders, the 11 capsaicin responders were characterized by higher scores of baseline pain and allodynia, and their thermal sensation in the affected skin was less impaired. When the intensity of capsaicin-induced pain in all 17 patients was plotted against sensory deficits, an inverse correlation was found. In other words, the better the sensory functions of small-diameter nerve fibers were preserved, the stronger was the capsaicin-induced response (Petersen et al. 2000).

The expansion of mechanical allodynia in some patients to previously unaffected skin would strongly point to central sensitization, driven by cap-saicin-induced increased activity in peripheral C fibers. Where there is a relative lack of functioning peripheral C fibers, such sensitization clearly will take place to a much lesser extent, if at all.

An alternative strategy involving blockade of peripheral afferents has yielded similar results. In some patients small amounts of lidocaine injected into the most painful area effectively eliminated the pain and allodynia for hours or days (Rowbotham and Fields 1989; Rowbotham et al. 1998). Topical lidocaine, either as a 5% gel or in the form of a self-adhesive patch, was superior to placebo in reducing pain without any evidence of systemic absorption, as shown by negligible lidocaine blood levels (Rowbotham et al. 1995). These results suggest that lidocaine relieves pain in PHN by a direct action on the skin. No studies have been published showing shrinkage of allodynic areas outside the topical application, i.e., reversal of central sensitization, though anecdotal reports of "disproportionate" amelioration of pain after cutaneous injections suggest that it in some patients is likely to occur.

While none of these studies proves conclusively that the peripheral dysfunctional afferent is the major mediator of PHN, it is clear that effective treatment aimed at blocking its activity can provide an effective means of treating PHN pain. The next logical step is to try to delineate the subclasses of neurons that act as substrates for the various types of pain and allodynia. One step further would be to link clinical characteristics with abnormalities of specific nerve fiber function, and develop treatments capable of targeting the given dysfunction.

Recent developments in the characterization of epidermal nerve fibers hold some hope in this regard. Skin punch biopsies have found slightly conflicting results in determining epidermal nerve fiber density in patients with PHN (Rowbotham et al. 1996b; Petersen et al. 2000; Oaklander 2001), but there seems to be no doubt that many afferent terminals have sustained considerable damage and undergone degeneration. As immunohistochemical methods improve, it should be possible to determine in great detail which receptors play an active role in maintaining the sensitized state of the nociceptor.

EVIDENCE FOR CENTRAL MECHANISMS

Some patients with PHN quickly become aware of a seeming paradox in that "the numb part of their body is hurting," the maximum area of pain showing pronounced sensory impairment. Several explanations are possible for this curious sensory paradox. Pain may be maintained by just a few surviving nociceptors, too few to contribute to normal sensitivity but enough to feed the afferent pain-mediating pathways and maintain central sensitization. Alternatively, pain may be due to increased activity in the deep (muscle, joint) nociceptors. However, pain may also be originating in the CNS independently of peripheral C fibers and may result from primary alterations in the functions of the neurons in the spinal cord or more rostrally.

In a selected group of 10 patients with chronic PHN and allodynia, Baron and Saguer (1993) used histamine iontophoresis to study the C-fiber-mediated axon reflex vasodilatation and flare. In all their patients these functions were diminished or abolished; none of the subjects reported increased pain or itch. The correlation between intensity of pain and impairment of these C-fiber functions was positive, suggesting a mechanism other than ongoing barrages in sensitized C nociceptors.

To support this view, Oaklander et al. (1998) reported a substantial reduction in the density of epidermal fibers within the affected skin in patients with PHN. Almost all epidermal neurites are capsaicin-sensitive nociceptors; other types of sensory neurons end in the dermis, and their density is not reflected in epidermal fiber counts. Skin punch biopsies were obtained from 38 patients, 19 with and 19 without pain after shingles, and were stained with the pan-neuronal marker PGP9.5. Light microscopy showed that epidermal fiber density in the pain-free subjects was over twice that seen in those with PHN. Moreover, Oaklander (2001) was able to suggest a specific threshold (650 neurites/mm^2) distinguishing subjects with and without PHN. The density in normal skin is approximately 2000 neurites/mm^2

(Oaklander et al. 1998). Reduced epidermal nerve fiber innervation was previously shown to correlate with impairment of cutaneous thermal sensitivity (Rowbotham et al. 1996b).

Previous psychophysical studies on patients with PHN provided indirect evidence that pain and allodynia may be present when cutaneous C-fiber functions are diminished or absent. In some patients undergoing quantitative sensory testing, thermal thresholds could not be detected, yet these patients complained of continuous pain and displayed tactile allodynia (Nurmikko and Bowsher 1990). In a subgroup of five patients with severe allodynia, blockade of the affected nerve with lidocaine abolished the pain and mechanical allodynia. Repeated sensory testing showed that by the time pain and allodynia returned, tactile thresholds had returned to near-normal levels, while thermal sensitivity was still absent (Nurmikko et al. 1991).

Examples in clinical practice indicate that pain originating in the CNS may project to the area in which cutaneous sensitivity is lost or impaired (e.g., central post-stroke pain [CPSP], brachial avulsion). Allodynia is a common finding in CPSP and syringomyelia and is occasionally seen in multiple sclerosis, or in purely central conditions. Animal models suggest that even in mechanical nerve injury, pain may be generated that is independent of any C-fiber activity (Liu et al. 2000). It is crucial to remember that in HZ there is evidence of direct viral invasion of the spinal cord (and the brainstem trigeminal complex), and that many (but not all) post mortem studies have shown major degenerative changes in the spinal cord in patients with PHN.

LACK OF A COMMON PATHOPHYSIOLOGY OF PHN

These observations and known pathoanatomical abnormalities found in both HZ and PHN suggest that a unifying theory of PHN pathophysiology is not attainable. Evidence is compelling for peripheral sensitization as the driving pathophysiological mechanism in a subset of patients. Such sensitization is likely to be associated with increased firing in the C nociceptors, leading to secondary central sensitization by any of the mechanisms implicated from experimental studies. Patients with the purest form of this type of PHN will have no or minimal sensory loss, but they do have hyperalgesia to heat and mechanical allodynia and show evidence of increased local blood flow. Their pain is accentuated by application of topical capsaicin and by cutaneous injection of an adrenergic agonist. The pain is relieved by cold, by local infiltration of the affected skin, and by topical lidocaine.

There is also good indirect evidence that in other subsets of patients, central mechanisms are dominant. Some patients show profound sensory loss, have no allodynia, and are unaffected by topical application of capsaicin or lidocaine. Skin punch biopsies show a complete lack of epidermal nerve fibers. In clinical practice, patients with this type of PHN are rarely seen. Another subset of patients has remained a source of some controversy. These are patients with moderate-to-severe sensory loss (with, perhaps, the exception of tactile sensation), and lack of vasodilatation even after topical capsaicin or histamine iontophoresis. Skin biopsies show a paucity of small-diameter epidermal nerve fibers. Drug challenges produce variable effects. In these patients the dominant feature is dynamic mechanical allodynia (with little or no static allodynia) that is abolished only by complete blockade with local anesthetics of all nerve fibers supplying the affected area (Nurmikko et al. 1991). The putative pathoanatomical change in this condition is reorganization at the level of the spinal cord in that preserved large-diameter Aβ fibers form abnormal connections with the dorsal horn nociceptive neurons. Alternatively, this subtype, or a very similar condition, could be caused by hyperactive afferents not connected to skin but maintaining central sensitization by ectopic firing; dynamic allodynia in these circumstances would represent secondary hyperalgesia rather than central reorganization.

It should be emphasized that the subtypes of PHN described here represent pathophysiological concepts and not well-defined entities. Few patients will fit one subtype category only; most will have different kinds of pain and allodynia, produced by a host of mechanisms. The challenge in the future will be to try to deal with individual patients on the basis of these mechanisms rather than forge them into the mold of a single etiological entity.

An example of how this might be done is provided by Petersen and coworkers (2000) in their elegant study evaluating the effect of topical capsaicin on PHN pain. Detailed sensory testing in a patient with PHN showed areas of relative preservation as well as clearly impaired thermal sensation, both within the affected skin. Skin punch biopsies were obtained from both areas, and capsaicin cream was applied. The authors showed a reduced number of epidermal nerve fibers coupled with a weaker capsaicin stimulation response in the area with impaired thermal sensation, compared to the area with preserved thermal sensation.

As our understanding of the pathophysiology increases, other subtypes may emerge. For example, the common phenomenon of itch in PHN (as opposed to other neuropathic pain conditions) has not been investigated. The role of mechano- and heat-insensitive C nociceptors has not been evaluated in PHN, but would seem a logical avenue to pursue, especially in cases deemed to represent the sensitized peripheral afferent subtype. It may be useful to remember that advances are being made in the prevention and treatment of this disease. As new nerve growth factors, more potent antivirals, vaccines, and new drugs that act to prevent neuroplastic changes become available, the manifestations of PHN—complex as they already are—may undergo many modifications.

Is PHN a good model for neuropathic pain? If the intention is to extrapolate from PHN to other neuropathic conditions, the answer will have to be no, given its diversity and unpredictability. If the intention is to maximally explore the mechanisms associated with its many extraordinary features, to pave the way for new targeted treatments, the answer will have to be yes. PHN remains one of the most intriguing pain conditions seen in the clinic and undoubtedly will attract many future generations of researchers.

ACKNOWLEDGMENTS

I wish to thank Prof. Michael Rowbotham and Dr. Karen Petersen for their review of the manuscript and helpful comments.

REFERENCES

Annunziato P, LaRussa P, Lee P, et al. Evidence of latent varicella-zoster virus in rat dorsal root ganglia. *J Infect Dis* 1998; 178(Suppl 1):S48–51.

Baron R, Saguer M. Postherpetic neuralgia: are C-nociceptors involved in signaling and maintenance of tactile allodynia? *Brain* 1993; 116:1477–1496.

Bhala BB, Ramamoorthy C, Bowsher D, Yelnoorker KN. Shingles and postherpetic neuralgia. *Clin J Pain* 1988; 4:160–174.

Bowsher D. The lifetime occurrence of Herpes zoster and prevalence of post-herpetic neuralgia: a retrospective survey in an elderly population. *Eur J Pain* 1999; 3:335–342.

Burgoon CF, Burgoon JS, Baldridge GD. The natural history of herpes zoster. *JAMA* 1957; 164:265–269.

Choi B, Rowbotham MC. Effect of adrenergic receptor activation on post-herpetic neuralgia pain and sensory disturbances. *Pain* 1997; 69:55–63.

Choo PW, Galil K, Donahue JG, et al. Risk factors for postherpetic neuralgia. *Arch Int Med* 1997; 157:1217–1224.

De Moragas JM, Kierland RB. The outcome of patients with herpes zoster. *Arch Dermatol* 1957; 75:193–196.

Denny-Brown D, Adams RD, Fitzgerald PJ. Pathologic features of herpes zoster. *Arch Neurol Psychiatry* 1944; 57:216–231.

Donahue JG, Choo PW, Manson JE, Platt R. The incidence of herpes zoster. *Arch Intern Med* 1995; 155:1605–1609.

Dworkin RH, Portenoy RK. Pain and its persistence in herpes zoster. *Pain* 1996; 67:241–251.

Fields HL, Rowbotham M, Baron R. Postherpetic neuralgia: irritable nociceptors and deafferentation. *Neurobiol Dis* 1998; 5:209–227.

Fleetwood-Walker SM, Quinn JP, Wallace C, et al. Behavioural changes in the rat following infection with varicella-zoster virus. *J Gen Virol* 1999; 80:2433–2436.

Gilden DH, Kleinschmidt-DeMasters BK, LaGuardia JL, Mahalingam R, Cohrs RJ. Medical progress: neurologic complications of the reactivation of varicella-zoster virus. *N Engl J Med* 2000; 342:635–645.

Haanpää M. *Herpes Zoster: A Clinical, Neurophysiological, Neuroradiological and Neurovirological Study.* Dissertation, University of Tampere, 1999.

Haanpää M, Häkkinen V, Nurmikko T. Motor involvement in acute herpes zoster. *Muscle Nerve* 1997; 20:1433–1438.

Haanpää M, Dastidar P, Weinberg A, et al. CSF and MRI findings in patients with acute herpes zoster. *Neurology* 1998; 51:1405–1411.

Haanpää M, Laippala P, Nurmikko T. Pain and somatosensory dysfunction in acute herpes zoster. *Clin J Pain* 1999; 15:78–84.

Haanpää M, Laippala P, Nurmikko T. Allodynia and pinprick hypoaesthesia in acute herpes zoster, and the development of postherpetic neuralgia. *J Pain Symptom Manage* 2000; 20:50–58.

Helgason S, Petursson G, Gudmundsson S, Sigurdsson JA. Prevalence of postherpetic neuralgia after a first episode of herpes zoster: prospective study with long follow up. *BMJ* 2000; 321:794–796.

Hope-Simpson RE. Postherpetic neuralgia. *J R Coll Gen Pract* 1975; 25:571–575.

Kennedy PGE, Grinfeld E, Bell JE. Varicella-zoster virus gene expression in latently infected and explanted human ganglia. *J Virol* 2000; 74:11893–11898.

Kress M, Fickenscher H. Infection by human varicella zoster virus confers norepinephrine sensitivity to sensory neurones from rat dorsal root ganglia. *FASEB J* 2001; 15:1037–1043.

Kruger L, Perl ER, Sedivec MJ. Fine structure of myelinated mechanical nociceptor endings in cat hairy skin. *J Comp Neurol* 1981; 198:137–154.

Lampl C, Neuner L, Klingler D. Possible postherpetic neuralgia first occurring seven years after herpes zoster. *Neurology* 1998; 192–193.

Liu C-N, Wall PD, Ben-Dor E, et al. Tactile allodynia in the absence of C-fiber activation: altered firing properties of DRG neurons following spinal nerve injury. *Pain* 2000; 85:503–521.

Nurmikko T, Bowsher D. Somatosensory findings in postherpetic neuralgia. *J Neurol Neurosurg Psychiatry* 1990; 53:135–141.

Nurmikko TJ, Räsänen A, Häkkinen V. Clinical and neurophysiological observations on acute herpes zoster. *Clin J Pain* 1990; 6:284–290.

Nurmikko T, Wells C, Bowsher D. Pain and allodynia in postherpetic neuralgia: role of somatic and sympathetic nervous systems. *Acta Neurol Scand* 1991; 84:146–152.

Oaklander AL. The density of nerve endings in human skin with and without postherpetic neuralgia after shingles. *Pain* 2001; 92:139–145.

Oaklander AL, Romans K, Horasek S, et al. Unilateral postherpetic neuralgia is associated with bilateral sensory neuron damage. *Ann Neurol* 1998; 44:789–795.

Pappagallo M, Oaklander AL, Quatrano-Piancentini AL, Clark MR, Raja SR. Heterogeneous patterns of sensory dysfunction in postherpetic neuralgia suggest multiple pathophysiologic mechanisms. *Anesthesiology* 2000; 92:691–698.

Petersen KL, Fields HL, Brennum J, Sandroni P, Rowbotham MC. Capsaicin evoked pain and allodynia in post-herpetic neuralgia. *Pain* 2000; 88:125–133.

Rowbotham MC, Fields HL. Post-herpetic neuralgia: the relation of pain complaint, sensory disturbance, and skin temperature. *Pain* 1989; 39:129–144.

Rowbotham MC, Fields HF. The relationship of pain, allodynia and thermal sensation in post-herpetic neuralgia. *Brain* 1996; 119:347–354.

Rowbotham MC, Davies PS, Fields HL. Topical lidocaine relieves postherpetic neuralgia. *Ann Neurol* 1995; 37:246–253.

Rowbotham MC, Davies PS, Verkempinck C, Galer BS. Lidocaine patch: double-blind controlled study of a new treatment method for post-herpetic neuralgia. *Pain* 1996a; 65:39–44.

Rowbotham MC, Yosipovitch G, Connolly MK, et al. Cutaneous innervation density in allodynic form of postherpetic neuralgia. *Neurobiol Dis* 1996b; 3:205–214.

Rowbotham MC, Petersen KL, Fields HL. Is postherpetic neuralgia more than one disorder? *Pain Forum* 1998; 7:231–237.

Sadzot-Delvaux C, Debrus S, Nikkels A, Piette J, Rentier B. Varicella-zoster virus latency in the adult rat is a useful model for human latent infection. *Neurology* 1995; 45(Suppl 18):S18–S20.

Sadzot-Delvaux C, Arvin AM, Rentier B. Varicella-zoster virus IE63, a virion component expressed during latency and acute infection, elicits humoral and cellular immunity. *J Infect Dis* 1998; 178(Suppl 1):S43–47.

Schott GD. Triggering a delayed-onset postherpetic neuralgia. *Lancet* 1998; 351:419–420.

Vafai A, Wellish M, Gilden D. Expression of varicella-zoster virus in blood mononuclear cells of patients with postherpetic neuralgia. *Proc Natl Acad Sci USA* 1998; 85:2767–2770.

Watson CPN, Deck JH, Morshead C, Van der Kooy D, Evans RJ. Postherpetic neuralgia: further post-mortem studies of cases with and without pain. *Pain* 1991a; 44:105–117.

Watson CPN, Watt VR, Chipman M, Birkett N, Evans RJ. The prognosis with postherpetic neuralgia. *Pain* 1991b; 46:191–195.

Watson CPN, Midha R, Devor M, et al. Trigeminal postherpetic neuralgia postmortem: clinically unilateral, pathologically bilateral. In: Devor M, Rowbotham MC, Wiesenfeld-Hallin Z (Eds). *Proceedings of the 9th World Congress on Pain,* Progress in Pain Research and Management, Vol. 16. Seattle: IASP Press, 2000, pp 733–739.

Zaal MJW, Völker-Dieben HJ, D'Amaro J. Risk and prognostic factors of postherpetic neuralgia and focal sensory denervation: a prospective evaluation in acute herpes zoster ophthalmicus. *Clin J Pain* 2000; 16:345–351.

Zacks, Langfitt TW, Elliott FA. Herpetic neuritis: a light and electron microscopic study. *Neurology* 1964; 14:744–750.

Correspondence to: Turo J. Nurmikko, MD, PhD, Pain Research Institute, Department of Neurological Science, University of Liverpool, Clinical Sciences Centre for Research and Education, Lower Lane, Liverpool L9 7LJ, United Kingdom. Tel: 44-151-529-5820; Fax: 44-151-529-5821; email: tjn@liv.ac.uk.

Neuropathic Pain: Pathophysiology and Treatment,
Progress in Pain Research and Management, Vol. 21,
edited by Per T. Hansson, Howard L. Fields, Raymond G.
Hill, and Paolo Marchettini, IASP Press, Seattle, © 2001.

9

Antidepressants in the Treatment of Neuropathic Pain

Søren H. Sindrup[a,b] and Troels S. Jensen[c]

*[a]Department of Neurology, Odense University Hospital, Odense, Denmark;
[b]Department of Clinical Pharmacology, University of Southern Denmark,
Odense, Denmark; [c]Department of Neurology, Aarhus University Hospital,
Aarhus, Denmark*

Drugs with a characteristic tricyclic structure (Fig. 1) have been used for many years to treat depression. Imipramine was the first drug in this class; only a few years after its introduction as an antidepressant (Kuhn 1958), its analgesic properties became apparent (Paoli et al. 1960) (Table I). Imipramine relieved pain in 14 of 20 patients treated with a daily dose of 75 mg; this positive response of around 70% corresponds to the response frequency observed in more recent controlled trials of antidepressants in neuropathic pain (Sindrup 1997). The patients who obtained relief all had neuropathic pain conditions, and tricyclic antidepressants are now the mainstay of treatment for this type of pain.

Although treatment of neuropathic pain with tricyclic antidepressants is evidence-based medicine (McQuay et al. 1996; Sindrup 1997), it is unclear how these drugs relieve pain. The first controlled trial of tricyclics in neuropathic pain was conducted in patients with diabetic neuropathy (Turkington 1980). Because all patients had substantial depression and pain relief was paralleled by alleviation of depression, the author suggested that depression was masquerading as painful neuropathy and that pain relief depended on successful treatment of depression. However, in a later study pain was relieved in diabetic neuropathy patients both with and without depression (Max et al. 1987). Further studies on diabetic neuropathy and other neuropathic pain conditions had similar findings (Max et al. 1988, 1991; Kishore-Kumar et al. 1990). Tricyclics also have an analgesic effect in experimental pain in animals (Biegon and Samuel 1980; Isenberg et al. 1984; Reichenberg et al. 1985) and humans (Bromm et al. 1986; Coquoz et al. 1991; Poulsen et al. 1995).

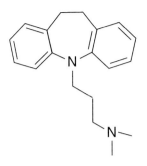

Fig. 1. The chemical structure of the tricyclic anti-depressant imipramine.

The analgesic effect of tricyclic antidepressants can be explained by several pharmacological mechanisms (Sindrup 1997; see Table I). Initially, research focused on their ability to inhibit presynaptic reuptake of norepinephrine and serotonin, but these drugs also act as NMDA-receptor antagonists and apparently block ion channels.

Whereas newer antidepressants have been tried in neuropathic pain, the tricyclics are still the drug class of choice. This chapter will discuss possible mechanisms of action of tricyclics in neuropathic pain conditions, compare

Table I
Tricyclic antidepressants through four decades

Clinical Development	Pharmacological Discoveries
1958 Report of antidepressant effect	
1960 First suggestion of analgesic effect	1960–1980 Presynaptic reuptake inhibition (norepinephrine and serotonin)
1970–1980 Observations of analgesic effect in painful diabetic neuropathy	Postsynaptic receptor blockade (α-adrenergic, cholinergic, histaminergic)
1980 First controlled trial in painful diabetic neuropathy	1980 μ-opioid receptor interaction
1984– Numerous controlled trials in neuropathic pain	
	1988 NMDA-antagonist-like effect
1990– Systematic reviews	1992 Calcium channel blockade
	1998 Sodium channel blockade

the efficacy of these agents with that of other drugs, outline guidelines for their use, and discuss future perspectives.

MECHANISMS OF ACTION

The pharmacological profile of various antidepressants is given in Table II. Several receptor actions and effects on ion channels are potentially analgesic. Inhibition of norepinephrine and serotonin reuptake may enhance the activity of neurons in the network comprising diffuse noxious inhibitory controls (DNIC), and the opioid activity of tricyclics may have the same effect (Fields and Basbaum 1984). The opioid effect is probably less important due to the low affinity of tricyclics for the μ-opioid receptor (Hall and Ögren 1981; Raffa et al. 1993). Reports that tricyclics have an NMDA-antagonist-like effect (Reynolds and Miller 1988; Watanabe et al. 1993; Eisenach and Gebhart 1995) point to a potential mechanism of pain relief because NMDA antagonists can relieve neuropathic pain, probably by inhibiting neuronal hyperexcitability (Max et al. 1995; Felsby et al. 1996; Nelson et al. 1997).

In peripheral neuropathy, the α-adrenergic-receptor blockade of the tricyclics may relieve pain generated or maintained by noradrenergic stimulation of highly sensitive receptors, which have been identified on sprouts from diseased peripheral nerves (Sanjue and Jun 1989; Sato and Perl 1991). The antihistaminergic action of the tricyclics may have a general analgesic effect, given reports that antihistamines can relieve pain (Rumore and Schlichting 1986).

Tricyclics change the electrocardiogram in a quinidine-like fashion (Giardina et al. 1979) due to blockade of sodium channels. Recent reports indicate that tricyclics also block sodium channels in neuronal tissue (Deffois et al. 1996; Pancrazio et al. 1998). Therefore, tricyclics may stabilize both diseased peripheral nerves and hyperexcitable neurons of the central nervous system. Blockade of calcium channels may be the mechanism of action of gabapentin, a newer drug in the treatment of neuropathic pain (Backonja et al. 1998; Rowbotham et al. 1998). Only a few studies have reported calcium channel blockade in tricyclics (Lavoie et al 1990, Shimizu et al. 1992).

The selective serotonin reuptake inhibitors (SSRIs) such as paroxetine, citalopram, and fluoxetine and the balanced serotonin-norepinephrine reuptake inhibitors (SNRIs) such as venlafaxine have a limited number of actions that can be linked to analgesic effect (Table II). Within the group of tricyclic antidepressants, some drugs are relatively noradrenergic, while others are balanced with respect to serotonergic and noradrenergic effects (Table II).

Table II
Pharmacodynamic profile of various antidepressants

	Reuptake Inhibition		Receptor Blockade			Opioid Receptor Interaction	Quinidine-like Effect
	Serotonin	Nor-epinephrine	α-Adrenergic†	H1-Histaminergic	Muscarinic Cholinergic		
Classical Tricyclics							
Imipramine	+	+‡	+	+	+	+	+
Clomipramine	+	+‡	+	+	+	+	?
Amitriptyline	+	+‡	+	+	+	+	+
Desipramine	−	+	(+)	(+)	(+)	+	+
Nortriptyline	−	+	+	(+)	+	+	+
Selective Serotonin Reuptake Inhibitors							
Paroxetine	+	−	−	−	(+)	?	−
Citalopram	+	−	−	−	−	?	−
Fluoxetine	+	−	−	−	−	(+)	−
Serotonin-Norepinephrine Reuptake Inhibitors							
Venlafaxine	+	+	−	−	−	?	−
Tetracyclics							
Mianserin	−§	(+)	+	+	−	(+)	−

† α₁- and α₂-adrenergic receptor interaction is not differentiated.
‡ Effect is mainly through metabolites, i.e. desipramine, desmethylclomipramine, and nortriptyline, respectively.
§ Mianserin appears to be antiserotonergic.

Thus, tricyclics have many actions that could be involved in their pain-relieving effect. Their multimodal mechanism of action could explain the superiority of this drug class compared to other agents with a more selective pharmacological effect.

EFFICACY

Randomized controlled trials confirm that tricyclic antidepressants relieve neuropathic pain conditions such as painful polyneuropathy, post-herpetic neuralgia, pain after peripheral nerve injuries, and central post-stroke pain. The literature on antidepressants as analgesics has been reviewed several times within the last decade (Magni 1991; Onghena and van Houdenhove 1992; Max 1994, McQuay et al. 1996; Sindrup 1997) and comprises 17 placebo-controlled trials, with 439 patients on antidepressants in different neuropathic pain conditions.

Taken together, controlled trials of the pain-relieving effect of tricyclics show that 60–70% of patients with neuropathic pain respond to these drugs. The size of the treatment effect can be estimated in a standardized manner by calculating the number needed to treat (NNT) in order to obtain one patient with more than 50% pain relief (NNT ≥ 50%) (Cook and Sackett 1995). The calculation of NNT is based on results from placebo-controlled trials and includes a correction for placebo responders:

$$NNT = \frac{1}{(goal\ achieved_{ACTIVE}/total_{ACTIVE}) - (goal\ achieved_{PLACEBO}/total_{PLACEBO})}$$

This calculation has been made for antidepressants in neuropathic pain by McQuay et al. (1996) and can be elaborated by performing further calculations based on previous and new studies (Sindrup and Jensen 1999).

The NNT for tricyclic antidepressants is very similar across different neuropathic pain conditions, with values of 2–3, which means that every second or third patient with neuropathic pain treated with a tricyclic will experience more than 50% pain relief (Fig. 2). In painful polyneuropathy, tricyclics with a balanced inhibition of norepinephrine and serotonin tend to have a better effect (lower NNT) than do the noradrenergic tricyclics. The difference may be more pronounced than the present data indicate because dosage regimens in some trials may have biased the results. One study shows the same effect for a balanced serotonergic/adrenergic drug (amitriptyline) and a noradrenergic drug (desipramine) (Max et al. 1992). However, the dosages were determined according to effect and side effects, which could have resulted in lower dosages of amitriptyline, the drug with the most

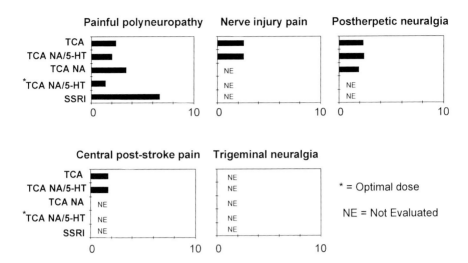

Fig. 2. Number needed to treat (NNT) to obtain one patient with ≥50% pain relief for antidepressants in five neuropathic pain conditions. TCA = tricyclic antidepressants; TCA NA/5-HT = tricyclics with balanced inhibition of norepinephrine and serotonin reuptake (imipramine, amitriptyline, and clomipramine); TCA NA = tricyclics with a relatively selective inhibition of norepinephrine reuptake (desipramine, nortriptyline, and maprotiline); SSRI = selective serotonin reuptake inhibitors (paroxetine, citalopram, and fluoxetine).

pronounced side effects. The interdrug comparison is therefore clinically relevant, but does not necessarily reflect the relative contribution of different pharmacological actions.

The SSRIs, which do not inhibit norepinephrine reuptake and have no postsynaptic effects and weaker ion-channel-blocking effects, clearly are less effective than the tricyclics; their NNT in painful polyneuropathy is about 7. The efficacy of balanced serotonin/norepinephrine reuptake inhibitors without postsynaptic effects has not yet been reported, but studies are in progress on one such drug, venlafaxine, in diabetic neuropathy and painful polyneuropathy in general.

Several studies of tricyclics in different neuropathic pain conditions have found a relationship between serum drug concentration and analgesic effect (Kvinesdal et al. 1984; Max et al. 1987; Leijon and Boivie 1989). In painful polyneuropathy a serum concentration-response relationship has been established for imipramine (Sindrup et al. 1990a). Most patients will have an individual maximal response if serum concentrations of imipramine plus its active metabolite desipramine are over 400 nM (Kvinesdal et al. 1984; Sindrup et al. 1990a). However, some patients have an individual maximal response at much lower concentrations of 100–200 nM. The importance of optimal dosage is supported by the NNT of 1.4 for imipramine in painful polyneuropathy in a study in which doses were adjusted according to serum concentrations (Sindrup et al. 1990b), as compared to the value of 2.4 for the entire group of tricyclics and 2 for the group of balanced noradrenergic/ serotonergic tricyclics.

No studies have tested the effect of antidepressants against that of other drugs used in neuropathic pain. NNT values from different trials can show the effect of antidepressants compared to that of other pharmacological treatments of painful polyneuropathy (Fig. 3). None of the drugs from other classes appear superior to the tricyclics, especially if the balanced noradrenergic/serotonergic tricyclics are used in optimal doses adjusted according to serum concentrations.

Carbamazepine was until recently the most often used alternative drug for neuropathic pain. In the single trial examining this drug in painful polyneuropathy (Rull et al. 1969) it appeared less effective (NNT = 3.3) than tricyclics; with respect to side effects it probably is tolerated no better than the tricyclics. The literature does not specify whether carbamazepine should be preferred in patients with lancinating pains or paroxysms, although this has become routine in clinical practice for many pain specialists. This strategy is indirectly supported by several trials reporting relief of trigeminal neuralgia with carbamazepine; pain relief with antidepressants has not been investigated in this condition.

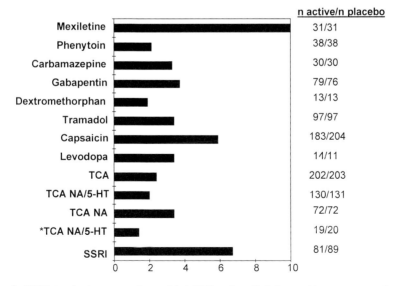

Fig. 3. NNT to obtain one patient with ≥50% pain relief for antidepressants and other drugs in painful polyneuropathy. *n* active/*n* placebo = total numbers of patients in the trials from which NNT was calculated. Abbreviations are as in Fig. 2.

Both the new antiepileptic gabapentin and the new analgesic tramadol relieve painful polyneuropathy quite effectively, with NNT values of 3.7 and 3.4, respectively, in trials with adequate samples (Backonja et al. 1998; Harati et al. 1998; Sindrup et al. 1999). Due to their better tolerability, these drugs may be the best alternative if tricyclics cannot be used due to contra-indications or intolerable side effects, although they seem to be slightly less effective. Tramadol probably relieves pain by a combined opioid and monoaminergic mechanism of action. The effect of pure opioids has not been tested in painful polyneuropathies, but in clinical practice they appear to provide at least some relief. In postherpetic neuralgia, the μ-opioid ago-nists morphine and oxycodone are clearly superior to placebo (Rowbotham et al. 1991; Watson and Babul 1998). However, the NNT for oxycodone is higher than that for tricyclics in this condition, and in Watson and Babul's study, oxycodone was used in combination with tricyclics in some patients.

Mexiletine is clearly less effective than the tricyclics (Oskarsson et al. 1997) and therefore should not be a first-line drug. Single small trials indi-cate that NMDA antagonists (Nelson et al. 1997) and L-dopa (Ertas et al. 1998) may be effective alternatives to tricyclics.

EFFECT OF TRICYCLICS ON ONGOING VERSUS STIMULUS-EVOKED PAIN

Data from several controlled studies indicate that tricyclics are effective for both steady and lancinating or brief pains (Max et al. 1987, 1991, 1992; Sindrup et al. 1990b,c), but it is more difficult to judge whether these drugs also relieve stimulus-evoked pain. An inherent problem with these studies is their failure to address the issue of specific effects on different pain types; they only show general pain relief for patients with different types of pain.

An indication of an effect of tricyclics on stimulus-evoked pain can be deduced from an experimental pain study in humans (Poulsen et al. 1995). Healthy volunteers were given a single oral dose of 100 mg imipramine. The threshold at which subjects experienced pain summation to repetitive (five stimulations at 3 Hz) transcutaneous electric sural nerve stimulation was increased by imipramine but not by placebo (Fig. 4). This effect of imi-pramine was reproduced in a recent study showing that the SSRI paroxetine does not alter the pain summation threshold (Enggaard et al., in press). The neuronal mechanism responsible for temporal pain summation may be simi-lar to the neuronal mechanism involved in some stimulus-evoked pains in neuropathic pain conditions. The effect of tricyclics and other antidepres-sants on stimulus-evoked pains cannot be reliably judged until controlled clinical trials focus on this issue.

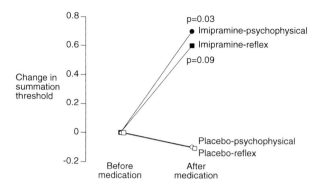

Fig. 4. The threshold at which subjective pain and the flexor reflex show temporal summation on repetitive electric stimulation of the sural nerve in humans before and after placebo and 100 mg imipramine (data from Poulsen et al. 1995).

PHARMACOKINETICS AND DOSAGE

Tricyclic antidepressants undergo hepatic oxidation and glucuronidation before they are excreted via the urine. Several tricyclics, including imipramine, desipramine, amitriptyline, nortriptyline, and clomipramine, are metabolized via the enzyme CYP2D6 (Brøsen and Gram 1989). This enzyme exhibits genetic polymorphism, with 90% of the white population having the enzyme (extensive metabolizers) and 10% lacking it (poor metabolizers) (Alván et al. 1990). This genetic polymorphism is responsible for the pronounced pharmacokinetic variability observed with these drugs. For imipramine,

Fig. 5. The relationship between imipramine (IP) dose and plasma concentration of IP plus its active metabolite desipramine (DMI) in two poor metabolizers (PM) and the range of extensive metabolizers (EM) of sparteine/debrisoquine/dextromethorphan. The suggested therapeutic range for treating neuropathic pain is shown by dashed lines (data from Sindrup et al. 1990d).

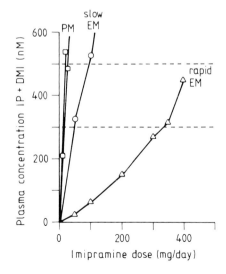

steady-state serum drug levels show a 30-fold variation among individuals on a daily dose of 100 mg (Reisby et al 1977). Another way to illustrate the variability is to look at individual dose-concentration relationships at relevant ranges, as shown in Fig. 5 (Sindrup et al. 1990d). It is clear from these plots that when taking a standard daily dose of 100 mg of imipramine, some individuals (poor metabolizers) will obtain toxic serum drug concentrations (>2000 nM) (Pedersen et al. 1982), while others (rapid extensive metabolizers) will be left at potentially inactive or suboptimal drug levels. For some of the tricyclics, the response variability is less pronounced. The metabolism of clomipramine exhibits saturation kinetics, and so the variability is diminished at steady state at medium or higher doses.

The SSRIs also exhibit pharmacokinetic variability; the metabolism of most drugs of this class partially depends on CYP2D6 (Brøsen 1993). The concentration-response relation for these generally nontoxic drugs is less clear.

It is unnecessary to dose every patient to drug levels of 400 nM of imipramine or 300 nM of amitriptyline, because some will have a completely satisfactory response on lower concentrations. Measurements of serum drug concentrations are advisable, mainly to avoid toxicity. Drug levels around 2000 nM, only five times higher than the therapeutic concentration for imipramine, are assumed to be toxic. It is impossible to know whether a poor response is due to inadequate dosing or to the fact that that the patient is a

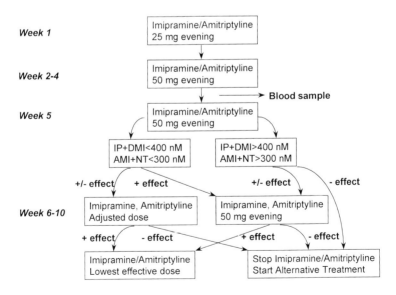

Fig. 6. Guidelines for use of tricyclic antidepressants in neuropathic pain. AMI = amitriptyline; DMI = desipramine; IP = imipramine; NT = nortriptyline.

non-responder (the response rate is 60–70%). In some cases the response can be enhanced by increasing the dose. Drug monitoring is recommended when using tricyclics for neuropathic pain, but it is unnecessary for the much less effective SSRIs.

GUIDELINES

Before treating neuropathic pain with a tricyclic antidepressant, clinicians must rule out important contraindications such as cardiac conduction disturbances (e.g., atrioventricular block), congestive heart failure, and convulsive disorders. Symptoms and signs of orthostatic phenomena are considered to be a relative contraindication. With no contraindications, patients can start a treatment regimen as detailed in Fig. 6. In cases with severe pain, the dose adjustment can be expedited to achieve an adequate effect faster and allow the clinician to decide whether to try alternative treatments in case of lack of effect or side effects.

When contraindications against tricyclics are present, the analgesic response is inadequate, or side effects are intolerable, the treatment regimen detailed in Fig. 7 is recommended. The sequence in which treatments such as gabapentin, tramadol, and SSRIs are tried is a matter of clinician preference.

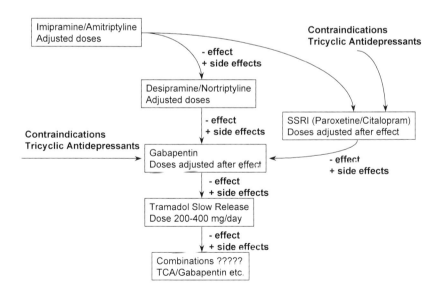

Fig. 7. Guidelines for use of alternative tricyclic antidepressants, other antidepressants, and other drug classes in neuropathic pain. SSRI = selective serotonin reuptake inhibitors; TCA = tricyclic antidepressants.

When the first-line tricyclic antidepressants are ineffective, it may be worth trying another antidepressant because patients in some trials respond better to the more selective compounds than to those with a broader spectrum of actions (Sindrup et al. 1990b; Watson et al. 1992; Vrethem et al. 1997).

PERSPECTIVES

The multiple pharmacological actions of tricyclics may be the key point of their efficacy in neuropathic pain, which may involve many different pain mechanisms for each patient. Therefore, in the search for new drugs for neuropathic pain, it may be wise to look for drugs with multiple actions or combinations of drugs, instead of focusing on agents with a selective pharmacological profile.

Tricyclic antidepressants are the standard against which to compare potential new treatments of neuropathic pain. Studies should incorporate both a placebo as an inactive control and a tricyclic as an active control, or NNT values for the new treatment should be compared with those for the tricyclics. Trials on tricyclics and other drugs in neuropathic pain should study their effect on specific pain phenomena to determine how to individualize each patient's pharmacological treatment.

The preemptive use of tricyclics to avoid the development of chronic pain conditions is an interesting new research direction. A controlled trial showed that low-dose amitriptyline during the acute phase of herpes zoster may reduce the risk of developing postherpetic neuralgia (Bowsher et al. 1997).

CONCLUSIONS

Firm evidence shows that tricyclic antidepressants relieve neuropathic pain. Across different neuropathic pain conditions, two to three patients must be treated for one to obtain more than 50% pain relief. The SSRIs, tested only in painful polyneuropathies, are much weaker than the tricyclics. The tricyclics probably act on many of the different pain phenomena experienced by patients with neuropathic pain, but because of the lack of detailed studies we do not know whether tricyclics relieve both ongoing and stimulus-evoked pain. Tricyclics should be considered the first choice in treatment of neuropathic pain, excluding the classical neuralgia of the face, oral cavity, and pharynx, because none of the other available and tested treatments is more effective or better documented.

REFERENCES

Alván G, Bechtel P, Iselius L, Gundert-Remy U. Hydroxylation polymorphisms of debrisoquine and mephenytoin in European populations. *Eur J Clin Pharmacol* 1990; 39:533–537.

Backonja M, Beydoun A, Edwards KR, et al. Gabapentin Diabetic Neuropathy Study Group. Gabapentin for the symptomatic treatment of painful neuropathy in patients with diabetes mellitus. *JAMA* 1998; 280:1831–1836.

Biegon A, Samuel D. Interaction of tricyclic antidepressants with opiate receptors. *Biochem Pharmacol* 1980; 29:460–462.

Bowsher D. The effects of pre-emptive treatment of postherpetic neuralgia with amitriptyline: a randomized, double-blind, placebo-controlled trial. *J Pain Symptom Manage* 1997; 13:327–331.

Bromm B, Meier W, Scharein E. Imipramine reduces experimental pain. *Pain* 1986; 25:245–257.

Brøsen K. The pharmacokinetics of the selective serotonin reuptake inhibitors. *Clin Invest* 1993; 71:1002–1009.

Brøsen K, Gram LF. Clinical significance of the sparteine/debrisoquine oxidation polymorphism. *Eur J Clin Pharmacol* 1989; 36:537–547.

Cook RJ, Sackett DL. The number needed to treat: a clinically useful measure of treatment effect. *BMJ* 1995; 310:452–454.

Coquoz D, Porchet HC, Dayer P. Effet analgésique central d'antidépresseurs à mode d'action distinct: désipramine, fluvoxamine et moclobémide. *Schweiz Med Wochenschr* 1991; 121:1843–1845.

Deffois A, Fage D, Carter C. Inhibition of synaptosomal veratridine-induced sodium influx by antidepressants and neuroleptics used in chronic pain. *Neurosci Lett* 1996; 220:117–120.

Eisenach JC, Gebhart GF. Intrathecal amitriptyline acts as an N-methyl-D-aspartate antagonist in the presence of inflammatory hyperalgesia in rats. *Anesthesiology* 1995; 83:1046–1054.

Enggaard T, Poulsen L, Arendt-Nielsen L, Gram LF, Sindrup SH. Paroxetine compared to imipramine and placebo in human experimental pain models. *Analgesia;* in press.

Ertas M, Sagduyu A, Arac N, Uludag B, Ertekin C. Use of levodopa to relieve pain from painful symmetrical diabetic polyneuropathy. *Pain* 1998; 75:257–259.

Felsby S, Nielsen J, Arendt-Nielsen L, Jensen TS. NMDA receptor blockade in chronic neuropathic pain: a comparison of ketamine and magnesium chloride. *Pain* 1996; 64:283–291.

Fields HL, Basbaum AI. Endogenous pain control mechanisms. In: Wall PD, Melzack R (Eds). *Textbook of Pain.* London: Churchill Livingstone, 1984, pp 142–152.

Giardina E-GV, Bigger JT, Glassman AH, Perel JM, Kantor SJ. The electrocardiographic and antiarrhythmic effects of imipramine hydrochloride at therapeutic plasma concentrations. *Circulation* 1979; 60:1045–1052.

Hall H, Ögren S-O. Effects of antidepressant drugs on different receptors in the brain. *Eur J Pharmacol* 1981; 70:393–407.

Harati Y, Gooch C, Swenson M, Edelman S, et al. Double-blind randomized trial of tramadol for the treatment of pain of diabetic neuropathy. *Neurology* 1998; 50:1842–1846.

Isenberg KE, Cicero TJ. Possible involvement of opiate receptors in the pharmacological profiles of antidepressant compounds. *Eur J Pharmacol* 1984; 103:57–63.

Kishore-Kumar R, Max MB, Schafer SC, et al. Desipramine relieves postherpetic neuralgia. *Clin Pharmacol Ther* 1990; 47:305–312.

Kuhn R. Treatment of depressive states with imipramine hydrochloride. *Am J Psychiatry* 1958; 115:459–464.

Kvinesdal B, Molin J, Frøland A, Gram LF. Imipramine treatment of painful diabetic neuropathy. *JAMA* 1984; 251:1727–1730.

Lavoie PA, Beauchamp G, Elie R. Tricyclic antidepressants inhibit voltage-dependent calcium channels and Na^+-Ca^{2+} exchange in rat brain synaptosomes. *Can J Physiol Pharmacol* 1990; 68:1414–1418.

Leijon G, Boivie J. Central post-stroke pain—a controlled trial of amitriptyline and carbamazepine. *Pain* 1989; 36:27–36.

Magni G. The use of antidepressants in the treatment of chronic pain. *Drugs* 1991; 42:730–748.

Max MB. Antidepressants as analgesics. In: Fields HL, Liebeskind JC (Eds). *Pharmacological Approaches to the Treatment of Chronic Pain: New Concepts and Critical Issues*, Progress in Pain Research and Management, Vol. 1. Seattle: IASP Press, 1994, pp 229–246.

Max MB, Culnane M, Schafer SC, et al. Amitriptyline relieves diabetic neuropathy pain in patients with normal or depressed mood. *Neurology* 1987; 37:589–596.

Max MB, Schafer SC, Culnane M, et al. Amitriptyline, but not lorazepam, relieves postherpetic neuralgia. *Neurology* 1988; 38:1427–1432.

Max MB, Kishore-Kumar R, Schafer SC, et al. Efficacy of desipramine in painful diabetic neuropathy: a placebo-controlled trial. *Pain* 1991; 45:3–9.

Max MB, Lynch SA, Muir J, et al. Effects of desipramine, amitriptyline, and fluoxetine on pain in diabetic neuropathy. *N Engl J Med* 1992; 326:1250–1256.

Max MB, Byas-Smith MG, Gracely RH, Bennett GJ. Intravenous infusion of the NMDA antagonist, ketamine, in chronic posttraumatic pain and allodynia: a double-blind comparison to alfentanil and placebo. *Clin Neuropharmacol* 1995; 18:360–368.

McQuay HJ, Tramér M, Nye BA, et al. A systematic review of antidepressants in neuropathic pain. *Pain* 1996; 68:217–227.

Nelson KA, Park KM, Robinovitz E, Tsigos C, Max MB. High-dose oral dextromethorphan versus placebo in painful diabetic neuropathy and postherpetic neuralgia. *Neurology* 1997; 48:1212–1218.

Onghena P, van Houdenhove B. Antidepressant-induced analgesia in chronic non-malignant pain: a meta analysis of 39 placebo-controlled studies. *Pain* 1992; 49:205–220.

Oskarsson P, Lins P-E, Ljunggren J-G, and the Mexiletine Study Group. Efficacy and safety of mexiletine in the treatment of painful diabetic neuropathy. *Diabetes Care* 1997; 20:1594–1597.

Pancrazio JJ, Kamatchi GL, Roscoe AK, Lynch C. Inhibition of neuronal Na$^+$ channels by antidepressant drugs. *J Pharmacol Exp Ther* 1998; 284:208–214.

Paoli F, Darcourt G, Corsa P. Note préliminaire sur l'action de l'imipramine dans les états douloureux. *Rev Neurol* 1960; 2:503–504.

Pedersen OL, Gram LF, Kristensen CB, et al. Overdosage of antidepressants: clinical and pharmacokinetic aspects. *Eur J Clin Pharmacol* 1982; 23:513–521.

Poulsen L, Arendt-Nielsen L, Brøsen K, Gram LF, Sindrup SH. The hypoalgesic effect of imipramine in different human experimental pain models. *Pain* 1995; 60:287–293.

Raffa RB, Friderichs E, Reimann W, et al. Complementary and synergistic interaction between enantiomers of tramadol. *J Pharmacol Exp Ther* 1993; 267:331–340.

Reichenberg K, Gaillard-Plaza G, Montastruc JL. Influence of naloxone on the antinociceptive effects of some antidepressant drugs. *Arch Int Pharmacodyn* 1985; 275:78–85.

Reisby N, Gram LF, Bech P, et al. Imipramine: clinical effects and pharmacokinetic variability. *Psychopharmacology* 1977; 54:263–272.

Reynolds IJ, Miller RJ. Tricyclic antidepressants block *N*-methyl-D-aspartate receptors: similarities to the action of zinc. *Br J Pharmacol* 1988; 95:95–102.

Rowbotham M, Reisner-Keller LA, Fields HL. Both intravenous lidocaine and morphine reduce pain of postherpetic neuralgia. *Neurology* 1991; 41:1024–1028.

Rowbotham M, Harden N, Stacey B, Bernstein P, Magnus-Miller L. Gabapentin Postherpetic Neuralgia Study Group. Gabapentin treatment of postherpetic neuralgia. *JAMA* 1998; 280:1837–1842.

Rull JA, Quibrera R, González-Millán H, Castañeda OL. Symptomatic treatment of peripheral diabetic neuropathy with carbamazepine (Tegretolâ): double blind crossover trial. *Diabetologia* 1969; 5:215–218.

Rumore MM, Schlichting DA. Clinical efficacy of antihistaminics as analgesics. *Pain* 1986; 25:7–22.

Sanjue H, Jun Z. Sympathetic facilitation of sustained discharges of polymodal nociceptors. *Pain* 1989; 38:85–90.

Sato J, Perl ER. Adrenergic excitation of cutaneous pain receptors induced by peripheral nerve injury. *Science* 1991; 251:1608–1611.

Shimizu M, Nishida A, Yamawaki S. Antidepressants inhibit spontaneous oscillations of intracellular Ca^{2+} concentration in rat cortical cultured neurons. *Neurosci Lett* 1992; 146:101–104.

Sindrup SH. Antidepressants as analgesics. In: Yaksh TL, Lynch C, Zapol WM, et al. (Eds). *Anesthesia: Biological Foundations.* Philadelphia: Lippincott-Raven, 1997, pp 987–997.

Sindrup SH, Jensen TS. Efficacy of pharmacological treatments of neuropathic pain: an update and effect related to mechanism of drug action. *Pain* 1999; 83:389–400.

Sindrup SH, Gram LF, Skjold T, Frøland A, Beck-Nielsen H. Concentration-response relationship in imipramine treatment of diabetic neuropathy symptoms. *Clin Pharmacol Ther* 1990a; 47:509–515.

Sindrup SH, Gram LF, Brøsen K, Eshøj O, Mogense EF. The selective serotonin reuptake inhibitor paroxetine is effective in the treatment of diabetic neuropathy symptoms. *Pain* 1990b; 42:135–144.

Sindrup SH, Gram LF, Skjold T, et al. Clomipramine vs desipramine vs placebo in the treatment of diabetic neuropathy symptoms: a double-blind cross-over study. *Br J Clin Pharmacol* 1990c; 30:683–691.

Sindrup SH, Brøsen K, Gram LF. Nonlinear kinetics of imipramine in low and medium plasma level ranges. *Ther Drug Monit* 1990d; 12:445–449.

Sindrup SH, Andersen G, Madsen C, et al. Tramadol relieves pain and allodynia in polyneuropathy. *Pain* 1999; 83:85–90.

Turkington RW. Depression masquerading as diabetic neuropathy. *JAMA* 1980; 243:1147–1150.

Vrethem M, Boivie J, Arnqvist H, et al. A comparison of amitriptyline and maprotiline in the treatment of painful polyneuropathy in diabetics and nondiabetics. *Clin J Pain* 1997; 13:313–323.

Watanabe Y, Saito H, Abe K. Tricyclic antidepressants block NMDA receptor-mediated synaptic responses and induction of long-term potentiation in rat hippocampal slices. *Neuropharmacology* 1993; 32:479–486.

Watson CPN, Babul N. Efficacy of oxycodone in neuropathic pain: a randomized trial in postherpetic neuralgia. *Neurology* 1998; 50:1837–1841.

Watson CPN, Chipman M, Reed K, Evans RJ, Birkett N. Amitriptyline versus maprotiline in postherpetic neuralgia: a randomized, double-blind, crossover trial. *Pain* 1992; 48:29–36.

Correspondence to: Søren H. Sindrup, MD, Department of Neurology, Odense University Hospital, DK-5000 Odense C, Denmark. Tel: 45-6541-2472; Fax: 45-6541-3389.

Neuropathic Pain: Pathophysiology and Treatment,
Progress in Pain Research and Management, Vol. 21,
edited by Per T. Hansson, Howard L. Fields, Raymond G.
Hill, and Paolo Marchettini, IASP Press, Seattle, © 2001.

10

Anticonvulsants and Antiarrhythmics in the Treatment of Neuropathic Pain Syndromes

Miroslav Backonja

*Department of Neurology, University of Wisconsin,
Madison, Wisconsin, USA*

Advances in the neuroscience of pain over the past two decades have revealed diverse pathophysiological processes involved in the genesis and maintenance of neuropathic pain. The involvement of many receptors and neurotransmitter systems offers an opportunity, at least on the conceptual level, to alleviate and even reverse the manifestations of neuropathic pain, or to prevent their development.

Although certain forms of neuropathic pain were recognized and described centuries ago (Mitchell 1864; Rey 1993), it was only in the later part of the 20th century that researchers began to apply the methods of modern neuroscience to the study of neuropathic pain. More than three and a half decades ago, even before peripheral and central sensitization had been defined in detail, the first controlled clinical trials with the anticonvulsant carbamazepine established its efficacy in relieving the pain of trigeminal neuralgia and diabetic neuropathy.

The next major therapeutic advance was the introduction of the newer anticonvulsants into clinical practice, with their wide range of pharmacological effects on various ion channels and neurotransmitters and their safer side effect profiles. Most anticonvulsants submitted recently to clinical trials have significantly alleviated the symptoms of neuropathic pain. In addition to these controlled trials, the literature includes many reports of open-label and retrospective studies, as well as abstracts of controlled randomized trials that describe positive results in treating neuropathic pain. This level of evidence is important as a guide for the design of randomized trials, but this chapter does not discuss anecdotal reports as they are reviewed elsewhere

(Tremont-Lukats et al. 2001). Systemic local anesthetics also have been used to treat neuropathic pain. Because they act primarily as sodium channel blockers and thus have a mechanism of action common to a few anticonvulsants, they are included in this discussion.

This chapter provides an evidence-based summary of randomized clinical trials published in peer-reviewed journals regarding the efficacy of anticonvulsants and systemic local anesthetics (frequently referred to as antiarrhythmics) in the treatment of neuropathic pain, based in part on three evidence-based reviews on the use of anticonvulsants for neuropathic pain (Kingery 1997; Sindrup and Jensen 1999; Wiffen et al. 2000). This chapter provides recommendations for using these agents to treat neuropathic pain disorders, following an overview of basic pathophysiological mechanisms that form the conceptual grounds for their use.

SIGNIFICANCE FOR THERAPY OF THE COMPLEXITY OF CHRONIC NEUROPATHIC PAIN

The clinical manifestation of neuropathic pain is very similar across most of the chronic neuropathic pain syndromes, regardless of the underlying etiological causes, which suggests that they share similar pathophysiological mechanisms. Neuropathic pain presents with a complex of symptoms, ranging from complete lack of sensation to severe hypersensitivity, and in most cases accompanied by ongoing pain. Lack of sensitivity or sensation is most commonly interpreted by patients as numbness. Extreme hypersensitivity to even the most innocuous stimulus, such as a slight movement, can be very disabling. Most puzzling to both patients and clinicians is the common simultaneous occurrence of symptoms from both ends of the spectrum, with wide variability in the range and severity of symptoms (Backonja and Galer 1998). This complexity has made neuropathic pain difficult to study, although progress was greatly facilitated by the development of animal models mimicking many aspects of human neuropathic pain (Bennett and Xie 1988; Chung et al. 1993).

Diseases affecting the peripheral nervous system create histological changes consisting of axonal loss and/or demyelination. A cascade of biochemical inflammatory and reparatory processes follows neuronal injury, as the injured neurons and surrounding tissues release glutamate, serotonin, epinephrine, adenosine, prostaglandins, bradykinin, and substance P as well as cytokines and neurotrophic growth factors (NGFs). Many receptors are activated on the neurons, including vanilloid receptors, receptors responding to protons (mDEG) (Bassilana et al. 1997), and many others that participate in inflammatory and reparatory processes. Novel channels also are expressed, such as TTX-resistant, sensory-neuron-specific PN3 sodium ion channels (Rabert et al. 1998; Cummins et al. 1999; Dib-Hajj et al. 1999).

Extensive animal studies have investigated the processes resulting from nociceptor activation that take place at the dorsal horn level. The initial release of glutamate from primary afferents is followed by activation of AMPA (α-amino-3-hydroxy-5-methyl-4-isoxazoleproprianic acid) receptors, and with continued release of glutamate from hyperexcited nociceptive primary afferents, as in the case of prolonged and severe pain, NMDA (*N*-methyl-D-aspartate) receptors are activated. Processes at the central terminals are further modulated and modified by the release of substance P and brain-derived neurotrophic factor (BDNF) from the primary afferents (Woolf and Salter 2000). Activated NMDA receptors lead to influx of calcium and activation of second messengers, nitric oxide (NO) systems, and phosphokinase (PK) systems, all of which are important steps in the intracellular transduction cascade. This cascade leads to protein phosphorylation, which alters the functional properties of nociceptive neurons. Consequences of persistent injury discharges from primary afferents include the phenotypic switch of Aβ fibers (Neumann et al. 1996), expansion of receptive fields (Mao et al. 1992), facilitatory modulation by locally released dynorphin and by cholecystokinin released from descending systems (Ossipov et al. 2000), and loss of inhibition (Fukuoka et al. 1998; Woolf and Salter 2000). These phenomena characterize the prolonged changes in synaptic nociceptive transmission due to nerve injury. The relationship of each of these processes to one another and in particular their relationship to clinical neuropathic pain conditions is far from clear. To solve the puzzle of pain it would be necessary to determine the hierarchy of these processes in generating and maintaining chronic neuropathic pain.

A further important step in improving pain diagnosis and therapy would be to translate the advances made at the basic science level to clinical practice and thus improve clinical management of chronic pain. Pathophysiological phenomena may be correlated with certain clinical findings. Examples include warm allodynia and heat hyperalgesia, which presumably result from peripheral sensitization of C fibers (Cline et al. 1989); dynamic mechanical allodynia, which is probably a result of NMDA-mediated synaptic activity and a phenotypic switch of Aβ fibers (Neumann et al. 1996); and exaggeration of pain with repeated stimuli, which is probably a wind-up-like phenomenon mediated by NMDA-receptor activity.

The complexity of the peripheral and central sensitization processes that underlie neuropathic pain makes it unlikely that an agent with a single mode of activity would reverse these processes and alleviate and resolve the pain, unless there is a crucial first step in a cascade of events that could be reversed. Patients with neuropathic pain generally require treatment with combinations of medications with varying modes of action that have effects on several different mechanisms. Such use of a combination of medications administered in a systematic way is termed rational polypharmacy. Only if and when a single process is discovered that controls the processes of peripheral and central sensitization, can a single agent be therapeutic and even curative.

ANTICONVULSANTS STUDIED IN RANDOMIZED CLINICAL TRIALS

The current pharmacopeia of anticonvulsants is relatively large, but the number of randomized trials for relief of pain is still very limited (Table I). Only carbamazepine, phenytoin, gabapentin, and lamotrigine have been studied in randomized clinical trials for relief of pain in neuropathic pain disorders. Thus far all of the studies with carbamazepine and gabapentin have been positive, but in the case of lamotrigine and phenytoin, results have been conflicting.

CARBAMAZEPINE

Carbamazepine was the first anticonvulsant used successfully in clinical trials to treat a neuropathic pain disorder. This iminostilbene derivative is chemically related to the tricyclic antidepressants. Its analgesic effect is probably due to both central and peripheral activity. Its ability to block ionic conductance appears to be frequency dependent, by suppressing spontaneous $A\delta$ and C-fiber activity (White 1999) without affecting normal nerve conduction.

Eleven randomized clinical trials have studied the use of carbamazepine to control neuropathic pain. All were double-blind, placebo-controlled, or comparator-controlled crossover trials. Three trials focused on trigeminal neuralgia (TN) (Campbell et al. 1966; Rockliff and Davis 1966; Nicol 1969), and one trial, in which carbamazepine was studied against placebo, included various neuralgias in addition to TN (Killian and Fromm 1968). Response rates for carbamazepine in these studies ranged from 70% to 89% after 5–14 days of treatment. The results are difficult to interpret because their methodology reflects the standard at the time they were conducted and reported: There was no washout period to prevent carry-over effects (Campbell et al. 1966; Rockliff and Davis 1966), concurrent interventions such as phenytoin or nerve blocks were continued, and reports about statistical analysis were lacking (Killian and Fromm 1968; Nicol 1969). Moreover, frequent side effects such as drowsiness, dizziness, ataxia, nausea, and vomiting were common to all these studies and may have unblinded the patients. Such limitations make it difficult to determine whether the data from these trials represent a specific and significant therapeutic effect of carbamazepine.

Only one randomized trial evaluated carbamazepine versus placebo in the treatment of painful diabetic neuropathy (PDN) using a double-blind crossover method (Rull et al. 1969). In this trial carbamazepine provided symptomatic relief of pain and paresthesias in 28 out of 30 patients after 2 weeks of therapy. Carry-over effects occurred during placebo administration.

Four double-blind trials have compared carbamazepine to active controls (Vilming et al. 1986; Lindstrom and Lindblom 1987; Lechin al. 1989; Gómez-Pérez et al. 1996). Carbamazepine was superior to tizanidine, an α_2-adrenergic agonist, in a small TN trial of 3 weeks' duration that included 12 patients (Vilming et al. 1986). Carbamazepine produced similar pain relief to tocainide, an antiarrhythmic agent, in a 4-week crossover study with the same number of TN patients (Lindstrom and Lindblom 1987). Carbamazepine was significantly less effective than pimozide, an antipsychotic agent, in relieving the pain of TN, but pimozide had a high frequency (83%) of adverse effects (Lechin et al. 1989). When carbamazepine was compared with a combination of nortriptyline (a tricyclic antidepressant) and fluphenazine (a neuroleptic drug), there were significant improvements from baseline with both therapies for PDN patients (Gómez-Pérez et al. 1996). Both treatments were equally effective, but side effects were more frequent with the nortriptyline-fluphenazine combination.

In one study, central post-stroke pain was partially relieved with carbamazepine in a number of patients, but the results were not statistically significant (Leijon and Boivie 1989), while for the same number of patients, amitriptyline provided statistically significant pain relief.

In summary, carbamazepine has an established efficacy in the treatment of neuropathic pain for patients with TN (Killian and Fromm 1968; Nicol 1969). The number of patients that needed to be treated in order for one patient to obtain at least 50% pain relief (NNT) was 2.6, with a range of 2.2–3.3. Carbamazepine also demonstrated efficacy in relieving the pain of patients with PDN, with an NNT of 3.3 (range 2–9.4) (Wilton 1974; Gómez-Pérez et al. 1996). Doses used in these studies ranged from 300 to 2400 mg per day in divided doses. The patient withdrawal rate due to adverse effects ranged from 0% to 11%, and up to 50% of patients experienced tolerable side effects, including somnolence, dizziness, and gait disturbance. In earlier studies hematological issues were a concern, and it is still advisable to monitor this possible complication of carbamazepine therapy.

Table I

Completed and fully published randomized trials of anticonvulsant drugs for neuropathic pain

Reference	Pain Disorder	n	Design	Dosage; Duration of Treatment	Results	Withdrawals and Adverse Effects
Carbamazepine						
Campbell et al. 1966	TN	77	CO	400–1200 mg/day; 2 weeks	CBZ > placebo	7 patients withdrew, 50% on CBZ had one or more AEs
Rockliff and Davis 1966	TN	9	CO	200 mg/day; 3 days	CBZ > placebo	No evaluable data
Killian and Fromm 1968	Various neuralgias	42	CO	400–1000 mg/day; 5 days	CBZ > placebo for TN only	3 patients withdrew, 23/36 had AEs
Rull et al. 1969	DN	30	CO	200–600 mg/day; 2 weeks	CBZ > placebo	3 patients withdrew, 16/30 had sonmolence, 12/30 dizziness
Nicol 1969	TN	54	Partial CO	100–2400 mg/day; duration not stated, follow-up up to 46 months	CBZ > placebo	2/37 patients withdrew, 4/37 died from other causes
Wilton 1974	DN	40	CO	600 mg/day; 1 week	CBZ > placebo	No withdrawals
Vilming et al. 1986	TN	12	P, AC	900 mg/day vs. tizanidine 3–6 mg/day; 3 weeks	CBZ > tizanidine	CBZ no withdrawals, tizanidine 3 withdrawals
Lindstrom and Lindblom 1987	TN	12	CO, MTD, AC	CBZ ~20 mg/kg/day, tocainide 20 mg/day; 2 weeks	CBZ = tocainide > placebo	1/10 patients on tocainide withdrew (rash)
Lechin et al. 1989	TN	59	CO, MTD, AC	CBZ 300–1200, pimozide 4–12 mg/day; 24 weeks	Pimozide > CBZ	40/48 patients had AEs on pimozide and 21/48 on CBZ
Leijon and Boivie 1989	Central PSP	15	CO, AC	CBZ 800 mg/day, amitriptyline 75 mg/day; 4 weeks	CBZ = placebo	1 patient withdrew
Gómez-Pérez et al. 1996	DN	16	CO, AC	CBZ 300–600 mg/day, nortriptyline 30–60 mg/day, fluphenazine 1.5–3.0 mg/day; 4 weeks	CBZ = nortriptyline = fluphenazine	2 withdrawals; 3/16 patients on CBZ and 8/16 on nortriptyline and fluphenazine had AEs

Phenytoin

Study	Condition	N	Design	Dose; Duration	Result	Adverse effects
Saudek et al. 1977	DN	30	PC, CO	300 mg/day; 23 weeks	PHN = placebo	10% had giddiness
Chadda and Mathur 1978	DN	40	PC, CO	300 mg/day; 2 weeks	PHN > placebo	4/38 patients reported giddiness; 2 dropouts

Gabapentin

Study	Condition	N	Design	Dose; Duration	Result	Adverse effects
Backonja et al. 1998	DN	165	PC, P, MC	Up to 3600 mg/day; 8 weeks	GBP > placebo	No difference in withdrawal rate between GBP and placebo; dizziness (23.8%), somnolence (22.6%)
Rowbotham et al. 1998	PHN	229	PC, P, MC	Up to 3600 mg/day; 8 weeks	GBP > placebo	Higher withdrawal rate for GBP (13.3%) vs. placebo (9.5%); somnolence (27.6%), dizziness (23.9%), peripheral edema (9.7%)
Morello et al. 1999	DN	25	DB, AC, CO	GBP 900–1800 mg/day, amitriptyline 25–75 mg/day; 6 weeks	GBP = amitriptyline	Sedation

Lamotrigine

Study	Condition	N	Design	Dose; Duration	Result	Adverse effects
Zakrzewska et al. 1997	Refractory TN	14	PC, CO	Up to 400 mg/day; 14 days	LTG > placebo	7/13 patients reported dizziness, constipation, nausea, somnolence, diplopia
Simpson et al. 2000	HIV neuropathy	42	MC, PC	Up to 300 mg/day; 14 weeks	LTG > placebo	5 patients had skin rash; high dropout rate (13/42)
Vestergaard et al. 2001	PSP	27	PC, CO	200 mg/day; 8 weeks	LTG > placebo	Skin, gastrointestinal symptoms

Abbreviations: AC = active comparator; CBZ = carbamazepine; CO = crossover; DB = double-blind; DN = diabetic neuropathy; GBP = gabapentin; HIV = human immunodeficiency virus; LTG = lamotrigine; MC = multicenter; MTD = maximum tolerated dose; P = parallel; PC = placebo-controlled; PB = placebo; PHN = postherpetic neuralgia; PHT = phenytoin; PSP = poststroke pain; TN = trigeminal neuralgia.

In contrast to the positive results obtained from randomized trials, clinical practice experience has been disappointing when carbamazepine has been used to relieve neuropathic pains other than TN. Carbamazepine is difficult to titrate, is associated with many side effects, interacts with many other drugs metabolized in the liver, and ultimately provides less than desirable pain relief for most patients. This is a good example of the discrepancy between scientific research and clinical experience.

GABAPENTIN

Clinical trials with gabapentin have set a new standard for studies in neuropathic pain. A thorough and systematic approach with a large number of patients and a parallel design has yielded positive results for this drug. A parallel design provides less uncertainty related to carry-over effects, which could be seen in a crossover type of design. Developed as a structural GABA analogue, gabapentin has no direct GABAergic action, nor does it affect GABA uptake or metabolism. Preliminary evidence points to the possible effect of gabapentin on $\alpha_2\delta$ type of Ca^{2+} channels (Taylor et al. 1998).

Two large randomized clinical trials established the efficacy of gabapentin for relief from neuropathic pain, one in patients with painful diabetic neuropathy (PDN; Backonja et al. 1998) and the other in patients with postherpetic neuralgia (PHN; Rowbotham et al. 1998). Both studies used a placebo-controlled parallel design with a large number of patients. Analysis was based on the intent-to-treat method. In our PDN study, which included 165 patients, up to 80% of patients were able to increase consumption from 900 mg to 3600 mg per day, in three divided doses, over 2 weeks. Pain relief was observed during the second week after the dose reached 1800 mg per day and was maintained after further dose increase and for the duration of the study (8 weeks). The PHN study by Rowbotham et al., with 229 patients, documented almost identical results. The comprehensive design of these studies allowed the investigators to assess other symptoms frequently associated with chronic severe pain. Not only was pain relieved, but patients also had better sleep and mood and improvement in their quality of life (Rowbotham et al. 1998; Vinik et al. 1998).

Morello et al. (1999) compared the analgesic efficacy of gabapentin with that of amitriptyline for peripheral diabetic neuropathy pain. In this double-blind randomized crossover trial, 21 of 25 patients enrolled completed 13 weeks of treatment that included a 1-week washout period between two 6-week treatment periods. There was no significant difference in analgesic efficacy between gabapentin, in doses of 900–1800 mg per day, and amitriptyline, in doses of 25–75 mg per day. Side effects were similar, except that six patients on amitriptyline gained weight, compared to none on gabapentin.

In summary, gabapentin has demonstrated its efficacy in relieving pain and associated symptoms for patients with PDN and PHN, with an NNT of 3.8 (2.4–8.7) for PDN and 3.2 (2.4–5.0) for PHN. Doses ranged from 900 mg to 3600 mg per day in three divided doses. Gabapentin was well tolerated and showed no significant difference from placebo regarding adverse effects in patients with PDN, while patients with PHN had a slightly higher rate of withdrawal due to adverse effects than with placebo (13.3% vs. 9.5% of patients, respectively). Dizziness and somnolence were the most frequent adverse effects, but were well tolerated. With easy tolerability, no significant interaction with other medications, and a safe side-effect profile, gabapentin could provide pain relief for patients with other types of neuropathic pain. This drug should therefore be studied in other painful neuropathic disorders such as central pain syndromes secondary to cerebrovascular disease, spinal cord injury, and phantom limb pain.

LAMOTRIGINE

Lamotrigine, a phenyltriazine derivative, is one of the newer antiepileptic agents, initially approved in the United States as an adjunct therapy for partial complex seizures. This drug blocks voltage-dependent Na^+ channels and inhibits glutamate release (McNamara 1996).

A clinical trial comparing lamotrigine with placebo in TN clearly showed greater benefit with lamotrigine (Zakrzewska et al. 1997). Another clinical trial with a small number of human immunodeficiency virus (HIV)-1-positive patients with painful sensory neuropathy showed that lamotrigine was more effective than placebo at reducing pain intensity, although the high withdrawal rate limited the reliability of the results (Simpson et al. 2000). A more recent randomized trial showed that 44% of central post-stroke pain patients responded favorably to 200 mg of lamotrigine per day (Vestergaard et al. 2001). A significant effect was observed in secondary outcomes such as physical pain and hypersensitivity to cold from a drop of acetone. In contrast to these positive results, a study with lamotrigine at doses up to 200 mg/day given to 100 patients with various neuropathic pain conditions in a randomized, double-blind, placebo-controlled fashion for 8 weeks showed that lamotrigine was no better than placebo (McCleane 1999a).

In summary, doses of 50–400 mg per day of lamotrigine have demonstrated efficacy in relieving pain in patients with TN refractory to other treatments, with an NNT of 2.1 (range 1.3–6.1), and the drug is beneficial for HIV neuropathy and central post-stroke pain. Adverse effects are common, including dizziness, ataxia, constipation, nausea, somnolence, and diplopia, and could be a significant limiting factor, as was revealed in the HIV neuropathy study. Another serious side effect is rash, which in rare instances can progress into Stevens-Johnson syndrome. Adverse effects are more pronounced in patients who are also taking valproate, a situation that is common in epilepsy but uncommon in the treatment of neuropathic pain.

PHENYTOIN

Current data indicate that the analgesic effect of phenytoin is achieved through blockage of Na^+ channels, inhibition of presynaptic glutamate release, and suppression of spontaneous neuronal ectopic discharges (White 1999).

Only three randomized clinical trials have been published regarding neuropathic pain, two for diabetic neuropathy (Saudek et al. 1977; Chadda and Mathur 1978) and one for various neuropathies (McCleane 1999b). The two studies conducted on PDN yielded opposite results, perhaps due to differences in study design including sample size and length of follow-up, but more likely due to lack of statistical power to detect differences between placebo and phenytoin. Based on these data, NNT was calculated to be 2.1 (1.5–3.6).

Saudek's randomized study demonstrated that phenytoin was no more effective than placebo while Chadda and Mathur showed that phenytoin was more effective than placebo. A recent study with intravenous (i.v.) phenytoin in doses of 15 mg/kg demonstrated analgesic efficacy when the drug was administered by bolus 2-hour infusion, suggesting its usefulness for treatment of neuropathic pain flare-ups (McCleane 1999b). The oral dose used in the studies by Saudek et al. (1977) and Chadda and Mathur (1978) was 300 mg per day, and the rate of adverse effects, most commonly dizziness, lightheadedness, and nausea, was around 10% in both trials.

LOCAL ANESTHETICS AND CONGENERS STUDIED IN RANDOMIZED CLINICAL TRIALS

There is a long tradition of using systemic local anesthetics for analgesia, and the best results have been demonstrated for neuropathic pain (see Chapter 12 for a detailed review). Unfortunately, the number of randomized controlled clinical trials is very small, and studies are limited to oral mexiletine, topical lidocaine, and i.v. bolus infusions of lidocaine (Table II). The primary mode of action of i.v. lidocaine is a dose-dependent blockade

Table II
Summary of the most relevant trials and reports in the literature using
anticonvulsants for different neuropathic painful disorders

Disease	Randomized Trials with Positive Results
Diabetic neuropathy	Rull et al. 1969 (CBZ)
	Wilton 1974 (CBZ)
	Chadda and Mathur 1978 (PHT)
	Gómez-Pérez et al. 1996 (CBZ)
	Backonja et al. 1998 (GBP)
	Morello et al. 1999 (GBP)
Trigeminal neuralgia	Campbell et al. 1966 (CBZ)
	Rockliff and Davis 1966 (CBZ)
	Killian and Fromm 1968 (CBZ)
	Nicol 1969 (CBZ)
	Vilming et al. 1986 (CBZ)
	Lindstrom and Lindblom 1987 (CBZ)
	Zakrzewska et al. 1997 (LTG)
Postherpetic neuralgia	Killian and Fromm 1968 (CBZ)
	Rowbotham et al. 1998 (GBP)
HIV polyneuropathy	Simpson et al. 2000 (LTG)
Central poststroke pain	Vestergaard et al. 2001 (LTG)

Abbreviations: CBZ = carbamazepine; GBP: gabapentin; HIV = human
immunodeficiency virus; LTG = lamotrigine; PHT: phenytoin.

of spontaneous ectopic activity in peripheral nerves and dorsal root ganglion cells (Tanelian and Brose 1991; Tanelian and MacIver 1991; Devor et
al. 1992). The relief of neuropathic pain with local anesthetics could be
explained in part by their actions on the central nervous system, such as
postsynaptic modification of NMDA-receptor activity and undescribed
mechanisms similar to opioid effects (Woolf and Wiesenfeld-Hallin 1985;
Kastrup et al. 1989; Biella and Sotgiu 1993).

A mechanism-based approach to neuropathic pain therapy would suggest that local anesthetics could be used for diagnostic and therapeutic pur-
poses. Systemically administered local anesthetics, in particular lidocaine,
provide prolonged relief of neuropathic pain, regardless of the route of
administration (Arnér et al. 1990; Marchettini et al. 1992; Biella and Sotgiu
1993); Marchettini and colleagues (1992) thus suggested that lidocaine be
used as a diagnostic test for neuropathic pain.

The use of pharmacological agents with firmly established mechanisms
of action to diagnose a neuropathic pain disorder and its components is
consistent with the concept of a mechanism-based approach. However, no
data support this concept in the case of neuropathic pain, and much more
basic scientific and clinical research is needed to establish this approach.
Until then, neuropathic pain and all its components can be diagnosed only

on the basis of clinical evaluation, medical history, and physical examination, with laboratory, psychophysical, and electrophysiological collaboration.

INTRAVENOUS LIDOCAINE

Studies of i.v. lidocaine, all using small samples, have shown efficacy, and some also have provided information about possible mechanisms of action. The first study to demonstrate the effects of i.v. lidocaine was conducted in patients with PDN (Kastrup et al. 1987). Pain relief was obtained with a dose of 5 mg/kg and lasted for 3–21 days after a single infusion. A follow-up study demonstrated that pain relief was correlated to an increase in serum β-endorphin (Kastrup et al. 1989). A study of 19 patients by Rowbotham et al. (1991) revealed that both i.v. lidocaine and morphine were effective in relieving PHN. Another study of 13 patients with various types of neuropathic pain by Ferrante et al. (1996) was performed with the goal of establishing a dose-response curve, but the authors were only able to conclude that the i.v. lidocaine response shows a characteristic "break in pain." However, a study by Wallace et al. (1996) using a computer-controlled infusion pump, did demonstrate a dose-response curve in patients with traumatic neuralgia. Patients suffering from complex regional pain syndrome type II (CRPS-II) experienced relief of spontaneous pain and pain from cool stimuli (Wallace et al. 2000). Attal et al. treated 16 patients with post-stroke pain and central pain from spinal cord injury, demonstrating that i.v. lidocaine was more effective than placebo in relieving spontaneous pain and mechanical allodynia and hyperalgesia, but not in relieving thermal allodynia and hyperalgesia (Attal et al. 2000).

Although the treatment of chronic pain by a single infusion is conceptually challenging, the fact remains that many patients experience prolonged relief. Continuous subcutaneous lidocaine infusion could be used in certain circumstances for appropriate patients (Brose and Cousins 1991).

MEXILETINE

Five randomized placebo-controlled trials have appeared, four in PDN (Dejgard et al. 1988; Stracke et al. 1992; Oskarsson et al. 1997; Wright et al. 1997) and one in central pain from spinal cord injury (Chiou-Tan et al. 1996). A large parallel design study of PDN showed no effect in the primary outcome when assessing global pain on a visual analogue scale, although there was relief of burning and stabbing pain, heat sensation, and formications (Oskarsson et al. 1997). Two studies with a smaller number of patients, one focusing on PDN (Wright et al. 1997) and the other on central pain from spinal cord injury (Chiou-Tan et al. 1996) were negative. A study by Galer et al. (1996) suggests that response to i.v. lidocaine positively predict continued response to mexiletine. In contrast to positive results in most studies on the drugs reviewed here, most studies with mexiletine have been negative (NNT = 10). Although the studies reviewed here suggest good tolerability, intolerable gastrointestinal adverse effects frequently observed in clinical practice limit the long-term use of this drug.

SUMMARY AND CONCLUSIONS

Advances in neuroscience have demonstrated the complexity of biochemical changes within the nervous system in animal models of neuropathic pain, which would strongly suggest similar changes in patients with chronic pain. Based on our current understanding of the underlying mechanisms of chronic neuropathic pain there are strong conceptual arguments for recommending the use of anticonvulsants and systemic local anesthetics in its treatment. Indeed, controlled randomized trials, though still limited in number, have demonstrated the efficacy of anticonvulsants in relieving chronic neuropathic pain. The available evidence supports the use of carbamazepine to treat TN and gabapentin to treat PDN and PHN. Carbamazepine could be considered for PDN and lamotrigine for post-stroke central pain syndrome, TN, and HIV neuropathy, although here the evidence is less convincing and clinical experience with carbamazepine has been disappointing. Evidence for the use of mexiletine is inconclusive because there are as many studies with negative outcomes as with positive ones. Intravenous lidocaine offers an interesting treatment option, but long-term i.v. administration presents a clinical challenge that research has not yet addressed.

We can draw many conclusions from this review. The main lesson we can learn from positive studies is that efficacy of anticonvulsants and systemic local anesthetics demonstrates the proof of the concept—these drugs have a significant effect and they probably work through the proposed mechanisms that are specific for each drug. Although these positive studies provide many answers, they also raise questions. For example, studies on systemic lidocaine suggest that the drug works via central postsynaptic mechanisms in addition to blocking peripheral Na channels, but this indication must be confirmed by further studies. Another conclusion that can be drawn from clinical trials is that adequate dosage is necessary to control chronic neuropathic pain—between 1800 and 3600 mg per day in the case of gabapentin. In addition, it is important to measure and assess secondary outcomes to obtain the full range of each drug's effects because chronic pain is a complex clinical phenomenon.

Lessons also can be learned from negative studies. A lamotrigine study with a relatively large number of patients with painful neuropathies suggested that inadequate dosing is likely to lead to a negative outcome, because doses of over 200 mg per day are used in daily clinical practice. With drugs such as mexiletine, a narrow therapeutic range is likely to yield negative results, so tolerability may be even more important than efficacy. Studies with a small number of patients, as in the case of phenytoin, are also likely to yield negative results.

Positive experience with anticonvulsants and systemic local anesthetics in the treatment of neuropathic pain should encourage further well-designed controlled clinical trials with a large enough number of patients to allow us to determine whether a drug is effective. Careful assessments of efficacy and adverse effects should allow us to establish therapeutic ratios for each of the drugs tested. Comparator studies are necessary to determine the specific role of each drug in the treatment algorithms for neuropathic pain. Most of the newer anticonvulsants have a wide dosing range that should be explored and utilized. Treatment concepts such as add-on therapy and rational polypharmacy should be studied in a systematic fashion in clinical trials. The new concept of mechanism-based diagnosis and therapy will help us make progress in treating chronic neuropathic pain.

REFERENCES

Arnér S, Lindblom U, Meyerson BA, Molander C. Prolonged relief of neuralgia after regional anesthetic blocks. A call for further experimental and systematic clinical studies. *Pain* 1990; 43:287–297.

Attal N, Gaude V, Brasseur L, et al. Intravenous lidocaine in central pain: a double-blind, placebo-controlled, psychophysical study. *Neurology* 2000; 54:564–574.

Backonja MM, Galer BS. Pain assessment and evaluation of patients who have neuropathic pain. *Neurol Clin* 1998; 16:775–790.

Backonja M, Beydoun A, Edwards KR, et al. Gabapentin for the symptomatic treatment of painful neuropathy in patients with diabetes mellitus: a randomized controlled trial. *JAMA* 1998; 280:1831–1836.

Bassilana F, Champigny G, Waldmann R, et al. The acid-sensitive ionic channel subunit ASIC and the mammalian degenerin MDEG form a heteromultimeric H^+-gated Na^+ channel with novel properties. *J Biol Chem* 1997; 272:28819–28822.

Bennett GJ, Xie YK. A peripheral mononeuropathy in rat that produces disorders of pain sensation like those seen in man. [Comment in *Pain* 1990; 42(2):253–255.] *Pain* 1988; 33:87–107.

Biella G, Sotgiu ML. Central effects of systemic lidocaine mediated by glycine spinal receptors: an iontophoretic study in the rat spinal cord. *Brain Res* 1993; 603:201–206.

Brose WG, Cousins MJ. Subcutaneous lidocaine for treatment of neuropathic cancer pain. *Pain* 1991; 45:145–148.

Campbell FG, Graham JG, Zilkha KJ. Clinical trial of carbamazepine (Tegretol) in trigeminal neuralgia. *J Neurol Neurosurg Psychiatry* 1966; 29:265–267.

Chadda VS, Mathur M. Double-blind study of the effects of diphenylhydantoin sodium diabetic neuropathy. *J Assoc Physicians India* 1978; 26:403–406.

Chiou-Tan FY, Tuel SM, Johnson JC, et al. Effect of mexiletine on spinal cord injury dysesthetic pain. *Am J Phys Med Rehabil* 1996; 75:84–87.

Chung K, Kim HJ, Na HS, Park MJ, Chung JM. Abnormalities of sympathetic innervation in the area of an injured peripheral nerve in a rat model of neuropathic pain. *Neurosci Lett* 1993; 162:85–88.

Cline MA, Ochoa J, Torebjork HE. Chronic hyperalgesia and skin warming caused by sensitized C nociceptors. *Brain* 1989; 112:621–647.

Cummins TR, Dib-Hajj SD, Black JA, et al. A novel persistent tetrodotoxin-resistant sodium current in SNS-null and wild-type small primary sensory neurons. *J Neurosci* (Online) 1999; 19:RC43.

Dejgard A, Petersen P, Kastrup J. Mexiletine for treatment of chronic painful diabetic neuropathy. *Lancet* 1988; 1:9–11.

Devor M, Wall PD, Catalan N. Systemic lidocaine silences ectopic neuroma and DRG discharge without blocking nerve conduction. *Pain* 1992; 48:261–268.

Dib-Hajj SD, Tyrrell L, Cummins TR, et al. Two tetrodotoxin-resistant sodium channels in human dorsal root ganglion neurons. *FEBS Lett* 1999; 462:117–120.

Ferrante FM, Paggioli J, Cherukuri S, Arthur GR. The analgesic response to intravenous lidocaine in the treatment of neuropathic pain. *Anesth Analg* 1996; 82:91–97.

Fukuoka T, Tokunaga A, Kondo E, et al. Change in mRNAs for neuropeptides and the GABA(A) receptor in dorsal root ganglion neurons in a rat experimental neuropathic pain model. *Pain* 1998; 78:13–26.

Galer BS, Harle J, Rowbotham MC. Response to intravenous lidocaine infusion predicts subsequent response to oral mexiletine: a prospective study. *J Pain Symptom Manage* 1996; 12:161–167.

Gómez-Pérez FJ, Choza R, Rios JM, et al. Nortriptyline-fluphenazine vs. carbamazepine in the symptomatic treatment of diabetic neuropathy. *Arch Med Res* 1996; 27:525–529.

Kastrup J, Petersen P, Dejgard A, Angelo HR, Hilsted J. Intravenous lidocaine infusion—a new treatment of chronic painful diabetic neuropathy? *Pain* 1987; 28:69–75.

Kastrup J, Bach FW, Petersen P, et al. Lidocaine treatment of painful diabetic neuropathy and endogenous opioid peptides in plasma. *Clin J Pain* 1989; 5:239–244.

Killian JM, Fromm GH. Carbamazepine in the treatment of neuralgia. *Arch Neurol* 1968; 19:129–136.

Kingery W. A critical review of controlled clinical trials for peripheral neuropathic pain and complex regional pain syndrome. *Pain* 1997; 73:123–139.

Lechin F, van der Dijs B, Lechin ME, et al. Pimozide therapy for trigeminal neuralgia. *Arch Neurol* 1989; 46:960–963.

Leijon G, Boivie J. Central post-stroke pain—a controlled trial of amitriptyline and carbamazepine. *Pain* 1989; 36:27–36.

Lindstrom P, Lindblom U. The analgesic effect of tocainide in trigeminal neuralgia. *Pain* 1987; 28:45–50.

Mao J, Price DD, Coghill RC, Mayer DJ, Hayes RL. Spatial patterns of spinal cord [^{14}C]-2-deoxyglucose metabolic activity in a rat model of painful peripheral mononeuropathy [published erratum appears in *Pain* 1992; 51(3):389]. *Pain* 1992; 50:89–100.

Marchettini P, Lacerenza M, Marangoni C, et al. Lidocaine test in neuralgia. *Pain* 1992; 48:377–382.

McCleane G. 200 mg daily of lamotrigine has no analgesic effect in neuropathic pain: a randomised, double-blind, placebo controlled trial. *Pain* 1999a; 83:105–107.

McCleane GJ. Intravenous infusion of phenytoin relieves neuropathic pain: a randomized, double-blinded, placebo-controlled, crossover study. *Anesth Analg* 1999b; 89:985–988.

McNamara J. Drugs acting on the central nervous system. In: Harman G, Limbird LE, Morinoff PB et al. (Eds). *Goodman and Gilman's The Pharmacological Basis of Therapeutics.* New York: McGraw-Hill, 1996:461–486.

Mitchell SW, Morehouse GR, Keen WW. *Gunshot Wounds, and Other Injuries of Nerves.* Philadelphia: J.B. Lippincott & Co., 1864.

Morello CM, Leckband SG, Stoner CP, Moorhouse DF, Sahagian GA. Randomized double-blind study comparing the efficacy of gabapentin with amitriptyline on diabetic peripheral neuropathy pain. *Arch Intern Med* 1999; 159:1931–1937.

Neumann S, Doubell TP, Leslie T, Woolf CJ. Inflammatory pain hypersensitivity mediated by phenotypic switch in myelinated primary sensory neurons. *Nature* 1996; 384:360–364.

Nicol C. A four year double blind randomized study of Tegretol in facial pain. *Headache* 1969; 9:54–57.

Oskarsson P, Ljunggren JG, Lins PE. Efficacy and safety of mexiletine in the treatment of painful diabetic neuropathy. The Mexiletine Study Group. *Diabetes Care* 1997; 20:1594–1597.

Ossipov MH, Lai J, Malan TP Jr, Porreca F. Spinal and supraspinal mechanisms of neuropathic pain. *Ann N Y Acad Sci* 2000; 909:12–24.

Rabert DK, Koch BD, Ilnicka M, et al. A tetrodotoxin-resistant voltage-gated sodium channel from human dorsal root ganglia, hPN3/SCN10A. *Pain* 1998; 78:107–114.

Rey R. *History of Pain.* Paris: La Decouverte, 1993.

Rockliff BW, Davis EH. Controlled sequential trials of carbamazepine in trigeminal neuralgia. *Arch Neurol* 1966; 15:129–136.

Rowbotham MC, Reisner-Keller LA, Fields HL. Both intravenous lidocaine and morphine reduce the pain of postherpetic neuralgia. *Neurology* 1991; 41:1024–1028.

Rowbotham MC, Davies PS, Fields HL. Topical lidocaine gel relieves postherpetic neuralgia. *Ann Neurol* 1995; 37:246–253.

Rowbotham MC, Davies PS, Verkempinck C, Galer BS. Lidocaine patch: double-blind controlled study of a new treatment method for post-herpetic neuralgia. *Pain* 1996; 65:39–44.

Rowbotham M, Harden N, Stacey B, Bernstein P, Magnus-Miller L. Gabapentin for the treatment of postherpetic neuralgia: a randomized controlled trial. *JAMA* 1998; 280:1837–1842.

Rull JA, Quibrera R, Gonzalez-Millan H, Lozano Castaneda O. Symptomatic treatment of peripheral diabetic neuropathy with carbamazepine (Tegretol): double blind crossover trial. *Diabetologia* 1969; 5:215–218.

Saudek CD, Werns S, Reidenberg MM. Phenytoin in the treatment of diabetic symmetrical polyneuropathy. *Clin Pharmacol Ther* 1977; 22:196–199.

Simpson DM, Olney R, McArthur JC, et al. A placebo-controlled trial of lamotrigine for painful HIV-associated neuropathy. *Neurology* 2000; 54:2115–2119.

Sindrup SH, Jensen TS. Efficacy of pharmacological treatments of neuropathic pain: an update and effect related to mechanism of drug action. *Pain* 1999; 83:389–400.

Stracke H, Meyer UE, Schumacher HE, Federlin K. Mexiletine in the treatment of diabetic neuropathy. *Diabetes Care* 1992; 15:1550–1555.

Tanelian DL, Brose WG. Neuropathic pain can be relieved by drugs that are use-dependent sodium channel blockers: lidocaine, carbamazepine, and mexiletine. *Anesthesiology* 1991; 74:949–951.

Tanelian DL, MacIver MB. Analgesic concentrations of lidocaine suppress tonic A-delta and C fiber discharges produced by acute injury. *Anesthesiology* 1991; 74:934–936.

Taylor CP, Gee NS, Su TZ, et al. A summary of mechanistic hypotheses of gabapentin pharmacology. *Epilepsy Res* 1998; 29:233–249.

Tremont-Lukats IW, Megeff C, Backonja MM. Anticonvulsants for neuropathic pain syndromes: mechanisms of action and place in therapy. *Drugs* 2001; 60:1029–1052.

Vestergaard K, Andersen G, Gottrup H, Kristensen BT, Jensen TS. Lamotrigine for central poststroke pain: a randomized controlled trial. *Neurology* 2001; 56:184–190.

Vilming ST, Lyberg T, Lataste X. Tizanidine in the management of trigeminal neuralgia. *Cephalalgia* 1986; 6:181–182.

Vinik A, Fonseca V, Lamoeaux L, Hes M, Edwards K. Neurontin (Gabapentin, GBP) improves quality of life (QOL) in patients with painful diabetic peripheral neuropathy. *Diabetes* 1998; 46:A374.

Wallace MS, Dyck JB, Rossi SS, Yaksh TL. Computer-controlled lidocaine infusion for the evaluation of neuropathic pain after peripheral nerve injury. *Pain* 1996; 66:69–77.

Wallace MS, Ridgeway BM, Leung AY, Gerayli A, Yaksh TL. Concentration-effect relationship of intravenous lidocaine on the allodynia of complex regional pain syndrome types I and II. *Anesthesiology* 2000; 92:75–83.

White HS. Comparative anticonvulsant and mechanistic profile of the established and newer antiepileptic drugs. *Epilepsia* 1999; 40(Suppl 5):S2–10.

Wiffen P, McQuay H, Carroll D, Jadad A, Moore A. Anticonvulsant drugs for acute and chronic pain. *Cochrane Database of Systematic Reviews* 2000; CD001133, available on the Internet.

Wilton T. Tegretol in the treatment of diabetic neuropathy. *S Afr Med J* 1974; 27:869–872.

Woolf CJ, Salter MW. Neuronal plasticity: increasing the gain in pain. *Science* 2000; 288:1765–1768.

Woolf CJ, Wiesenfeld-Hallin Z. The systemic administration of local anesthetics produces a selective depression of C-afferent fibre evoked activity in the spinal cord. *Pain* 1985; 23:361–374.

Wright JM, Oki JC, Graves L. Mexiletine in the symptomatic treatment of diabetic peripheral neuropathy. *Ann Pharmacother* 1997; 31:29–34.

Zakrzewska JM, Chaudhry Z, Nurmikko TJ, Patton DW, Mullens EL. Lamotrigine (Lamictal) in refractory trigeminal neuralgia: results from a double blind placebo controlled crossover trial. *Pain* 1997; 73:223–230.

Correspondence to: Miroslav Backonja, MD, Department of Neurology, University of Wisconsin, 600 Highland Avenue, Madison, WI 53792, USA. Email: backonja@neurology.wisc.edu.

Neuropathic Pain: Pathophysiology and Treatment,
Progress in Pain Research and Management, Vol. 21,
edited by Per T. Hansson, Howard L. Fields, Raymond G.
Hill, and Paolo Marchettini, IASP Press, Seattle, © 2001.

11

Efficacy of Opioids in Neuropathic Pain

Michael C. Rowbotham

Pain Clinical Research Center, University of California,
San Francisco, California, USA

It is not unusual for heated debates to be fueled by a lack of definitive data. This is clearly the case for the controversy over using opioids for managing chronic neuropathic pain. As recently as a decade ago, many considered it axiomatic that neuropathic pain was rarely relieved by opioids, that any initial subjective pain reduction would soon be lost through development of tolerance, and that addiction would occur in a high proportion of patients (Maruta et al. 1979; Pagni 1984; Portenoy et al. 1990; Wall 1990). This view was challenged using mostly retrospective data suggesting that opioids were effective as long-term therapy for nonmalignant pain (including neuropathic pain), with a low risk of addiction (Porter and Jick 1980; Taub 1982; France et al. 1984; Portenoy and Foley 1986; Urban et al. 1986; Watson et al. 1988).

Arnér and Meyerson (1988a) set off a lively debate with an article entitled "Lack of analgesic effect of opioids on neuropathic and idiopathic forms of pain." They reported on the effectiveness of opioid infusion as compared with placebo in three groups of patients who had nociceptive visceral pain, neuropathic pain, or idiopathic pain, respectively. The 12 patients with neuropathic pain, all scheduled for placement of electrodes for deep brain stimulation, received opioid and placebo infusions to help plan the stimulation target and to see whether opioids should be instituted as an alternative or supplementary therapy. These patients had long histories of "severely incapacitating pain which had resisted all previous treatments," including nerve blocks, peripheral pain surgery, opioids (four patients were still taking high doses), and in most cases anticonvulsants and tricyclic antidepressants. The patients received 15 mg of morphine or placebo on at least four occasions. If they reported significant pain reduction, the effect was reversed with intravenous (i.v.) naloxone. The 21 patients suffering from idiopathic pain received several different opioids, with a total of between 4 and 13 active or placebo infusions. The 15 patients with nociceptive pain reported dramatic pain reduction with opioid infusion (87% reduction in pain intensity on a visual analogue scale [VAS]) compared to saline placebo (17% reduction), but the neuropathic and idiopathic pain groups reported no pain relief from opioid infusions. Doses were not increased for neuropathic patients already taking opioids, and the doses used did not produce side effects. As the neuropathic patients were candidates for deep brain stimulation by virtue of being unresponsive to nearly every treatment tried, including opioids, the group could not be considered fully representative of the large and heterogenous group of neuropathic pain patients. As pointed out by Howard L. Fields (1988), while it may be correct that neuropathic pain is less responsive to opioids or that many patients with neuropathic pain do not respond to opioids, Arnér and Meyerson's study did not exclude the possibility that opioids are effective for neuropathic pain. Fields warned that the results of the study should not encourage physicians to withhold opioid therapy. In a response to Fields' critique, Arnér and Meyerson (1988b) agreed that it would be unfortunate if opioids were withheld from patients in whom they produced analgesia. They further replied: "It may seem premature to base a conclusion concerning the lack of effect of opioids in chronic neuropathic pain on such a small group of patients. We would have hesitated to do so were it not for the fact that the outcome of the tests just confirmed our experience over the years with a larger number of such patients—an experience that we share with others."

In 1988, Max and colleagues reported the results of a four-session crossover study comparing single oral doses of codeine (120 mg), clonidine, ibuprofen, and placebo in patients with postherpetic neuralgia. Codeine produced side effects but was no better than placebo at relieving pain. The only drug that relieved pain, clonidine, also had the highest incidence of side effects. Even though codeine is a well-established analgesic, a dose of 120 mg produces relatively modest pain reduction when given to patients with other disorders.

In 1990, Portenoy, Foley, and Inturrisi published a comprehensive review of the concept of opioid responsiveness as supported by data from uncontrolled infusions of various opioids in patients with neuropathic pain, primarily of malignant origin. They proposed a continuum of opioid responsiveness in which patients with neuropathic pain may simply require higher drug doses to experience analgesia. Arnér and Meyerson (1991), commenting on Portenoy et al.'s paper, noted that while the authors found little evidence to support the resistance of neuropathic pain to opioids, they failed to admit that no systematic, controlled study had demonstrated that such pain does respond to opioids. *Pain* editor Ronald Dubner (1991) summarized the state of affairs in the same issue through an editorial comment entitled: "A call for more science, not more rhetoric, regarding opioids and neuropathic pain." He called for prospective, controlled trials of opioids in homogeneous groups of neuropathic pain patients, drawing an analogy with the chronology of research on the analgesic efficacy of antidepressants in pain associated with diabetic neuropathy and postherpetic neuralgia. Early anecdotal observations and open-trial studies had suggested that tricyclic antidepressants were clinically effective, but it was not known whether these effects were related to analgesia, mood changes, or sedative effects. Subsequent blinded trials with active and inactive placebos had been able to satisfactorily answer these questions by studying relatively homogeneous populations of patients.

RHETORIC GIVES WAY TO SCIENCE: CONTROLLED TRIALS OF INTRAVENOUS OPIOIDS

The first prospective placebo-controlled opioid trial in a homogenous group of patients with neuropathic pain appeared almost immediately. Rowbotham, Reisner-Keller, and Fields (1991) reported the results of a three-session, double-blind, crossover study comparing 1-hour i.v. infusions of 0.3 mg/kg of morphine (average total dose of 19.2 mg), 5 mg/kg of lidocaine (average total dose of 316 mg), and matching saline placebo in 19 patients with established postherpetic neuralgia. Pre-infusion VAS ratings of pain intensity declined by 33% during the morphine sessions, significantly more than the 13% decline during the placebo sessions. Relief ratings were higher during the morphine infusion than during either lidocaine or placebo infusions. Eleven subjects chose the morphine session as providing the best relief. Ten of these subjects also experienced either a normalization of subjective cutaneous sensation or a loss of painful hypersensitivity following the morphine infusion. The change in pain intensity ratings was correlated with blood levels of morphine at the end of the infusion. Side effects were *not* correlated with pain relief for either active drug.

Subsequently, Kupers and colleagues (1991) reported the effect of i.v. morphine at a dose of 0.3 mg/kg and saline placebo in a two-session crossover study comparing patients with pain associated with central and peripheral neuropathic conditions to a small group of "idiopathic" pain patients. The authors hypothesized that the primary reason why patients with pain consumed opioids over the long term was for their mood-changing effects. Therefore, they used a modification of the McGill Pain Questionnaire to train subjects to separately rate the affective (unpleasantness) and sensory (intensity) components of ongoing pain. Their subjects consisted of six patients with neuropathic pain of central nervous system (CNS) origin, eight with neuropathic pain of peripheral nervous system (PNS) origin, and six with idiopathic chronic pain. The patients with neuropathic pain of PNS origin were somewhat atypical; two had low back pain for which surgical and other treatments had failed, and two had brachial plexus avulsions. Affective pain ratings decreased significantly in both groups of neuropathic pain patients, but sensory pain ratings were unchanged. The group with idiopathic pain demonstrated no change in either aspect of pain.

The largest study to date is the two-session crossover trial reported by Dellemijn and Vanneste (1997). In 50 patients with different types of pain, they compared the analgesic effect of i.v. fentanyl with either saline placebo or the benzodiazepine diazepam. Diazepam was included as a control agent in the belief that it would modulate the subject's emotional experience of pain without producing intrinsic analgesic effects. Each infusion lasted a total of 5 hours, fentanyl at a rate of 5 µg/kg/h and diazepam at 0.2 µg/kg/h. Fentanyl reduced both the affective and sensory dimensions of pain, providing a maximum pain reduction of 65% compared to 15–20% during the placebo and diazepam control infusions. Diazepam produced sedation that was nearly as great as that produced by fentanyl, but the drug was no more effective than saline placebo in relieving pain. Dellemijn and Vanneste's study is especially important because they specifically controlled for the sedating effects of opioids by including a benzodiazepine.

Together, these studies provide compelling evidence in favor of a specific analgesic effect of opioids on both the intensity and the unpleasantness of neuropathic pain. The studies of Rowbotham et al. and Dellemijn and Vanneste were primarily designed to test the hypothesis that opioids could relieve neuropathic pain. They were not intended to answer other important questions about opioid therapy, such as the relative opioid responsivity of different types of neuropathic pain, and whether opioids are equal to or better than other medication therapies for chronic neuropathic pain.

SUSTAINED RELIEF OF NEUROPATHIC PAIN DURING ORAL OPIOID ADMINISTRATION

The results of two prospective, placebo-controlled trials of oral opioids (oxycodone and tramadol) for neuropathic pain appeared in the same issue of *Neurology* in 1998 (Harati et al. 1998; Watson and Babul 1998). Oxycodone and tramadol are widely used for outpatient pain control in the United States.

Oxycodone is a typical μ-opioid agonist of moderate potency. Tramadol is an atypical drug; the parent drug and its major metabolite combine to produce low-affinity binding to μ-opioid receptors and to inhibit norepinephrine and serotonin reuptake, so it remains unsettled to what extent mechanisms other than μ-opioid-receptor binding contribute to overall pain reduction. Tramadol is approved for use in the United States for "moderate to moderately severe" pain.

Watson and Babul described a random-order crossover trial of twice-daily controlled-release oxycodone in 50 patients with postherpetic neuralgia (1998). The 45% of subjects with prior opioid experience (typically combinations of acetaminophen with either codeine or oxycodone) abstained from all opioid use for at least 7 days before study entry. At randomization, subjects began with either placebo or 10 mg oxycodone twice a day and were titrated at weekly intervals up to a maximum of 30 mg twice a day. A total of 38 subjects completed the trial (dropout rate = 24%). Outcome data for efficacy in the 12 dropouts were not reported, and the statistical analysis was carried out on data from completing subjects only. Opioid-experienced subjects were not separated from opioid-naive subjects in the data analysis. Completing subjects achieved a mean total daily oxycodone intake of 45 mg. Daily diary pain intensity scores were significantly lower during oxycodone treatment than during placebo treatment by the second week of the 4-week treatment period. Overall pain intensity during the last week of treatment was 54 mm on a 100-mm VAS during treatment with placebo and 35 mm during treatment with oxycodone ($P = 0.0001$). VAS scores for steady pain, brief pain, and skin pain were all significantly lower during the last week of oxycodone treatment than during placebo treatment. Similarly, pain relief category ratings and disability scores significantly favored oxycodone. Mean pain relief ratings on a six-point scale were "moderate" with oxycodone compared to "slight" with placebo. Not surprisingly, reports of adverse events increased significantly during oxycodone therapy, particularly constipation, nausea, and sedation. Despite the greater reduction of pain during oxycodone therapy, there were no treatment differences on the Beck Depression Inventory or on any of the six scales of the Profile of Mood States. Given the steady dose escalation during a treatment period of only 4 weeks, tolerance was not expected and was not evident.

Harati and coworkers (1998) reported the results of a multicenter, randomized, placebo-controlled trial of parallel design in 131 subjects with chronic neuropathic pain due to distal symmetric diabetic neuropathy. After 21 days off tricyclic antidepressants or anticonvulsants and 7 days off shorter-acting analgesics, subjects were treated with either tramadol or placebo for 6 weeks. Subjects were allowed to titrate up to a maximum of 400 mg/day, and were required to use a minimum of 100 mg/day during the last 4 weeks of the treatment period. A total of 82 subjects completed the study (dropout rate = 37%), taking a mean dose of 210 mg/day of tramadol. There were more "adverse event" dropouts in the tramadol group, and more "lack of efficacy" dropouts in the placebo group. In contrast to Watson and Babul's study, the data analysis was based on all drug-exposed subjects not lost to follow-up (n = 127). Subjects treated with tramadol had significantly less pain and greater pain relief at all time points from day 14 of treatment to day 42 at the end of the treatment period. Pain intensity on a five-point Likert scale was reduced from 2.5 to 1.4, compared to a change from 2.6 to 2.2 for those subjects assigned to placebo (P < 0.001). Pain relief ratings were similar to those in Watson and Babul's study. Tramadol produced "moderate" relief, compared to "slight" relief with placebo. Sleep, current health perception, psychological distress, and overall role functioning scales were not improved with tramadol therapy, but scales of physical and social functioning showed significant improvement in the tramadol group. Compared to Watson and Babul's study, Harati et al.'s results provide more convincing proof of efficacy because of the larger sample, a more conservative efficacy analysis using all drug-exposed subjects, and a longer treatment period.

Sindrup and coworkers (1999) reported a crossover study of tramadol in 45 patients with polyneuropathy of diverse etiologies. The total noncompletion rate was 25%, with seven of nine adverse event dropouts during tramadol treatment. Data analysis on the 34 subjects completing the trial showed that tramadol reduced pain by approximately 33% (compared to no change in pain during placebo treatment) at a mean dose of 347 mg/day. Reductions in spontaneous and touch-evoked pain were significant and were positively correlated with each other during tramadol treatment.

DO DIFFERENT TYPES OF NEUROPATHIC PAIN DIFFER IN OPIOID RESPONSIVITY?

At least for neuropathic pain of peripheral nerve origin in the form of postherpetic neuralgia and diabetic neuropathy, we now have the same chronology of proof for opioid efficacy that was described for antidepressants by Dubner in his 1990 editorial. Case reports have been followed by controlled trials demonstrating longer-term efficacy of oral opioids. Furthermore, the i.v. infusion studies have demonstrated that opioid analgesia is not simply due to sedation and other side effects. Paradoxically, opioid responsivity is now better validated for chronic neuropathic pain of PNS origin than for any other type of chronic nonmalignant pain. For example, longer-term opioid trials for chronic musculoskeletal pain have had mixed results. A prospective controlled trial of codeine in osteoarthritis of the hip showed no benefit over a 4-week treatment period and had a high dropout rate (Kjaersgaard-Andersen et al. 1990). A controlled trial of oral morphine for chronic musculoskeletal pain showed modest benefit that was almost completely lost by the end of the 9-week treatment period (Moulin et al. 1996). This is an important point because animal research has indirectly promoted the belief that chronic neuropathic pain is somehow less opioid responsive than is non-neuropathic chronic pain. In fact, we lack data comparing groups of patients with chronic neuropathic and non-neuropathic pain of nonmalignant origin who are matched for disease chronicity, age, and pain severity and are treated with oral opioids under identical double-blind conditions.

In his landmark book, *The Management of Pain,* Bonica (1953) observed that thalamic pain and other central pain states appeared unresponsive to opioids. Pagni and others have presented anecdotal evidence in favor of this view (Pagni 1984; Hammond 1991). Preliminary data from double-blind, placebo-controlled studies conducted in our laboratory indicate that pain of CNS origin is indeed less responsive to opioids than is pain of PNS origin. The unresolved problem of how to treat central pain could be an important source of long-held negative views about opioids and neuropathic pain in general. Some patients with thalamic pain, for example, make a strong impression on the pain practitioner with their strikingly abnormal neurological examinations, profound suffering, and utter failure to respond to all therapies. Leijon and Boivie (1989) were able to demonstrate that amitriptyline was effective in a very small group of patients with post-stroke pain. Otherwise, no controlled evidence has been published in favor of *any* oral drug category for this type of central pain.

HOW SHOULD OPIOID EFFICACY BE JUDGED?

Testing individual patients is very different than demonstrating efficacy in a particular syndrome. What criteria should be used for determining opioid responsiveness? Conversely, what evidence is needed to convincingly demonstrate that an individual's pain is opioid resistant? If the goal is to demonstrate that neuropathic pain can be transiently reduced in intensity, an i.v. infusion study with an appropriate control should suffice, although the positive and negative predictive power of such testing is unknown. For longer-term therapy, judgments of pain relief and adverse effects need to be balanced, and outcome measures must be appropriate for the larger question being tested. Is subjective reduction in pain intensity a sufficient reason to prescribe opioids, or should an objectively verified increase in activity tolerance or a return to work be expected in order to justify long-term opioid therapy? Expecting patients with chronic neuropathic pain to lead better, more productive lives as a precondition for continued opioid therapy holds this form of treatment to a standard not expected of other oral medication classes, but this is perhaps the understandable consequence of fears of addiction and of diversion of drugs to the illicit market.

As tolerance is a major concern of clinicians, more data must be gathered prospectively on the importance of this issue in clinical practice. Except for a study of chronic musculoskeletal pain by Moulin et al. (1996), the blinded trials either have used short treatment periods of 4–6 weeks or did not search for evidence of tolerance development. Although animal studies can demonstrate near-complete loss of antinociceptive effects in as little as 24–48 hours during continuous opioid administration, the clinical implications of this finding are uncertain. If humans with chronic pain showed loss of analgesia comparable to the animal studies, opioids would be useless as long-term therapy. In clinical practice, analgesia appears to be sustained. Although tolerance develops at varying rates compared to other effects of opioids, analgesic tolerance has not been proven to exist in medically stable patients with chronic nonmalignant pain.

The larger question then is how effective opioids are overall compared to other therapies for neuropathic pain. The answer remains to be determined—no large-scale, random assignment studies have directly compared opioids with proven non-opioid therapies (such as gabapentin and tricyclic antidepressants) to look for meaningful differences in long-term efficacy, side-effect profiles, and risks of long-term use. For postherpetic neuralgia and diabetic neuropathy, three medication classes—tricyclic antidepressants, opioids, and the anticonvulsant gabapentin—have proven effective in double-blind controlled studies with sufficiently large groups of subjects for adequate statistical power and with treatment periods of 4–8 weeks (McQuay et al. 1996; Backonja et al. 1998; Harati et al. 1998; Rowbotham et al. 1998; Watson and Babul 1998). For all three medication types, the results seem roughly equivalent. With active therapy, overall pain intensity reduction averages about 30–40%, pain relief is "moderate," and about half of drug-exposed subjects experience satisfactory pain relief. Crossover studies in which subjects were given all three types of medications in random order would be particularly useful in showing what proportion of patients who fail to respond to antidepressants and gabapentin will have a satisfactory response to opioids, and vice versa.

MONOTHERAPY VERSUS POLYPHARMACY

Only half of subjects achieve "satisfactory" or "moderate" pain relief from a drug proven effective (compared to placebo) in clinical trials, and only about 10% achieve "complete" or near-complete relief. Thus many (if not most) patients will require multiple medication trials and will probably be managed with a polypharmacy regimen that combines different drug classes. As shown in Fig. 1, the value of each drug added to the regimen will pay diminishing returns as the total number of medications used in combination increases. Where do opioids belong in a polypharmacy regimen? In a pain clinic setting, most patients taking three or more drugs for pain relief will be taking an opioid. The benefit of including opioids in a polypharmacy regimen is uncertain, as synergy, antagonism, or simple additivity has not been proven in well-designed studies of chronic pain patients for essentially any combination drug regimen. The only data come from studies of healthy volunteers subjected to experimental pain. Gabapentin enhances morphine analgesic efficacy in healthy volunteers (Eckhardt et al. 2000), and is suggested to be a useful "add-on" therapy in neuropathic cancer pain patients who are only partially responsive to opioids (Caraceni et al. 1999). Tricyclic antidepressants have produced mixed results (Levine et al. 1986; O'Neill and Valentino 1986) when given before or added to opioids.

As long as physicians fear scrutiny by regulatory agencies (Joranson 1995) and feel pressure from other physicians and health insurance organizations not to prescribe opioids, these drugs will continue to be used only when other medications fail. For opioids, more than any other type of pain

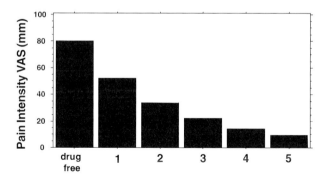

Fig. 1. Theoretical plot of change in pain with the addition of up to five drugs in a polypharmacy regimen. Each drug added produces an additional 35% reduction in pain intensity. In a population study, the incremental benefit from adding a fourth or fifth drug is likely to be too small to be statistically significant. As shown, pain will not be completely eliminated in a polypharmacy regimen.

therapy, the attitudes and beliefs of the patient and his or her social network, the prescribing physician, and society must all be taken into account. It is not enough to simply demonstrate that pain is reduced. For opioids to become a first-line medication for chronic neuropathic pain (as monotherapy or in a polypharmacy regimen), research must prospectively demonstrate that the ratio of risks to benefits of chronic opioid therapy is *at least* as favorable as for any other therapy.

ACKNOWLEDGMENTS

The author is supported by NINDS Program Project NS21445 and NINDS K24 award NS02164.

REFERENCES

Arnér S, Meyerson BA. Lack of analgesia effect of opioids on neuropathic and idiopathic forms of pain. *Pain* 1988a; 33:11–23.

Arnér S, Meyerson BA. Reply to Howard L. Fields on 'Can opiates relieve neuropathic pain?' *Pain* 1988b; 35:366–367.

Arnér S, Meyerson BA. Genuine resistance to opioids—fact or fiction? *Pain* 1991; 47:116–118.

Backonja M, Beydoun A, Edwards KR, et al. Gabapentin Diabetic Neuropathy Study Group. Gabapentin for the symptomatic treatment of painful neuropathy in patients with diabetes mellitus. *JAMA* 1998; 280:1831–1836.

Bonica JJ. *The Management of Pain*. Philadelphia: Lea & Febiger, 1953.

Caraceni A, Zecca E, Martini C, De Conno F. Gabapentin as an adjuvant to opioid analgesia for neuropathic cancer pain. *J Pain Symptom Manage* 1999; 17:441–445.

Dellemijn PL, Vanneste JA. Randomized double-blind active-placebo-controlled crossover trial of intravenous fentanyl in neuropathic pain. *Lancet* 1997; 349:753–758.

Dubner R. A call for more science, not more rhetoric, regarding opioids and neuropathic pain. *Pain* 1991; 47:1–2.

Eckhardt K, Ammon S, Hofmann U, et al. Gabapentin enhances the analgesic effect of morphine in healthy volunteers. *Anesth Analg* 2000; 91:185–191.

Fields HL. Can opiates relieve neuropathic pain? *Pain* 1988; 35:365.

France RD, Urban BJ, Keefe FJ. Long-term use of narcotic analgesics in chronic pain. *Soc Sci Med* 1984; 19:1379–1382.

Hammond DL. Do opioids relieve central pain? In: Casey KL (Ed). *Pain and Central Nervous System Disease: The Central Pain Syndromes*. New York: Raven Press, 1991, pp 233–241.

Harati Y, Gooch C, Swenson M, et al. Double-blind randomized trial of tramadol for the treatment of the pain of diabetic neuropathy. *Neurology* 1998; 50(6):1842–1846.

Joranson DE. State medical board guidelines for treatment of intractable pain. *Am Pain Soc Bull* 1995; 5:1–4.

Kjaersgaard-Andersen P, Nafei A, Skov O, et al. Codeine plus paracetamol versus paracetamol in longer-term treatment of chronic pain due to osteoarthritis of the hip. A randomised, double-blind, multi-centre study. *Pain* 1990; 43:309–318.

Kupers RC, Konings H, Adriaensen H, Gybels JM. Morphine differentially affects the sensory and affective pain ratings in neurogenic and idiopathic forms of pain. *Pain* 1991; 47:5–12.

Leijon G, Boivie J. Central post-stroke pain: a controlled trial of amitriptyline and carbamazepine. *Pain* 1989; 36:27–36.

Levine JD, Gordon NC, Smith KR, McBryde RK. Desipramine enhances opiate postoperative analgesia. *Pain* 1986; 27:45–49.

Maruta T, Swanson DW, Finlayson RE. Drug abuse and dependency in patients with chronic pain. *Mayo Clin Proc* 1979; 54:241–244.

Max MB, Schafer SC, Culnane M, Dubner R, Gracely RH. Association of pain relief with side effects in postherpetic neuralgia: a single-dose study of clonidine, codeine, ibuprofen and placebo. *Clin Pharm Ther* 1988; 43:363–371.

McQuay HJ, Tramèr M, Nye BA, et al. A systematic review of antidepressants for neuropathic pain. *Pain* 1996; 68:217–227.

Moulin DE, Iezzi A, Amireh R, et al. Randomized trial of oral morphine for chronic non-cancer pain. *Lancet* 1996; 347:143–147.

O'Neill KA, Valentino D. Chronic desipramine attenuates morphine analgesia. *Pharmacol Biochem Behav* 1986; 24:155–158.

Pagni CA. Central pain due to spinal cord and brainstem damage. In: Wall PD, Melzack R (Eds). *Textbook of Pain.* Edinburgh: Churchill Livingstone, 1984, pp 481–496.

Portenoy RK, Foley KM. Chronic use of opioid analgesics in non-malignant pain: report of 38 cases. *Pain* 1986; 25:171–186.

Portenoy RK, Foley KM, Inturrisi CE. The nature of opioid responsiveness and its implications for neuropathic pain: new hypotheses derived from studies of opioid infusions. *Pain* 1990; 43:273–286.

Porter J, Jick H. Addiction rare in patients treated with narcotics. *N Engl J Med* 1980; 302:123.

Rowbotham MC, Reisner-Keller LA, Fields HL. Both intravenous lidocaine and morphine reduce the pain of postherpetic neuralgia. *Neurology* 1991; 41:1024–1028.

Rowbotham MC, Harden N, Stacey B, Bernstein P, Magnus-Miller L. Gabapentin for the treatment of post-herpetic neuralgia. *JAMA* 1998; 280:1837–1842.

Sindrup SH, Andersen G, Madsen C, et al. Tramadol relieves pain and allodynia in polyneuropathy: a randomised, double-blind, controlled trial. *Pain* 1999; 83:85–90.

Taub A. Opioid analgesics in the treatment of chronic intractable pain of non-neoplastic origin. In: Kitihata LM, Collins JD (Eds). *Narcotic Analgesics in Anesthesiology.* Baltimore: Williams & Wilkins, 1982, pp 199–208.

Urban BJ, France RD, Steinberger EK, Scott DL, Maltbie AA. Long-term use of narcotic/ antidepressant medication in the management of phantom limb pain. *Pain* 1986; 24:191–196.

Wall PD. Neuropathic pain. *Pain* 1990; 43:267–268.

Watson CPN, Babul N. Efficacy of oxycodone in neuropathic pain: a randomized trial in postherpetic neuralgia. *Neurology* 1998; 50:1837–1841.

Watson CPN, Evans RJ, Watt VR, Birkett N. Post-herpetic neuralgia: 208 cases. *Pain* 1988; 35:289–297.

Correspondence to: Michael C. Rowbotham, MD, UCSF Pain Clinical Research Center, 1701 Divisadero Street, Suite 480, San Francisco, CA 94115, USA. Tel: 415-885-7899; Fax: 415-885-7855; email: mcrwind@itsa.ucsf.edu.

Neuropathic Pain: Pathophysiology and Treatment,
Progress in Pain Research and Management, Vol. 21,
edited by Per T. Hansson, Howard L. Fields, Raymond G.
Hill, and Paolo Marchettini, IASP Press, Seattle, © 2001.

12

Topical Local Anesthetics
for Neuropathic Pain

C. Peter N. Watson

Department of Medicine, University of Toronto, Toronto, Canada

> *Pure cocaina ... leaves upon the tongue a peculiar
> numbness, followed by a sensation of cold.*
> Albert Niemann (1860)

Scientifically proven pharmacological approaches, principally some of the antidepressants, anticonvulsants, and opioids, are effective in treating some chronic neuropathic pain conditions. However, none of these agents has better than a modest effect, and adverse effects are problematic, particularly in older patients. Furthermore, many patients with neuropathic pain receive little, if any, benefit from these agents. Simple, effective approaches without significant adverse effects are needed for use alone or as adjunctive therapy. Topical agents offer the promise of such a treatment.

Topical agents for neuropathic pain include local anesthetics, capsaicin, and nonsteroidal anti-inflammatories. The most extensively studied are capsaicin and local anesthetics, particularly lidocaine. Capsaicin has significant limitations; its effect is modest at best, and clinical trials cannot be adequately blinded due to the burning sensation the compound almost always elicits when applied to affected areas. Local anesthetics thus appear to be the most practical of the topical agents; the most extensive research has been done with lidocaine. This chapter will focus on randomized controlled trials (RCTs) showing the benefit of lidocaine used alone and in combination with prilocaine, particularly in postherpetic neuralgia (PHN). PHN, along with painful diabetic neuropathy, is one of the best models for the clinical investigation of neuropathic pain because numbers of patients are adequate and the condition provides a stable chronic pain state and a contralateral control.

MECHANISM OF ACTION OF TOPICAL LOCAL ANESTHETICS IN NEUROPATHIC PAIN

Local anesthetics act on cell membranes to prevent the generation and spread of nerve impulses (Catterall and Mackie 1996). They act by blocking voltage-gated sodium channels, which are responsible for the transient increase in the permeability of excitable membranes to Na^+ that is normally produced by depolarization of the membrane. This anesthetic effect elevates the threshold and slows the rate of rise of the action potential; at lower concentrations it slows conduction velocity. The $A\delta$ and C fibers that subserve pain are more susceptible to local anesthetics than are large fibers; they are blocked earlier and to a greater degree. This greater susceptibility is thought to be related to such factors as the shorter internodal distances of smaller fibers. An important factor in the action of local anesthetics is pH, as I will discuss regarding research with topical lidocaine. Because these agents are only slightly soluble as unprotonated amines, they are marketed as water-soluble hydrochlorides, which causes them to be mildly acidic and thus more stable. The unprotonated form is necessary for diffusion across cell membranes, but the cationic (basic) form seems to act preferentially with sodium channels. Both forms, however, have anesthetic activity.

The action of topical local anesthetics in neuropathic pain could depend on an effect on peripheral factors such as ectopic discharges from sensitized cutaneous nerves bombarding the dorsal horn of the spinal cord. These damaged or regenerating sensitized fibers undergo changes in the number and location of sodium channels. Ectopic impulses from injured peripheral nerves may be sensitive to lower concentrations of local anesthetic than are required for blocking normal impulse conduction (Chabal et al. 1989).

Normal, intact skin is a significant barrier to the action of topical agents. Areas of greater skin thickness, such as the palm of the hand, have a slower onset of analgesia. Highly vascular skin, such as facial skin, is associated with a more rapid onset but a shorter duration of anesthetic effect. The damaged skin in such neuropathic pain conditions as PHN may also influence the action of topical agents, although it is not clear in which direction.

TREATMENT OF NEUROPATHIC PAIN WITH TOPICAL LOCAL ANESTHETICS

Cocaine, the first local anesthetic, has the topical effect of numbness on the mucous membrane of the tongue, as noted by Albert Niemann in 1860 when he first isolated the drug. Since then, local anesthetics have been given to countless patients by various routes to control acute and chronic neuropathic pain.

Local peripheral nerve, epidural, or sympathetic anesthetic blocks appear to relieve acute herpes zoster pain, but no good RCT has shown prevention of PHN. For established PHN, such blocks appear to provide only transient relief for most patients.

Subcutaneous lidocaine infiltration was reported to relieve PHN as long ago as 1941 (Secunda et al. 1941). Rowbotham and Fields (1989a) found that 9 of 12 patients with PHN had at least 50% relief (7 patients had 90% relief) lasting up to several weeks from a single subcutaneous infiltration into the area of maximum pain.

The skin is better penetrated by base forms of local anesthetics than by the mildly acidic hydrochloride forms commonly used (Dalili and Adriani 1971). New formulations such as EMLA Cream (Astra Pharmaceuticals; 2.5% lidocaine and 2.5% prilocaine) and Lidoderm (ENDO Pharmaceuticals; 5% lidocaine), were developed to improve transdermal delivery. Uncontrolled trials have reported a benefit of EMLA in PHN (Milligan et al. 1989; Stow et al. 1989; Litman et al. 1996; Attal et al. 1999). Two of these references are single case reports of refractory cases (Milligan et al. 1989; Litman et al. 1996). The uncontrolled study of Stow et al. (1989) reported significant pain reduction in a trial of EMLA Cream in 12 patients with both spinal and trigeminal PHN under an occlusive dressing for 24 hours. Attal et al. (1999) studied 11 patients with spontaneous or evoked PHN, using a series of daily applications of EMLA for 5 hours per day over 6 consecutive days. Repeated applications significantly reduced paroxysmal pain and both dynamic and static subtypes of mechanical allodynia, but the effects on spontaneous, ongoing pain were more variable. A parallel RCT of topical EMLA versus placebo under occlusive dressing was conducted at two Canadian centers in 77 patients with chronic, nonfacial PHN refractory to other approaches (Lycka et al. 1996). For 13 consecutive days patients received the cream for 10 hours. Pain was evaluated before treatment, after 6 hours of treatment, and prior to cream removal. The patients were seen at 7, 14, and 28 days. Of 71 evaluable patients, only 33 completed the study according to the protocol. No significant difference was seen between treatment groups with regard to several outcome measures for pain and pain relief. Although occasional patients may benefit from EMLA topically, its current method of use does not appear to help most patients.

Rowbotham and coworkers have reported a randomized, double-blind, vehicle-controlled study of 5% lidocaine in gel form in PHN (Rowbotham et al. 1995). A total of 39 out of 46 patients entering the study completed the three-session crossover study. The 16 patients with facial or upper cervical PHN had gel applied without an occlusive dressing during the 8-hour sessions, and the 23 patients with PHN of the torso and limbs had gel applied under Tegaderm dressings for 24 hours. To analyze gel effects and systemic absorption of lidocaine through normal and postherpetic skin, the investigators treated both the painful area and the matching contralateral area of skin during each session. One session was a double-placebo session, one session consisted of application of lidocaine gel to the painful area and of vehicle to contralateral normal skin, and one session consisted of application of lidocaine gel to the matching contralateral normal skin (a control for systemic absorption of lidocaine as the basis of pain relief) and of vehicle on the painful area. A significant decrease in pain intensity and a significant increase in pain relief scores were measured on a visual analogue scale (VAS) with lidocaine gel compared to vehicle at 8 and 24 hours in the torso/limb group. In the facial/upper cervical group there were no significant differences between active drug and vehicle in pain intensity VAS scores, but pain relief scores significantly favored the active drug at nearly all time points. A difference in facial skin thickness and vascularity may account for this difference. Forty-two of 50 patients recruited were followed for up to 30 months after choosing lidocaine gel treatment. Thirty-one patients used this treatment for more than 2 months, and 23 of 31 (55% of the 42 patients followed) reported moderate or better relief. Thirteen of the 16 patients in the facial/upper cervical group requested open-label treatment with lidocaine gel. Follow-up for this group for up to 14 months indicated that 10 of the 13 patients continued to use it as needed.

Occlusive dressings used with topical agents are poorly tolerated and are impractical for many PHN sufferers. A gel of 5% lidocaine has been incorporated into adhesive patches with a nonwoven, polyethylene adhesive backing that can be used to cover the area of pain. A further randomized, placebo-controlled trial (Rowbotham et al. 1996a) has demonstrated the benefit of the lidocaine patch form. Thirty-five of 40 recruited subjects with PHN affecting the torso or extremities completed a four-session, crossover, random-order, double-blind, vehicle-controlled study of the analgesic effects of this patch. Lidocaine patches were applied in two of four 12-hour long sessions; in another session, vehicle patches were applied, and the remaining session was a no-treatment observation session. Lidocaine patches significantly reduced pain intensity at all time points from 30 minutes to 12 hours compared to the observation session and at all time points at 4–12 hours compared to vehicle patches. Lidocaine patches were superior to both no-treatment observations and vehicle patches in averaged category pain relief scores. Minimal systemic absorption was documented. No systemic side effects occurred, and patches were well tolerated on allodynic skin for 12 hours. The majority (24 of 35 subjects) reported partial pain relief, with

10 of 35 subjects (28%) noting moderate or better relief. The vehicle patch alone had a significant pain-reducing effect compared with no treatment, presumably by protecting painful, sensitive skin from contact with clothing and gentle touch. The patch itself appeared to be a significant advance in this study because it was so well tolerated and exerted its own protective effect.

A longer RCT of parallel design of the lidocaine patch was conducted in 150 patients with PHN affecting the torso or limbs who were treated with the lidocaine ($n = 100$) or vehicle patch ($n = 50$) for 4 weeks. On entering the study, patients participated in two laboratory sessions to assess acute pain-relieving effects, blood levels, and sensory effects of patch application (Rowbotham et al. 1996b). More than 60% of subjects in the lidocaine patch group achieved moderate or better pain relief.

A randomized, vehicle-controlled trial (Galer et al. 1999) addressed the contribution of the patch alone versus the lidocaine patch in providing relief in PHN because of the protective effect of the patch observed in previous work. This study had an enriched enrollment design as all 33 subjects had experienced moderate or better relief with topical lidocaine patches on a regular basis for at least a month prior to study enrollment. This was a crossover study with two treatment periods. The primary efficacy variable was "time to exit"; subjects were allowed to discontinue either treatment period if their pain relief score decreased by two or more categories on a pain relief scale for two consecutive days. Patients participated from home and received a telephone assessment at least 6 days per week. The median time to exit with the lidocaine patch phase was greater than 14 days, whereas the vehicle patch exit time was 3.8 days. Twenty-five of 32 subjects (78%) preferred the lidocaine patch as compared with 3/32 (9.4%) for the vehicle patch. No difference in adverse events was noted. The most common untoward effect was "application site reaction" (skin redness or rash), which occurred in about 30% of patients in each group. The authors concluded that the topical lidocaine patch gave significantly better pain relief than did the vehicle patch.

An open-label study (Devers et al. 2000) has shown benefit for the lidocaine patch in several neuropathic pain states including incisional neuralgia, painful diabetic neuropathy, complex regional pain syndrome, and post-amputation stump pain. Sixteen such patients were treated with the lidocaine patch. Moderate or greater pain relief was reported in 13 patients (81%), with mean duration of patch use of 6 weeks and no adverse effects. RCTs are necessary to further evaluate the benefit of lidocaine patches in these conditions.

CONCLUSIONS

The topical lidocaine patch holds significant promise for the treatment of PHN and other neuropathic pain conditions. Side effects are minor, and blood levels of topical lidocaine are low (Rowbotham and Fields 1989; Stow et al. 1989; Rowbotham et al. 1996a). Follow-up assessment in published RCTs reveals that 30–53% of patients with PHN report at least moderate benefit from this approach. The patch itself appears to be an advance over occlusive "food wrap" type dressings because it seems better tolerated, it can be cut to fit the area of pain, and it protects against the light tactile stimuli that so often provoke pain in PHN. The patch may have limitations if the pain is in the distribution of the ophthalmic division of the trigeminal nerve (one of the most common sites for intractable PHN) because patients may have severe pain in the scalp areas (to which the patch cannot easily be affixed). However, the lidocaine patch can be recommended in PHN as monotherapy or, if a partial effect occurs, as an adjunct to oral agents such as antidepressants, anticonvulsants, or opioids. Further studies of the lidocaine patch are necessary in other neuropathic pain conditions.

REFERENCES

Attal N, Brasseur L, Chauvin M, et al. Effects of single and repeated application on a eutectic mixture of local anaesthetics (EMLA) cream on spontaneous and evoked pain in post-herpetic neuralgia. *Pain* 1999; 81(1–2):203–209.

Catterall W, Mackie K. Local anaesthetics. In: Hardman JG, Limbird LE, Morinoff PB, et al. (Eds). *Goodman and Gilman's The Pharmacologic Basis of Therapeutics,* 9th ed. New York: McGraw-Hill, 1996.

Chabal C, Russell LC, Burchiel K. The effect of intravenous lidocaine, tocainide, and mexiletine on spontaneously active fibers arising in rat sciatic nerve neuromas. *Pain* 1989; 38:333–338.

Dalili H, Adriani J. The efficacy of local anaesthetics in blockading the effects of itch, burning and pain in normal and "sunburned" skin. *Clin Pharmacol Ther* 1971; 12:913–919.

Devers A, Galer BS. Topical lidocaine patch relieves a variety of neuropathic pain conditions: an open label study. *Clin J Pain* 2000; 16:205–208.

Galer BS, Rowbotham MC, Perander J, Friedman E. Topical lidocaine patch relieves postherpetic neuralgia more effectively than a vehicle topical patch: results of an enriched enrollment study. *Pain* 1999; 80:533–538.

Litman SJ, Vikun SA, Poppers PJ. Use of EMLA cream in the treatment of post-herpetic neuralgia. *J Clin Anesth* 1996; 8:54–57.

Lycka BA, Watson CPN, Nevin K. EMLA cream for treatment of postherpetic neuralgia. In: *American Pain Society 15th Annual Meeting—Abstracts.* Washington, DC: American Pain Society, Nov 14–17, 1996, A-III.

Milligan KA, Atkinson RE, Schofield PA. Lignocaine-prilocaine cream in postherpetic neuralgia. *BMJ* 1989; 298:253.

Niemann A. On the alkaloid and other constituents of coca leaves. *Am J Pharmacy* 1860; 122–126.

Rowbotham MC, Fields HL. Topical lidocaine reduces pain in post-herpetic neuralgia. *Pain* 1989a; 38:297–301.

Rowbotham MC, Fields HL. Post-herpetic neuralgia: the relation of pain complaint, sensory disturbance, and skin temperature. *Pain* 1989b; 39:129–144.

Rowbotham MC, Reisner LA, Fields HL. Both intravenous lidocaine and morphine reduce the pain of postherpetic neuralgia. *Neurology* 1991; 41:1024–1028.

Rowbotham MC, Davies PS, Fields HL. Topical lidocaine gel relieves postherpetic neuralgia. *Ann Neurol* 1995; 37:246–253.

Rowbotham MC, Davies PS, Verkernpinck C, et al. Lidocaine patch: double-blind controlled study of a new treatment method for post-herpetic neuralgia. *Pain* 1996a; 65:39–44.

Rowbotham MC, Davies PS, Galer BS. Multicenter, double-blind, vehicle-controlled trial of long term use of lidocaine patches for postherpetic neuralgia. In: *Abstracts: 8th World Congress on Pain*. Seattle: IASP Press, 1996b, p 274.

Secunda L, Wolf W, Price J. Herpes zoster: local anaesthetics in the treatment of pain. *N Engl J Med* 1941; 224:501–503.

Stow PJ, Glynn CJ, Minor B. EMLA cream in the treatment of post-herpetic neuralgia: efficacy and pharmacokinetic profile. *Pain* 1989; 39:301–305.

Correspondence to: C. Peter N. Watson, MD, FRCPC, 1 Sir Williams Lane, Toronto, Ontario, Canada, M9A 1T8.

Neuropathic Pain: Pathophysiology and Treatment,
Progress in Pain Research and Management, Vol. 21,
edited by Per T. Hansson, Howard L. Fields, Raymond G.
Hill, and Paolo Marchettini, IASP Press, Seattle, © 2001.

13

Central Nervous System Stimulation for Neuropathic Pain

Bengt Linderoth and Björn A. Meyerson

*Department of Neurosurgery, Karolinska Hospital/Institute,
Stockholm, Sweden*

Severe neuropathic pain remains a treatment challenge because few pharmacological therapies offer significant benefits and nerve blocks rarely provide long-term pain relief. Neurosurgical methods to treat neuropathic pain date back to lesional strategies used in the early 1900s, followed by neurostimulation methods developed in the early 1960s. These treatments, sometimes referred to as "neuroaugmentation" or "neuromodulation," are still based on vague theories about pain pathophysiology and the involvement of endogenous pain controls.

The history of neurostimulation therapy is often believed to have begun with the presentation of the gate control theory by Melzack and Wall (1965), but Mazars and colleagues (1973, 1975) had begun conducting trials of electric stimulation in Paris in about 1962, using implanted electrodes in the sensory thalamus to treat severe neuropathic pain. This treatment approach was based on the theory of Head and Holmes (1911) that chronic pain originates from an imbalance between the "epicritic" and "protopathic" components of the afferent systems. These authors postulated that a nervous system lesion could diminish epicritic (non-nociceptive) afference, leading to a relative overflow of protopathic (nociceptive) influx that could cause persistent pain.

The gate control concept generated new research aiming to manipulate endogenous pain controls. Early trials introduced low-intensity stimulation of peripheral nerves via implanted electrodes (reported by Sweet 1976), followed by spinal cord stimulation (SCS) (Shealy et al. 1967). Transcutaneous electric nerve stimulation (TENS), introduced at the same time, was used at that time merely to screen patients for SCS treatment. A more specialized strategy, designed to activate selected groups of large-diameter fibers, was stimulation of the trigeminal ganglion and rootlets in cases of painful trigeminal neuropathy (Steude 1978; Meyerson and Håkanson 1986; Young 1995). The gate control theory has been much criticized, but it provides a general conceptual base for most of the stimulation pain treatments currently in use.

A second major breakthrough in pain research was the demonstration by Reynolds (1969) of an endogenous pain-modulatory system in the periaqueductal gray (PAG). This discovery triggered the first attempts to activate this region by implanting electrodes (Richardson and Akil 1977) in an effort to reproduce the powerful analgesia observed in animal experiments.

A third approach, reminding us of the complexity of the endogenous control systems of the central nervous system (CNS), began with a report by Tsubokawa et al. (1991) that electrical activation of the cortical motor region could induce pain relief in post-stroke pain, one of the most therapy-resistant neuropathic pain conditions. The "classical" neurophysiological literature had already established that stimulation of the sensory-motor cortex may inhibit nociceptive dorsal horn neurons (e.g., Lindblom and Ottosson 1957), and more recent studies have demonstrated that abnormally enhanced neuronal discharge in the brainstem following deafferentation is also attenuated by such stimulation (Namba et al. 1988). These effects may reflect the functional background to the beneficial effects of motor cortex stimulation.

This chapter discusses the possible neurophysiological mechanisms underlying the pain-relieving effects of various techniques of CNS stimulation and reviews the clinical applications of these methods in various neuropathic pain conditions.

SPINAL CORD STIMULATION

Antidromic stimulation of the large fibers in the dorsal columns (also referred to as dorsal column stimulation [DCS]) is thought to activate the proposed gating mechanisms in the dorsal horn (DH). Accordingly, SCS should also be effective in suppressing nociceptive pain, both acute and chronic. Paradoxically, however, SCS has a *direct* effect on neuropathic forms of pain (e.g., Gybels and Sweet 1989). Reported SCS effects on other types of pain are probably secondary to stimulation-induced alterations in the cardiovascular system.

More than 15,000 SCS implantations are performed each year worldwide, reflecting a growing awareness of the effectiveness of SCS for neuropathic pain, for which there are few alternative therapies. A further reason for the renewed interest in SCS is its application for indications other than neurogenic pain. For example, it is used to treat nociceptive pain in peripheral vascular disease (PVD) and in refractory angina pectoris. However, in these conditions the pain relief obtainable with SCS is presumably due to its effect on tissue ischemia (for these applications of SCS see Linderoth and Foreman 1999; Meyerson and Linderoth 2000a; Linderoth and Meyerson 2001.)

Two consensus documents specify indications for SCS and guidelines for its implementation (North and Levy 1994; Gybels et al. 1998; for reviews see Simpson 1994; Barolat 1995; Shetter 1997; Meyerson and Linderoth 1999; North and Linderoth 2000).

Comments on the surgical technique. Implantation of SCS systems has become a routine procedure at many pain centers. Percutaneous leads are implanted under local anesthesia with the patient in a prone, or sometimes in a sitting position. Perioperative fluoroscopy is always used to guide the lead to the intended position, where stimulation evokes paresthesiae throughout the painful region. The electrode is then anchored subcutaneously. A period of trial stimulation usually follows that may last from a few days up to several weeks. If the lead has a tendency to migrate or if it is difficult to obtain complete paresthesia coverage of the painful region, a plate electrode may be implanted via a small laminotomy under local or general anesthesia. In some cases multiple leads or leads with complex arrays of poles may be preferred (for reviews, see Meyerson and Linderoth 2000a; North and Linderoth 2000).

PHYSIOLOGICAL MECHANISMS

SCS in neuropathic pain

Despite extensive use of SCS for more than 30 years, the mechanisms involved in its pain-relieving effect are still poorly understood. The technical advancement of stimulation devices and of implantation techniques is in sharp contrast to the lack of stringent indications and validated prognostic factors. Extensive reviews on the mode of action of SCS have recently been published (Roberts and Rees 1994; Linderoth 1995; Linderoth and Foreman 1999; Meyerson and Linderoth 2000c; Linderoth and Meyerson 2001).

Neurophysiological and behavioral studies. In the 1970s and 1980s, numerous animal experiments employing acute, noxious stimuli (heat, pinch, pressure, electrical stimuli, algogenic substances) were performed to elucidate the mechanisms of SCS (e.g., Handwerker et al. 1975, Shetter and Atkinson 1977). These experiments demonstrated that neuronal activity in the DH and spinothalamic tract evoked by peripheral noxious stimuli could be inhibited by concomitant antidromic activation of the dorsal columns (DC) (e.g., Foreman et al. 1976; Dubuisson 1989).

Some studies suggest that the SCS effect is at least partially dependent on supraspinal mechanisms. In a series of experiments, Saadé and his group (1985, 1999) found that the inhibitory effect of SCS persisted after DC transection caudal to the stimulating electrode, whereas it was abolished by a DC lesion rostral to the stimulation site.

Most of the early studies have limited clinical relevance because they used intact animals and acute nociceptive peripheral stimuli. Moreover, SCS generally was applied for short periods of time and with high intensity; in most studies the observed effects were short-lasting. To mimic a type of neuropathic pain that often responds well to SCS, we performed a series of studies on rats with mononeuropathy produced by partial injury of the sciatic nerve according to Bennett and Xie (1988) or Seltzer et al. (1990). These rats display hypersensitivity to tactile stimulation of the nerve-lesioned hindpaw, resembling the hypersensitivity to innocuous stimulation (allodynia) sometimes present in patients with neuropathic pain. SCS delivered via an implanted miniature electrode system can suppress this hypersensitivity (Meyerson et al. 1995). This effect outlasts a stimulation period of 20 minutes by up to an hour. The findings from our behavioral studies are supported by recordings from sensitized wide-dynamic-range (WDR) neurons in the dorsal horns of "allodynic" rats responsive to stimulation therapy. During and after SCS their firing patterns were normalized (Yakhnitsa et al. 1999). It was reported in 1975 that SCS may effectively suppress allodynia and hyperalgesia to both tactile and thermal stimuli in patients with peripheral nerve injury (Lindblom and Meyerson 1975). Our animal experiments led us to conclude that SCS may have a selective inhibitory effect on the abnormal functioning of the spinal projection of Aβ fibers on WDR neurons (Yakhnitsa et al. 1999).

Neurochemical mechanisms. Data from human studies on biochemical correlates to SCS are sparse and partly contradictory. In an experimental study from 1985, Duggan and Foong reported that the SCS-induced inhibition of spinothalamic tract neurons could be counteracted by the $GABA_A$ (γ-aminobutyric acid) antagonist bicuculline. In a series of studies we have explored the possible role of GABA in SCS. Using microdialysis we demonstrated that the basal DH release of GABA was significantly lower in rats displaying tactile allodynia after sciatic nerve injury than in intact animals. Moreover, SCS increased GABA release in animals that had responded to SCS in preceding behavioral experiments with a normalization of the withdrawal thresholds in the nerve-injured hindpaw (Stiller et al. 1996). In another microdialysis study, we showed that rats with nerve injury and tactile allodynia have an increased basal DH release of the excitatory amino acids (EAAs) glutamate and aspartate; SCS reduces release of these EAAs and increases release of GABA (Cui et al. 1997a). In behavioral studies, we observed that intrathecal (i.t.) administration of GABA or its agonists in nerve-injured rats markedly enhances the effect of SCS on tactile allodynia. There are indications that the effect is partially mediated via $GABA_B$ receptors (Cui et al. 1996). It was also found that intrathecal administration of the adenosine A1 agonist R-PIA transformed rats that did not respond to SCS into responders, even at low doses that were ineffective when used alone (Cui et al. 1997b). Furthermore, R-PIA and baclofen seemed to have a synergistic effect (Cui et al. 1998). Fig. 1 illustrates a simplified model of putative biochemical mechanisms involved in the pain-relieving effect of SCS.

The synergistic effects we observed in rats of administration of baclofen and/or adenosine along with SCS encouraged us to conduct clinical trials with patients who were receiving insufficient therapeutic effect from SCS treatment (Meyerson et al. 1997). Adenosine sometimes induces severe pain when administered i.t., so we have postponed further trials with this drug. On the other hand, 6 of 30 patients studied responded positively to the addition of low i.t. doses of baclofen to SCS. We are treating four patients with both SCS and continuous baclofen infusion via an implanted, programmable pump. These patients originally received only slight pain relief from SCS, but the addition of baclofen, in a dose that was ineffective when given alone, has produced an estimated 75–100% alleviation of pain (B. Linderoth, G. Lind, and B.A. Meyerson, unpublished data).

SCS in ischemic pain and in pain conditions involving dysautonomia/dystrophy

It is well known that SCS can induce pronounced peripheral vasodilatation in both the macrocirculation (e.g., Augustinsson et al. 1985) and microcirculation (Jacobs et al. 1988); this effect is a plausible reason why SCS can alleviate ischemic pain in peripheral vascular disease (PVD). Evidence suggests that the beneficial SCS effect in PVD is primarily due to a modulation of autonomic activity, and that the peripheral vasodilatation following SCS is secondary to a decreased sympathetic tone associated with the vasodilatory effect (for discussion, see Linderoth 1995; Linderoth and Meyerson 1995; Linderoth and Foreman 1999). This hypothesis is partly based on experimental findings showing that cutting of the ventral roots, sectioning of the sciatic nerve, or bilateral lumbar sympathectomy abolished the vasodilatory effect of SCS (Linderoth et al. 1991). In pain conditions associated with signs of sympathetic dysfunction, which may be the case in

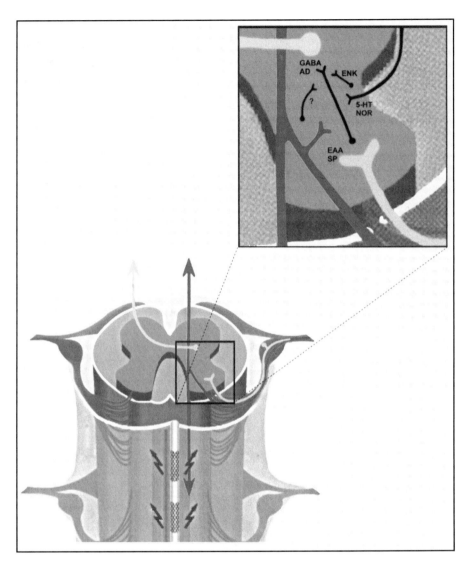

Fig. 1. Schematic illustration of the spinal cord with a dorsal epidural multipolar electrode. The activation of dorsal column axons transmits impulses antidromically via collaterals to the target regions in the dorsal horns. The schematic insert figure (top right) depicts the increased release of GABA from dorsal horn interneurons, which decreases the release of the excitatory amino acids (EAAs) glutamate and aspartate following SCS in nerve-lesioned rats with tactile "allodynia." Adenosine (AD) may play a role similar to that of GABA. Norepinephrine (NOR) and serotonin (5-HT), possibly emanating from descending inhibitory pathways, may also be involved in producing the beneficial effects. (ENK = enkephalin; SP = substance P). (Original drawing by A. Röhl; redrawn after Cui 1999, with permission).

both types of complex regional pain syndrome (CRPS-I, formerly reflex sympathetic dystrophy, and CRPS-II, sometimes known as causalgia), a sympathicolytic action of SCS may contribute to the pain-relieving effect (see, e.g., Baron et al. 1999; Wasner et al. 1999; Kemler 2000a). However, these effects are only partially understood and are still a matter of controversy (see Max et al. 1999; Kemler et al. 2000b). Some investigators have proposed that antidromic activation of large afferents may stimulate the release of vasoactive substances; interest has focused on SCS-induced peripheral release of calcitonin gene-related peptide (CGRP) (e.g., Croom et al. 1997).

The beneficial effect of SCS in pain syndromes that are partly related to sympathetic dysfunction also may result either from inhibitory influences on pathological adrenergic-somatosensory couplings or from effects on the peripheral ischemia that activates damaged afferents (the indirect coupling hypothesis) (e.g., Michaelis 2000; Häbler et al. 2000). However, as yet we lack firm data to support these ideas.

CLINICAL APPLICATION

As is the case for other forms of electric stimulation in pain treatment, SCS requires the active participation of the patient in operating the stimulation equipment. The patient should be instructed to differentiate true pain relief from the possible masking effect of the stimulation-induced paresthesiae.

The special features of SCS, particularly when applied for neuropathic pain, create heavy demands on the treating physician. Physicians who undertake the responsibility of giving patients SCS treatment must be prepared to supply almost lifelong support because patients suitable for SCS typically suffer from a chronic multifactorial disease with pain as the major, but not the only, reason for their incapacity.

A further prerequisite for SCS treatment is a thorough pain analysis. It is of particular importance to establish the relative importance of neuropathic pain components in "mixed pain conditions," a term used to imply the coexistence of neuropathic and nociceptive pains.

We strongly recommend that the pretreatment evaluation should include examination by a psychologist or a pain-oriented psychiatrist. Psychological factors correlate highly with the outcome of SCS (e.g., Kupers et al. 1994; Burchiel et al. 1995; for discussion, see Simpson 1994). A psychological examination can exclude patients with major personality disorders, those with deficient capacity to collaborate with caregivers and to communicate their pain problems, those with drug-seeking behavior or drug abuse, and those with poor pain-coping ability ("chronic pain behavior"). The fact that a patient is on regular opioid medication does not constitute an exclusion criterion provided that the medication provides a true analgesic effect and that there is no history of rapid dose escalation that would suggest tolerance or drug seeking. Contrary to arguments proposed in several studies, we feel that ongoing litigation is not by itself a contraindication.

INDICATIONS AND RESULTS

Neuropathic pain conditions likely to respond to SCS are listed in Table I.

Pain due to peripheral nerve injury. Many specialists regard this type of pain as the prime indication for SCS, with the best chances of obtaining satisfactory and long-lasting pain relief (e.g., Siegfried 1991; Simpson 1994; Barolat 1995; Lazorthes et al. 1995). However, others have reported relatively modest results in such cases as compared to spinal root pain (e.g., North et al. 1993).

Nerve injury associated with pain, both spontaneous and evoked, may follow trauma, surgery, entrapment, inflammation, and metabolic disorders (polyneuropathy). This form of pain may result from injury to one major nerve, e.g., ulnar nerve entrapment, or from partial injury to distal nerve branches, e.g., incisional pain. CRPS types I and II constitute a special form of peripheral nerve injury pain; they also may respond to SCS.

The most extensive study, with regard to both number of cases and length of follow-up, on SCS in pain due to peripheral nerve injury is a cooperative study from Toulouse and Zürich (Lazorthes et al. 1995). Of the 132 patients from Zürich, 90% had a positive long-term result (over 2–20 years). The outcome assessment included degree of pain relief, daily life functioning, and consumption of analgesics. In our experience a positive effect of SCS may be retained for long periods of time; in a retrospective study with a mean follow-up of 6.8 years we found that 27 out of 38 patients with peripheral nerve injury pain still regularly used their stimulators (Meyerson et al. 1991). Fig. 2 shows the radiograph of the thoracic spine of a patient with postsurgical inguinal neuralgia; SCS had provided good pain relief for 25 years. Another relatively large study was reported by Sanchez-Ledesma et al. (1989). Out of 49 patients characterized as having "peripheral deafferentation pain," 36 responded favorably to trial stimulation. They were followed for 5.5 years, and 57% of the patients reported substantial pain relief (>75%). In a meta-analysis of 11 studies from the 1980s on SCS treatment of pain due to peripheral nerve injury, often termed reflex sympathetic dystrophy (RSD) or causalgia, 70% of the patients originally subjected to trial stimulation had a favorable long-term outcome (Spiegelmann and Friedman 1991; see also Barolat 1989). In contrast to these relatively

Table I
Indications for spinal cord stimulation (SCS) in neuropathic pain

Peripheral Nerve Lesion (Preganglionic)

Trauma
Surgery (including incisional scar pain)
Entrapment
CRPS types I and II*
Brachial and lumbosacral plexus pain†
    Trauma, radiation, malignancy
Polyneuropathy
    Diabetic
Deafferentation pain
    Anesthesia dolorosa (nonfacial)
    Stump pain
    Phantom pain

Spinal Root or Ganglion Lesion

Cervical or thoracic rhizopathy
Lumbosacral rhizopathy, including cauda equina syndrome
Surgery, trauma, spondylosis with foraminal obliteration
Postherpetic neuralgia

Spinal Cord Lesion

Incomplete lesion with preservation of dorsal column function‡
Complete lesion with segmental pain at lesion level
Multiple sclerosis
Postcordotomy dysesthesia

Questionable

Pain confined to the neck, thoracic spine, and low back
Pain confined to midline parts of the trunk (thorax, abdomen)
Perineal, rectal, and genital pain
Pain of supraspinal origin

---

* Complex regional pain syndrome (CRPS) type I, according to the International Association for the Study of Pain's definition (Merskey and Bogduk 1994), develops after an initiating noxious event, is not limited to the distribution of a single peripheral nerve, and is disproportionate to the inciting event. There may be edema, changes in skin blood flow, abnormal sudomotor activity, and allodynia/hyperalgesia. Previously this condition was often referred to as reflex sympathetic dystrophy. The syndrome may be sympathetically maintained or sympathetically independent. In CRPS type II, previously often referred to as causalgia, pain appears after partial injury of a nerve or one of its major branches, usually in the hand or foot.
† Pain due to complete avulsion of spinal roots does not respond.
‡ Pain in extensive spinal cord disease such as syringomyelia or myelopathy that may be caused by spinal stenosis or myelitis is less likely to respond.

favorable results, in a series of 30 patients with pain associated with peripheral neuropathy only 14 patients enjoyed long-term pain relief (Kumar et al. 1996). However, the same group recently reported that out of 12 patients diagnosed as having RSD, eight had excellent pain relief and four described good results, with a mean follow-up of 41 months (Kumar et al. 1997).

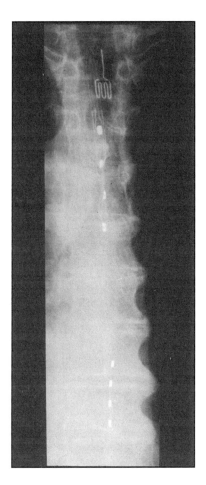

Fig. 2. Radiograph of the thoracic spine of a patient who has had SCS treatment for severe chronic inguinal neuralgia for 25 years. The most rostral electrode was implanted in 1976; when it ceased to function after several years, a second plate electrode was inserted via a small laminectomy. This electrode was later changed to a percutaneous four-polar electrode (the caudal lead). The earlier, rostral electrodes produced paresthesiae in the entire lower body while the caudal electrode more selectively targeted the painful region. The patient contacted the clinic again in the spring of 2000 because of a broken extension, which was replaced. She was still dependent on daily stimulation sessions.

The most recent study is that of Kemler et al. (2000a), who randomized 54 RSD patients to SCS plus physiotherapy or to conventional treatment with physiotherapy alone. Six months after the implant there were significant differences in favor of the SCS-treated group ($n = 36$) in pain intensity rated on a visual analogue scale and in a global measure of perceived effect of the therapy. Differences between the two groups were nonsignificant in other measures including functional status and perceived quality of life.

Painful diabetic peripheral neuropathy was the subject of a well-conducted study that included placebo stimulation using a stimulator without a battery (Tesfaye et al. 1996). At the end of the study (14 months' follow-up), 6 of the 10 patients receiving genuine stimulation gained significant pain relief and improved exercise tolerance. No patients reported pain relief with placebo "stimulation."

Pain after spinal root injury. Lumbosacral rhizopathy is regarded by many authors to be the best indication for SCS treatment. The literature often refers to this condition as "failed back surgery syndrome" (FBSS) or "postlaminectomy syndrome," which are misnomers because the condition is neither a disease nor a pain diagnosis. In fact, these patients often present with a mixture of both nociceptive and neuropathic pain components. Most authors contend that SCS predominantly influences the "radiating pain components" or "pain in the leg," which conceivably may correspond to the neuropathic pain associated with lumbosacral rhizopathy.

Turner et al. (1995) performed a meta-analysis of publications (1967–1994) on SCS for chronic "low back pain." All 39 studies included were case series because no randomized trials could be retrieved. An average of 74% of patients screened with trial stimulation were permanently implanted. At a mean follow-up of 16 months, an average of 59% of patients reported >50% pain relief. In another prospective, multicenter study comprising 219 patients with "chronic back and extremity pain" who received trial stimulation, 83% were permanently implanted. After a year, 55% of these patients were successfully managing their pain (Burchiel et al. 1996). Preliminary results have been reported from an ongoing prospective, randomized study comparing the outcome of SCS to reoperation in patients suffering from "FBSS" (North et al. 1994). Twenty-seven patients in this series followed for more than 6 months showed a statistically significant advantage for SCS over reoperation.

One of the most detailed and well-performed studies is that of North et al. (1993), with a mean follow-up of 7 years. Of 153 patients classified as having "FBSS," 133 received permanent electrode implants. Of particular interest is that in this study follow-up assessments were performed by a "disinterested third party." About 50% of the patients were classified as having a successful outcome with regard to pain relief, consumption of analgesics, and level of functioning. It should be emphasized that the patients were carefully selected; only those with a predominant radiating pain in the leg(s) were included.

Lumbosacral rhizopathy is doubtless a good indication for SCS treatment, but most published studies fail to precisely define the selection criteria. Insufficient information is provided on patients, and the relative severity of pain in the lower back and pain due to rhizopathy is often poorly analyzed and described.

CONCLUSIONS: SCS FOR NEUROPATHIC PAIN

SCS is not evidence based in a strict sense because of the paucity of prospective controlled studies. Moreover, because paresthesiae are a prerequisite for pain relief, genuine double-blind study designs are impossible. Nevertheless, over the past two decades numerous studies have documented the efficacy of SCS in treating certain pain conditions that are otherwise notoriously difficult to manage; the results of these studies are surprisingly concordant with regard to pain relief. Experienced pain clinicians generally agree that SCS is an indispensable treatment modality for many patients with certain forms of chronic neuropathic pain. There is no evidence yet that SCS *directly* influences nociceptive forms of pain. However, beneficial effects may be obtained via indirect routes, e.g., by influencing the microcirculation.

We believe that SCS is presently underused. To promote the dissemination of this technique we recommend that it should be adopted by pain specialists outside the neurosurgical profession. However, it should only be used within the context of a multidisciplinary pain team in centers with extensive experience in managing difficult pain cases (cf. Kupers et al. 1994). SCS treatment is time consuming and requires long-term doctor-patient contact and expensive equipment. Nevertheless, recent studies indicate that SCS treatment is highly cost-effective (Bell et al. 1997).

The lack of a thorough understanding of the physiological and biochemical mechanisms involved in the pain-relieving effect of SCS has hampered its further dissemination and development. Continuing investigation of its mode of action is greatly needed.

INTRACRANIAL STIMULATION

In the late 1970s several clinical studies provided evidence that intracerebral stimulation (ICS) (often referred to as deep brain stimulation [DBS]) would be useful in managing pain otherwise resistant to any therapeutic modality (for review, see Gybels and Sweet 1989; Gybels and Kupers 1995; Richardson 1995; Meyerson and Linderoth 2000b). Some recent retrospective studies have established the long-lasting positive effects of stimulation applied in the medial thalamus to treat mixed nociceptive-neuropathic pain, predominantly in the condition generally referred to as "low back pain" (Kumar et al. 1997; Young and Rinaldi 1997).

ICS has evolved along two lines, corresponding to the two major target regions for stimulation: the sensory thalamic nuclei (the ventroposterior medial nucleus [VPM] and the ventroposterior lateral nucleus [VPL]) and the periaqueductal-periventricular gray region (PAG/PVG) (Fig. 3). Stimulation in these two regions may influence pain by activating different mechanisms or systems. Robust evidence indicates that stimulation in the sensory thalamus is selectively effective for neuropathic pain, often referred to as deafferentation pain, whereas PAG/PVG stimulation appears preferentially to affect nociceptive forms of pain.

Recent years have seen great interest in a novel mode of CNS stimulation targeting the precentral motor area (Brodmann's area 4). This treatment, pioneered by Tsubokawa and colleagues (1991) has proven particularly effective for central post-stroke pain, which is otherwise notoriously difficult to manage. Motor cortex stimulation also appears to be a promising treatment for painful trigeminal neuropathy, including facial anesthesia dolorosa (Meyerson et al. 1993; Nguyen et al. 1999).

INTRACEREBRAL STIMULATION

Basic mechanisms

Sensory thalamic stimulation. The first trials with stimulation in the sensory thalamic nucleus were performed in Paris by Mazars in the early 1960s (Mazars et al. 1973, 1975). It is unlikely that those who pioneered this new treatment approach in the United States, Hosobuchi et al. (1973) and Adams et al. (1974), were aware of the earlier experiments in Paris.

Only a few experimental studies have attempted to elucidate the mechanisms by which sensory thalamic stimulation relieves pain. In view of the similarities between this form of stimulation and SCS, it was natural to postulate supraspinal gating mechanisms. Experiments in monkeys have shown

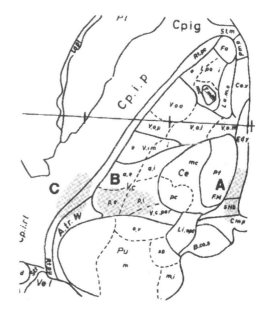

Fig. 3. Approximate location and extent of stimulation-susceptible regions in (A) the periventricular gray matter (PVG), (B) the sensory thalamic nuclei, and (C) the internal capsule (midline to the right of the figure). Note that the PVG comprises the endymalis nucleus and at least part of the parafascicular nucleus. The internal capsular target region is located in the most posterior and medial portion and comprises part of the area triangularis and nucleus reticularis pulvinaris. This target was earlier selected to treat central pain syndromes. (Horizontal section 2 mm above the intercommissural plane; distances between marks on the horizontal lines represent 10 mm.) Adapted from Schaltenbrand and Bailey's stereotactic atlas (1959), with permission.

that stimulation of the ventrobasal complex of the thalamus can inhibit spinothalamic tract WDR neurons in the dorsal horn that are activated by both innocuous and noxious peripheral stimuli (Gerhart 1983).

In an electrophysiological study designed to mimic the neuropathic pain, cats were subjected to trigeminal deafferentation, which increased spontaneous neuronal discharge in the spinal trigeminal nucleus (Namba and Nishimoto 1988). Stimulation of both the sensory thalamus and the internal capsule inhibited this deafferentation hyperactivity in about 40% of neurons, with long-lasting post-stimulatory effects. Kupers and Gybels (1993) performed an interesting behavioral study on a rat model of mononeuropathy. Following partial sciatic nerve injury, these animals displayed signs of neuropathy in the form of tactile hypersensitivity in the hindpaw of the nerve-ligated leg; stimulation applied to the sensory thalamus markedly suppressed this hypersensitivity.

Ample evidence indicates that conditions of neuropathic pain, in particular central pain, create profound functional changes in the sensory thalamus. A series of crucial studies using microstimulation and microrecording in patients during stereotactic interventions have demonstrated thalamic somatotopic reorganization and marked signs of neural hyperexcitability in patients with neuropathic pain (e.g., Tasker et al. 1992; Lenz et al. 1993; Lenz and Dougherty 1997; for review, see Gybels and Kupers 1995).

Periaqueductal/periventricular stimulation. The observation that stimulation of the periaqueductal gray matter in rats could produce powerful analgesia marked a major breakthrough in modern pain research (Reynolds 1969). However, most of the experimental data on pain suppression by PAG/PVG stimulation may not be relevant for clinical applications because these experiments were designed to study acute nociceptive events. Experimental studies with obvious clinical relevance have been performed on an animal model of chronic nociceptive pain (De Castro-Costa et al. 1981; Kupers et al. 1988). The scratching and biting behavior interpreted as signs of ongoing pain in rats with chronic arthritis was suppressed by stimulation in the periventricular area.

The analgesic effect of PAG/PVG stimulation in experimental animals is associated with the activation of endogenous opioid systems (Basbaum et al. 1976; Yaksh et al. 1976). The involvement of opioid mechanisms is substantiated by the observation that stimulation-induced analgesia can be reversed with naloxone (Akil et al. 1976), and by the subsequent demonstration in patients that such stimulation increases the release of β-endorphin in the cerebrospinal fluid (Akil et al. 1978). For further discussion on the physiological background of PAG/PVG stimulation, see Young and Chambi (1987) and Richardson (1995).

Clinical application

Choice of stimulation target. Despite more than two decades of clinical use, ICS still cannot be regarded as an established treatment modality for routine usage. Therefore, it should be practiced only in centers with extensive experience in dealing with difficult pain problems and with a thorough knowledge of stereotactic procedures.

Much evidence indicates that stimulation applied to the sensory thalamus is effective only for pain identified as neuropathic. Therefore, the indications for this target are in principle the same as for SCS, in addition to similar pain conditions of supraspinal etiology. Some forms of neuropathic pain are associated with extensive degeneration of the primary afferent fibers projecting into the dorsal columns, and these conditions are generally not amenable to SCS but may respond to ICS. Examples are deafferentation pain (phantom limb pain, trigeminal neuropathic pain, and facial anesthesia dolorosa). Sensory thalamic stimulation has also been applied for lumbosacral rhizopathy as part of the mixed condition of "low back pain" or "failed back surgery syndrome" (e.g., Hosobuchi 1986).

PAG/PVG stimulation is mostly efficacious for pain components characterized as nociceptive, although there are reports of successful outcomes in neuropathic pain as well. The great majority of patients who receive PAG/PVG stimulation suffer from "low back pain." This "syndrome" often represents both nociceptive and neuropathic pain components. The relative importance of these components must be evaluated, and a thorough pain analysis is mandatory for the proper selection of stimulation targets.

Comments on the surgical technique. The implantation procedure is always performed under local anesthesia to enable perioperative stimulation with verbal reports from the patient. Nowadays stereotactic magnetic resonance imaging (MRI) is usually used, but some centers still use ventriculography to calculate the target. After test stimulation with a stiff semi-microelectrode, the surgeon inserts a permanent electrode into the target region and fixes it to the calvarium. The technique differs between centers. Sometimes microelectrodes are used both for recording along the trajectories and for stimulation at the target site. Usually there is a period of trial stimulation with a percutaneous extension for several weeks before the final implantation of the subcutaneous stimulator (for details, see Meyerson and Linderoth 2000b).

Clinical results. Several reviews have summarized the literature on ICS (Gybels and Kupers 1987; Duncan et al. 1991; Kumar et al. 1997; Young and Rinaldi 1997). Bendok and Levy (1998) conducted a thorough meta-analysis of all studies that included more than 15 patients. In 13 studies, comprising 1114 patients, the results varied between 19% and 79% of patients who received long-term pain relief. The results of several of the major ICS stud-ies with long-term follow-up clearly show a more favorable outcome in patients with nociceptive than with neuropathic forms of pain. Young and Rinaldi (1997) report 70% and 50% success for the two types of pain, re-spectively. The most recent study concluded that "low back pain" is the best indication for ICS (Kumar et al. 1997). With PAG/PVG stimulation, sometimes combined with sensory thalamic stimulation, 71% (35 out of 49 patients) reported excellent or good pain relief (>50%), considerable reduc-tion of analgesic intake, and improvement in work capacity. According to Bendok and Levy's meta-analysis (1998), PAG/PVG stimulation may also be effective for neuropathic pain; no less than 23% of patients with long-term success had been treated for such pain. On the other hand, sensory thalamic stimulation seems to be completely ineffective for nociceptive forms of pain. Some of the major studies provide data for the different types of neuropathic pain treated with sensory thalamic stimulation. However, the results are extremely variable and inconsistent. Conversely, the results in lumbosacral rhizopathy with stimulation in the same target have been suc-cessful in about 70% of cases, although only a few studies have reported this diagnosis separately from "low back syndrome."

Conclusions: ICS for neuropathic pain

As in the case of other invasive procedures, most studies on the use of ICS to treat neuropathic pain are open to criticism. Physician bias due to the lack of third party evaluation and the lack of placebo controls (which would be possible only with PAG/PVG stimulation, which can be applied without evoking any subjective sensations) are factors that preclude the classifica-tion of ICS as evidence-based medicine. Moreover, the reported results are highly variable, with success rates ranging from 30% to 70%. Nevertheless, a thorough examination of the few recent publications with long-term re-sults reveals that a comparatively large proportion of patients with pain conditions that have failed to respond to any other treatment modality have enjoyed useful and sustained alleviation of their pain with ICS treatment. It is regrettable that medicolegal regulations in the United States have de-prived many patients of this therapy. Many patients who have benefitted from ICS on a long-term basis for pain in the lower part of the back may also be candidates for long-term intraspinal morphine administration. Intraspinal morphine (alone and in combination with adjuvant drugs) has gained popu-larity in recent years, but tolerance may develop and serious side effects are not uncommon. We strongly recommend that ICS should be considered as a therapeutic option for such patients.

MOTOR CORTEX STIMULATION

Basic mechanisms

Motor cortex stimulation (MCS) has been in use for about a decade, but the underlying mechanisms of its pain-relieving effect are still poorly understood, and there are few experimental data pertaining to its mode of action.

An experimental study in cats showed that stimulation of the motor, but not the sensory, cortex could suppress the increased neuronal spontaneous discharge of thalamic neurons rendered hyperactive following spinothalamic tractotomy (Tsubokawa et al. 1991). However, Namba and Nichimoto (1988) had previously investigated deafferentation hyperactivity in the spinal trigeminal nucleus of cats subjected to trigeminal denervation. In their experiments, hyperactive WDR neurons could be inhibited by stimulation of *both* the sensory and motor cortices. Sensory-motor interconnections form the basis of a theory that may explain the pain-relieving effect of MCS (Tsubokawa et al. 1993; Tsubokawa 1995). Tsubokawa hypothesized that pain following a cerebral lesion is the result of deficient inhibitory pain control. Ortho- or antidromic activation of large-fiber reciprocal connections between the motor and sensory cortices by MCS would in turn activate non-noxious fourth-order sensory neurons and thus restore inhibitory pain control. However, Nguyen et al. (1999) reported that a parietal lobe infarction including the sensory cortex does not exclude a positive response to MCS. Positron emission tomography (PET) studies of patients undergoing MCS have demonstrated a significant increase in cerebral blood flow in the ipsilateral thalamus, cingulate gyrus, orbitofrontal cortex, and brainstem (Garcia-Larrea et al. 1999). At variance with Tsubokawa's theory, these authors concluded that the integrity of the somatosensory cortex and the lemniscal system does not constitute a condition for MCS-produced pain relief. Instead, there is reason to believe that MCS directly activates both the thalamus and the brainstem, which serve as relays for pain control

Clinical application

Selection of patients. Substantial evidence indicates that MCS is efficacious only for certain forms of neuropathic pain; no clinical observations suggest that it may also influence nociceptive pain. Particularly when applied for central pain, the outcome of MCS is variable and reliable outcome predictors are lacking. In a thorough study in patients with central pain, Yamamoto et al. (1997) conducted pharmacological tests to investigate the relationship of the analgesic potency of a barbiturate (thiamylal), of morphine, and of ketamine with the outcome of MCS. A positive response to MCS treatment correlated with sensitivity to thiamylal and ketamine and with resistance to morphine, but this finding could not be confirmed in a later study by Saitosh et al. (2000). Katayama et al. (1998) observed a much more favorable long-term outcome in central pain patients without or with only mild motor weakness than in those with more pronounced deficits. An interesting report describes a patient with central pain in whom repetitive magnetic coil stimulation of the motor cortex for 30 minutes produced 30% pain relief. Subsequent long-term MCS proved effective for that patient, while another patient failed to respond to either type of stimulation (Migita et al. 1995).

Clinical results. Both central pain and painful trigeminal neuropathy are notoriously difficult to manage, and sensory thalamic or internal capsular stimulation rarely provide long-term beneficial results (Tsubokawa et al. 1993) (a typical case is illustrated in Fig. 4). The largest series of patients with central pain are those reported by Yamamoto et al. (1997; see also Tsubokawa et al. 1991, 1993), Katayama et al. (1998), and Nguyen et al. (1999). The overall positive results vary between 40% and 70% of patients receiving trial stimulation (with a total of approximately 100 patients studied). An analysis of the clinical records reveals no clear relationship between the outcome and the site of the lesion.

Although only about 30 patients with trigeminal neuropathy have been studied, the results tend to be somewhat better than in cases with central pain (Meyerson and Linderoth 2000b). In a recent study, Nguyen et al. (1999) reported that 10 out of 12 patients with trigeminal neuropathy experienced good relief (>50%), with a mean follow-up of 27 months. The alternative treatments for this condition are stimulation of the trigeminal ganglion or rootlets and sensory thalamic stimulation, which provide a satisfactory outcome in only 30–40% of patients. Most patients with central pain, as well as painful trigeminal neuropathy, also experience various forms of evoked pain such as allodynia and dysesthesia. Several studies have reported that MCS markedly relieves these evoked pain components as well (e.g., Meyerson et al. 1993).

Comments on the surgical technique. The surgical procedure can be performed under local anesthesia with slight sedation, or under general anesthesia. Formerly the epidural space was approached via an enlarged burr hole, but today most surgeons open a bone flap to gain access to a wider epidural area, to enable the use of grid electrodes, and to ensure epidural hemostasis.

The crucial part of the implantation procedure is not only to localize the precentral motor gyrus but also to identify the appropriate portion of the

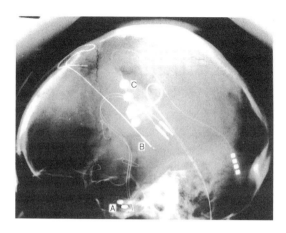

Fig. 4. Lateral radiograph of the skull of a patient who received motor cortex stimulation because of severe painful trigeminal neuropathy. She had previously received stimulation of the trigeminal ganglion and rootlets and the sensory thalamus, but the treatment had provided only short-lasting relief. A four-polar plate electrode has been placed epidurally over the motor strip on the contralateral side; the electrode must be placed over the part of the motor cortex corresponding to the face.

gyrus according to its somatotopic organization. To ensure optimal electrode placement it is not possible to rely on bony landmarks. Tsubokawa and collaborators (1991) described a preoperative examination using somatosensory evoked potentials to identify the central sulcus. Herregodts et al. (1994, 1995) introduced an elegant method of using preoperative 3-D MRI images of the cortical surface to localize the motor cortex. Nguyen et al. (1999) developed this approach by using a neuronavigator system that permits perioperative visualization and localization of the cortical gyri. Surgeons can further localize the central sulcus and motor cortex by recording somatosensory evoked potentials and by using high-intensity, low-frequency stimulation to produce peripheral muscle contractions. These techniques permit detailed mapping of the somatotopy of the motor cortex. It is reasonable to assume that functional MRI may further improve the localization and delineation of the functional subdivisions of the motor cortex (for review, see Meyerson and Linderoth 2000b).

Conclusions: MCS for neuropathic pain

MCS must be regarded as a treatment modality under development and cannot yet be recommended for routine usage. Evidence indicates that it has about a 50% chance of providing greater than 50% alleviation of central, supraspinal (post-stroke) pain. Its efficacy seems to be somewhat better in painful trigeminal neuropathy (presumably including anesthesia dolorosa), with a success rate of about 70–80%. The positioning of the electrode is critical and should preferably be performed with the aid of computerized tomography and magnetic resonance visualization of the precentral gyrus and with a perioperative electrophysiological control. The optimal stimulation regime and parameters remain to be determined. Although no serious side effects have been reported, the possible risk of producing permanent focal epilepsy cannot be disregarded (cf. Bezard et al. 1999). Because MCS usually is not accompanied by subjective sensations, researchers can assess the effect of neurostimulation for pain using a double-blind procedure. In view of the promising results obtained in treating pain conditions for which there is otherwise little to offer, a systematic exploration of the possible efficacy of MCS seems warranted for other difficult pain conditions, such as pain of spinal origin and cervical root avulsion.

CONCLUDING REMARKS: CNS STIMULATION FOR NEUROPATHIC PAIN

The various electric neuromodulation techniques offer minimally invasive and reversible therapeutic options in cases of neuropathic pain where conventional treatments have failed. SCS should be regarded as a routine therapy in selected neuropathic pain conditions. Supraspinal electric stimulation should at present be restricted to centers with special experience and interest in these types of strategies and with extensive knowledge of pain analysis and patient selection.

The further development of microcomputer techniques will enable more sophisticated stimulation regimens and miniaturization of the equipment. During the last decade the paresthesiae evoked during SCS have been controlled by using more complicated electrode designs and devices with many stimulating poles and multiple leads. The development of these new devices has partly been based on computer models of SCS (Holsheimer et al. 1997, 1998). The design of such equipment will be simpler in the future, and rapid shifting among various stimulation programs should enhance a diversity of effects. Rectangular pulses with fairly high, constant frequency are still routinely used. With increased knowledge about the modulatory pathways in the CNS, researchers will be able to develop more sophisticated stimulation patterns.

It is general clinical experience that patients who present with almost identical symptoms of painful neuropathy following peripheral nerve injury may respond differently to stimulation therapy; one patient may enjoy almost complete alleviation of both spontaneous and evoked pain, whereas another may not respond to the stimulation in spite of technically adequate treatment (i.e., complete paresthesia coverage of the entire painful region with SCS). The same situation seems to occur in nerve-lesioned rats exhibiting marked signs of painful neuropathy; SCS completely suppresses these signs in some rats, whereas in others the treatment has no effect whatsoever. It would presumably be of clinical relevance to explore the biochemical background to the differential effect of SCS in these animals with the aim of designing a laboratory work-up by which the response to SCS can be predicted in patients. We have already shown that SCS applied to nonresponding rats does *not* increase GABA release (Stiller et al. 1996); this finding suggests that in these animals the GABA system may be more disturbed than in those responding. However, it is highly likely that the involvement of the GABAergic and adenosine-related systems are just examples of biochemical correlates to the effect of SCS, and that numerous other transmitter/modulator systems are influenced by the stimulation. We have hitherto focused on tactile allodynia, but both threshold and suprathreshold functions of thermal allodynia and hyperalgesia may give clues to the differential response to SCS. Further research is also warranted on the possible role of the NMDA-receptor system and of the calcium and sodium channel controls in SCS.

A major spin-off of our research has been the possibility of enhancing the SCS effect by concomitant administration of baclofen and adenosine. In recent experiments (J. Wallin et al., unpublished manuscript) we have found that gabapentin can also depress the hyperexcitability of dorsal horn WDR neurons and suppress behavioral signs of tactile allodynia. This drug can also potentiate SCS when administered intrathecally or intravenously, in normally inactive doses. Numerous substances are candidates for a possible SCS-potentiating effect. We believe that a more diversified, adjuvant pharmacological treatment regimen may enhance the efficacy of SCS in patients who initially do not respond or who receive insufficient pain relief.

With improved knowledge about the biochemical background of the beneficial effects of SCS, could pharmacological therapy replace stimulation treatment? Conventional routes of administration necessarily imply the distribution of drugs to large areas of the body with the hope that some molecules will find their way to the target cells. In situ drug delivery close to the target cells is a strategy that eventually could compete with SCS. However, SCS probably releases a cascade of biochemical substances in the CNS and in the periphery, some of which are critical for the technique's beneficial effect on neuropathic pain. Conceivably, the composite of substances is not the same for all patients or animal subjects, as demonstrated by experiments and clinical studies where different individuals require different substances and doses to maximize the effect. Furthermore, as demonstrated by the studies described above, the adjuvant drugs, when combined with SCS, may be delivered at doses far too low to induce effects per se or to result in disturbing side effects.

Electrical stimulation of the CNS is an artificial way of exciting nervous tissue that requires expensive equipment and close follow-up. However, electric neuromodulation has the attractive features of being reversible and harmless when applied with moderate intensity, and it enables the activation of endogenous pain controls. We therefore strongly believe that electrical CNS stimulation deserves further methodological development and increased research efforts to discover the underlying mechanisms, and we recommend the continued dissemination of these treatment strategies for neuropathic pain.

ACKNOWLEDGMENTS

Studies from our laboratory referred to in this chapter were supported by grants from the Karolinska Institutet, Magn. Bergvalls Stiftelse, Åke Wibergs Stiftelse, Kapten Arthur Erikssons Stiftelse, Medtronic Europe S.A., and the Swedish Medical Research Council (14X-122 10-01A and K1999-04X-012210-03A).

REFERENCES

Adams JE, Hosobuchi Y, Fields HS. Stimulation of internal capsule for relief of central pain. *J Neurosurg* 1974; 41:740–744.

Akil H, Mayer DJ, Liebeskind JC. Antagonism of stimulation-produced analgesia by naloxone, a narcotic antagonist. *Science* 1976; 191:961–962.

Akil H, Richardson DE, Hughes DE, Barchas JD. Enkephalin-like material elevated in ventricular cerebrospinal fluid of pain patients after analgesic focal stimulation. *Science* 1978; 201:463–465.

Augustinsson LE, Carlsson CA, Holm J, Jivegård L. Epidural electrical stimulation in severe limb ischemia. *Ann Surg* 1985; 202:104–110.

Barolat G. Current status of epidural spinal cord stimulation. *Neurosurg Q* 1995; 5:98–124.

Barolat G, Schwartzman R, Woo R. Epidural spinal cord stimulation in the management of reflex sympathetic dystrophy. *Sterotact Funct Neurosurg* 1989; 53:29–39.

Baron R, Blumberg H, Jänig W. Clinical characteristics of patients with complex regional pain syndrome in Germany with special emphasis on vasomotor function. In: Jänig W, Stanton-Hicks M (Eds). *Reflex Sympathetic Dystrophy: A Reappraisal,* Progress in Pain Research and Management, Vol. 6. Seattle: IASP Press, 1996, pp 25–48.

Baron R, Levine JD, Fields H. Causalgia and reflex sympathetic dystrophy: does the sympathetic nervous system contribute to the generation of pain? *Muscle Nerve* 1999; 22:678–695.

Basbaum AL, Clanton CH, Fields HL. Opiate and stimulus-produced analgesia: functional anatomy of a medullospinal pathway. *Proc Natl Acad Sci USA* 1976; 73:4685–4688.

Bell GK, Kidd D, North RB. Cost-effectiveness analysis of spinal cord stimulation I treatment of failed back surgery syndrome. *J Pain Symptom Manage* 1997; 13:286–295.

Bendok B, Levy RM. Brain stimulation for persistent pain management. In: Gildenberg PL, Tasker RR (Eds). *Textbook of Stereotactic and Functional Neurosurgery.* New York: McGraw-Hill, 1998, pp 1539–1546.

Bennett GJ, Xie YK. A peripheral mononeuropathy in rat produces disorders of pain sensation like those seen in man. *Pain* 1988; 33:87–107.

Bezard E, Boraud T, Nguyen JP, et al. Cortical stimulation and epileptic seizure: a study of the potential risk in primates. *Neurosurgery* 1999; 45:346–350.

Burchiel KJ, Anderson VC, Wilson BJ, et al. Prognostic factors of spinal cord stimulation for chronic back and leg pain. *Neurosurgery* 1995; 36:1101–1111.

Burchiel KJ, Anderson VC, Brown FD, et al. Prospective, multicenter study of spinal cord stimulation for relief of chronic back and extremity pain. *Spine* 1996; 21:2786–2794.

Croom JE, Foreman RD, Chandler MJ, Barron KW. Cutaneous vasodilatation during dorsal column stimulation is mediated by dorsal roots and CGRP. *Am J Physiol* 1997; 272:H950–H957.

Cui JG. Spinal cord stimulation in neuropathy: experimental studies of neurochemistry and behaviour. Thesis. Karolinska Institutet, Stockholm, 1999, p 80.

Cui JG, Linderoth B, Meyerson BA. Effects of spinal cord stimulation on touch-evoked allodynia involve GABAergic mechanisms. An experimental study in the mononeuropathic rat. *Pain* 1996; 66:287–295.

Cui JG, O'Connor WT, Ungerstedt U, Linderoth B, Meyerson BA. Spinal cord stimulation attenuates augmented dorsal horn release of excitatory amino acids in mononeuropathy via a GABAergic mechanism. *Pain* 1997a; 73:87–95.

Cui J-G, Sollevi A, Linderoth B, Meyerson BA. Adenosine receptor activation suppresses tactile hypersensitivity and potentiates effect of spinal cord in mononeuropathic rats. *Neurosci Lett* 1997b; 223:173–176.

Cui JG, Meyerson BA, Sollevi A, Linderoth B. Effects of spinal cord stimulation on tactile hypersensitivity in mononeuropathic rats is potentiated by $GABA_B$ and adenosine receptor activation. *Neurosci Lett* 1998; 247:183–186.

De Castro-Costa M, De Sutter P, Gybels J, Van Hees J. Adjuvant-induced arthritis in rats: a possible animal model of chronic pain. *Pain* 1981; 10:173–185.

Dubuisson D. Effect of dorsal-column stimulation on gelatinosa and marginal neurons of cat spinal cord. *J Neurosurg* 1989; 70:257–265.

Duggan AW, Foong FW. Bicuculline and spinal inhibition produced by dorsal column stimulation in the cat. *Pain* 1985; 249–450.

Duncan GH, Bushnell MC, Marchand S. Deep brain stimulation: a review of basic research and clinical studies. *Pain* 1991; 45:49–59.

Foreman RD, Beall JE, Applebaum AE, Coulter JD, Willis WD. Effects of dorsal column stimulation on primate spinothalamic tract neurons. *J Neurophysiol* 1976; 39:534–546.

Garcia-Larrea L, Peyron R, Mertens P, et al. Electrical stimulation of motor cortex for pain control: a combined PET-scan and electrophysiological study. *Pain* 1999; 83:259–273.

Gerhart KD, Yeziersky RP, Fang ZR, et al. Inhibition of primate spinothalamic tract neurons by stimulation in ventral posterior lateral (VPL) thalamic nucleus: possible mechanisms. *J Neurophysiol* 1983; 49:406–423.

Gybels J, Kupers R. Central and peripheral electrical stimulation of the nervous system in the treatment of chronic pain. *Acta Neurochir Suppl* 1987; 38:64–75.

Gybels JM, Kupers RC. Brain stimulation on the management of persistent pain. In: Schmidek HH, Sweet WH (Eds). *Operative Neurosurgical Techniques.* Philadelphia: W.B. Saunders, 1995, pp 1389–1398.

Gybels JM, Sweet WH. *Neurosurgical Treatment of Persistent Pain.* Basel: Karger, 1989.

Gybels J, Erdine S, Maeyaert J, et al. Neuromodulation of pain: a consensus statement. *Eur J Pain* 1998; 2:203–210.

Häbler H-J, Eschenfelder S, Brinker H, et al. Neurogenic vasoconstriction in the dorsal root ganglion may play a crucial role in sympathetic-afferent coupling after spinal nerve injury. In: Devor M, Rowbotham MC, Wiesenfeld-Hallin Z (Eds). *Proceedings of the 9th World Congress on Pain*, Progress in Pain Research and Management, Vol. 16. Seattle: IASP Press, 2000, pp 661–667.

Handwerker HO, Iggo A, Zimmermann M. Segmental and supraspinal actions on dorsal horn neurons responding to noxious and non-noxious skin stimuli. *Pain* 1975; 1:147–165.

Head H, Holmes G. Sensory disturbances from cerebral lesions. *Brain* 1911; 34:102–254.

Herregodts P, Stadnik T, D'Haens J. Easy preoperative planning of deeply located brain lesions using external skin reference and 3-dimensional surface MRI. *Stereotact Funct Neurosurg* 1994; 63:26–30.

Herregodts P, Stadnik T, De Ridder F, D'Haens J. Cortical stimulation for central neuropathic pain: 3-D surface MRI for easy determination of the motor cortex. In: Meyerson BA, Ostertag C (Eds). *Advances in Stereotactic and Functional Neurosurgery*, Vol. 11. Vienna: Springer-Verlag, 1995, pp 132–135.

Holsheimer J, Wesselink WA. Effect of anode-cathode configuration on paresthesia coverage in spinal cord stimulation. *Neurosurgery* 1997; 41:654–659.

Holsheimer J, Nuttin B, King GW. Clinical evaluation of paresthesia steering with a new system for spinal cord stimulation. *Neurosurgery* 1998; 42:541–547.

Hosobuchi Y. Subcortical electrical stimulation for control of intractable pain in humans. *J Neurosurg* 1986; 64:543–553.

Hosobuchi Y, Adams JE, Rutkin B. Chronic thalamic stimulation for the control of facial anaesthesia dolorosa. *Arch Neurol* 1973; 29:158–161.

Jacobs MJHM, Jörning PJG, Joshi SR, et al. Epidural spinal cord electrical stimulation improves microvascular blood flow in severe limb ischemia. *Ann Surg* 1988; 207:179–183.

Katayama Y, Fukaya C, Yamamoto T. Poststroke pain control by chronic motor cortex stimulation: neurological characteristics predicting a favourable response. *J Neurosurg* 1998; 89:585–591.

Kemler M, Barendse GAM, van Kleef M, et al. Effects of spinal cord stimulation in patients with chronic reflex sympathetic dystrophy—a randomized trial. *N Engl J Med* 2000a; 343(9):618–624.

Kemler M, Barendse GAM, van Kleef M, et al. Pain relief in reflex sympathetic dystrophy due to spinal cord stimulation does not depend on vasodilatation. *Anesthesiology* 2000b; 92:1653–1660.

Kumar K, Toth C, Nath RK. Spinal cord stimulation for chronic pain in peripheral neuropathy. *Surg Neurol* 1996; 46:363–369.

Kumar K, Toth C, Nath R. Deep brain stimulation for intractable pain: a 15-year experience. *Neurosurgery* 1997; 40:736–747.

Kupers R, Gybels J. Electrical stimulation of the ventroposterolateral thalamic nucleus (VPL) reduces mechanical allodynia in a rat model of neuropathic pain. *Neurosci Lett* 1993; 150:95–98.

Kupers RC, Vos BPJ, Gybels JM. Stimulation of the nucleus paraventricularis thalami suppresses scratching and biting behaviour of arthritic rats and exerts a powerful effect on tests for acute pain. *Pain* 1988; 32:115–125.

Kupers RC, Van den Oever R, Van Houdenhove B, et al. Spinal cord stimulation in Belgium: a nation-wide survey on the incidence, indications and therapeutic efficacy by the health insurer. *Pain* 1994; 56:211–216.

Lazorthes Y, Siegfried J, Verdie JC, Casaux J. La stimulation médullaire chronique dans le traitement des douleurs neurogènes. *Neurochirurgie* 1995; 41:73–88.

Lenz F, Dougherty P. Pain processing in the human thalamus. In: Seriade M, Jones E, McCormick D (Eds). *Thalamus*, Vol. 2. Oxford: Elsevier Press, 1997, pp 617–651.

Lenz FA, Seike M, Richardson RT, et al. Thermal and pain sensations evoked by microstimulation in the area of human ventrocaudal nucleus. *J Neurophysiol* 1993; 70:200–212.

Lindblom U, Meyerson BA. Influence on touch, vibration and cutaneous pain of dorsal column stimulation in man. *Pain* 1975; 1:257–270.

Lindblom U, Ottosson J-O. Influence of pyramidal stimulation upon the relay of coarse cutaneous afferents in the dorsal horn. *Acta Physiol Scand* 1957; 38:309–318.

Linderoth B. Spinal cord stimulation in ischemia and ischemic pain: possible mechanisms of action. In: Horsch S, Claeys L (Eds). *Spinal Cord Stimulation II. An Innovative Method in the Treatment of PVD and Angina.* Darmstadt: Steinkopff Verlag, 1995, pp 19–35.

Linderoth B, Foreman RD. Physiology of spinal cord stimulation. review and update. *Neuromodulation* 1999; 2:150–164.

Linderoth B, Meyerson BA. Dorsal column stimulation: modulation of somatosensory and autonomic function. *Seminar Neurosci* 1995; 7:263–277.

Linderoth B, Meyerson BA. Spinal cord stimulation: mechanisms of action. In: Burchiel KJ (Ed). *Pain Surgery.* New York: Thieme, 2001, in press.

Linderoth B, Gunasekera L, Meyerson BA. Effects of sympathectomy on skin and muscle microcirculation during dorsal column stimulation: animal studies. *Neurosurgery* 1991; 29:874–879.

Mazars GJ. Intermittent stimulation of nucleus ventralis posterolateralis for intractable pain. *Surg Neurol* 1975; 4:93–95.

Mazars G, Merienne S, Cioloca C. Stimulations thalamiques intermittentes antalgiques. *Rev Neurol (Paris)* 1973; 128:273–279.

Max MB, Gilron I. Sympathetically maintained pain: has the emperor no clothes? *Neurology* 1999; 52:905–907.

Melzack R, Wall PD. Pain mechanisms: a new theory. *Science* 1965; 150:971–978.

Merskey H, Bogduk N. *Classification of Chronic Pain: Descriptions of Chronic Pain Syndromes and Definitions of Pain Terms,* 2nd ed. Seattle: IASP Press, 1994.

Meyerson B, Håkanson S. Suppression of pain in trigeminal neuropathy by electric stimulation of the Gasserian ganglion. *Neurosurgery* 1986; 18:59–66.

Meyerson BA, Linderoth B. Electric stimulation of the central nervous system. Max M (Ed). *Pain 1999—An Updated Review.* Seattle: IASP Press, 1999, pp 269–280.

Meyerson BA, Linderoth B. Spinal cord stimulation. In: Loeser JD (Ed). *Bonica's Management of Pain,* 3rd ed. Philadelphia: Lippincott, 2000a, pp 1857–1876.

Meyerson BA, Linderoth B. Brain stimulation: intracerebral and motor cortex stimulation. In: Loeser JD (Ed). *Bonica's Management of Pain,* 3rd ed. Philadelphia: Lippincott, 2000b, pp 1877–1889.

Meyerson BA, Linderoth B. Mechanisms of spinal cord stimulation in neuropathic pain. *Neurol Res* 2000c; 22:285–292.

Meyerson BA, Linderoth B, Lind G. Ryggmärgsstimulering vid kronisk neuropatisk smärta. *Läkartidningen* 1991; 88:727–732.

Meyerson BA, Lindblom U, Linderoth B, Lind G, Herregodts P. Motor cortex stimulation as treatment of trigeminal neuropathic pain. In: Meyerson, Ostertag C (Eds). *Advances in Stereotactic and Functional Neurosurgery,* Vol. 11. Vienna: Springer-Verlag, 1993, pp 150–153.

Meyerson BA, Ren B, Herregodts P, Linderoth B. Spinal cord stimulation in animal models of mononeuropathy: effects on the withdrawal response and the flexor reflex. *Pain* 1995; 61:229–243.

Meyerson BA, Cui JG, Yakhnitsa V, et al. Modulation of spinal pain mechanisms by spinal cord stimulation and the potential role of adjuvant pharmacotherapy. *Stereotact Funct Neurosurg* 1997; 68:129–140.

Michaelis M. Coupling of sympathetic and somatosensory neurons following nerve injury: mechanisms and potential significance for the generation of pain. In: Devor M, Rowbotham MC, Wiesenfeld-Hallin Z (Eds). *Proceedings of the 9th World Congress on Pain,* Progress in Pain Research and Management, Vol. 16. Seattle: IASP Press, 2000, pp 645–656.

Migita K, Uozumi T, Arita K, Monden S. Transcranial magnetic coil stimulation of motor cortex in patients with central pain. *Neurosurgery* 1995; 36:1037–1040.

Namba S, Nishimoto A. Stimulation of internal capsule, thalamic sensory nucleus (VPM) and cerebral cortex inhibited deafferentation hyperactivity provoked after gasserian ganglionectomy in cat. *Acta Neurochir* 1988; (Suppl 42):243–247.

Nguyen JP, Lefaucheur JP, Decq P, et al. Chronic motor cortex stimulation in the treatment of central and neuropathic pain. Correlations between clinical, electrophysiological and anatomical data. *Pain* 1999; 82:245–251.

North RB, Levy RM. Consensus conference on the neurosurgical management of pain. *Neurosurgery* 1994; 34:756–761.

North RB, Linderoth B. Spinal cord stimulation for chronic pain. In: Schmidek HH (Ed): *Schmidek and Sweet's Operative Neurosurgical Techniques,* 4th ed. Philadelphia: Saunders, 2000, pp 2407–2422.

North RB, Kidd DH, Zahurak M, James CS, Long DM. Spinal cord stimulation for chronic, intractable pain: experience over two decades. *Neurosurgery* 1993; 32:384–395.

North RB, Kidd DH, Lees MS. A prospective, randomized study of spinal cord stimulation versus reoperation for failed back surgery syndrome: initial results. *Stereotact Funct Neurosurg* 1994; 62:267–272.

Reynolds DV. Surgery in the rat during electrical analgesia induced by focal brain stimulation. *Science* 1969; 164:444–445.

Richardson DE, Akil H. Pain reduction by electrical brain stimulation in man. Part 2: chronic self administration in the periventricular gray matter. *J Neurosurg* 1977; 47:184–194.

Richardson DR. Deep brain stimulation for the relief of chronic pain. *Neurosurg Clin N Am* 1995; 6:135–144.

Roberts MHT, Rees H. Physiological basis of spinal cord stimulation. *Pain Reviews* 1994; 1:184–198.

Saadé NE, Tabet MS, Banna NR, Atweh SF, Jabbur SJ. Inhibition of nociceptive evoked activity in spinal neurons through a dorsal column-brainstem-spinal loop. *Brain Res* 1985; 339:115–158.

Saadé NE, Atweh SF, Privat A, Jabbur SJ. Inhibitory effects from various types of dorsal column and raphe magnus stimulations on nociceptive withdrawal flexion reflexes. *Brain Res* 1999; 846:72–86.

Saitosh Y, Shibata M, Hirano S-I, et al. Motor cortex stimulation for central and peripheral deafferentation pain. *J Neurosurg* 2000; 92:150–155.

Sanchez-Ledesma MJ, Garcia-March G, Diaz-Cascajo P, Gomez-Moreta J, Broseta J. Spinal cord stimulation in deafferentation pain. *Stereotact Funct Neurosurg* 1989; 53:40–55.

Schaltenbrand G, Bailey P. *Introduction to Stereotaxis with an Atlas of the Human Brain.* Stuttgart: Georg Thieme Verlag, 1959.

Seltzer Z, Dubner R, Yoram S. A novel behavioral model of neuropathic pain disorders produced in rats by partial sciatic nerve injury. *Pain* 1990; 43:205–218.

Shealy CN, Mortimer JT, Reswick JB. Electrical inhibition of pain by stimulation of the dorsal columns: preliminary clinical report. *Anesth Analg* 1967; 46:489–91.

Shetter AG. Spinal cord stimulation in the treatment of chronic pain. *Curr Rev Pain* 1997; 1:213–222.

Shetter AG, Atkinson JR. Dorsal column stimulation: its effect on medial bulboreticular unit activity evoked by noxious stimuli. *Exp Neurol* 1977; 54:185–198.

Siegfried J. Therapeutical neurostimulation: indications reconsidered. *Acta Neurochir* 1991; 52:112–117.

Simpson BA. Spinal cord stimulation. *Pain Rev* 1994; 1:199–230.

Spiegelmann R, Friedman W. Spinal cord stimulation: a contemporary series. *Neurosurgery* 1991; 28:65–71.

Steude U. Percutaneous electrostimulation of the trigeminal nerve in patients with atypical trigeminal neuralgia. *Neurochir* 1978; 21:66–69.

Stiller C-O. *Neurotransmission in CNS Regions Involved in Pain Modulation.* Stockholm: Karolinska Institute, 1997, p 61.

Stiller C-O, Cui J-G, O'Connor WT, et al. Release of GABA in the dorsal horn and suppression of tactile allodynia by spinal cord stimulation in mononeuropathic rats. *Neurosurgery* 1996; 39:367–375.

Sweet W. Control of pain by direct electrical stimulation of peripheral nerves. *Clin Neurosurg* 1976; 19:103–111.

Tasker RR, de Carvalho GTC, Dolan EJ. Intractable pain of spinal cord origin: clinical features and implications for surgery. *J Neurosurg* 1992; 77:373–378.

Tesfaye S, Watt J, Benbow SJ, et al. Electrical spinal-cord stimulation for painful diabetic peripheral neuropathy. *Lancet* 1996; 348:1698–1701.

Tsubokawa T. Motor cortex stimulation for deafferentation pain relief in various clinical syndromes and its possible mechanism. In: Besson JM, Guilbaud G, Ollat H (Eds). *Forebrain Areas Involved in Pain Processing.* Paris: John Libbey Eurotext, 1995, pp 261–276.

Tsubokawa T, Katayama Y, Yamamoto TEA. Chronic motor cortex stimulation for the treatment of central pain. In: Hitchcock ER, Broggi G, Burzaco JEA (Eds). *Advances in Stereotactic and Functional Neurosurgery,* Vol. 9. Vienna: Springer-Verlag, 1991, pp 137–139.

Tsubokawa T, Katayama Y, Yamamoto TEA, Hirayama T, Koyama S. Chronic motor cortex stimulation in patients with thalamic pain. *J Neurosurg* 1993; 78:393–401.

Turner JA, Loeser JD, Bell KG. Spinal cord stimulation for chronic low back pain: a systematic literature synthesis. *Neurosurgery* 1995; 37:1088–1096.

Wasner G, Heckmann K, Maier C, et al. Vascular abnormalities in acute reflex sympathetic dystrophy (CRPS I). *Arch Neurol* 1999; 56:613–620.

Yakhnitsa V, Linderoth B, Meyerson BA. Effects of spinal cord stimulation on dorsal horn neuronal activity in a rat model of mononeuropathy. *Pain* 1999; 79:223–233.

Yaksh TL, Yeung JC, Rudy TA. Systematic examination in the rat of brain sites sensitive to direct application of morphine: observations of differential effects within the periaqueductal gray. *Brain Res* 1976; 114:83–103.

Yamamoto T, Katayama Y, Hirayama TEA. Pharmacological classification of central post-stroke pain: comparison with the results of chronic motor cortex stimulation therapy. *Pain* 1997; 72:5–12.

Young RF. Electrical stimulation of the trigeminal nerve root for the treatment of chronic facial pain. *J Neurosurg* 1995; 83:72–78.

Young RF, Chambi VI. Pain relief by electrical stimulation of the periaqueductal and periventricular gray matter: evidence for a non-opioid mechanism. *J Neurosurg* 1987; 66:364–371.

Young RF, Rinaldi PC. Brain stimulation. In: North RB, Levy RM (Eds). *Neurosurgical Management of Pain.* New York: Springer, 1997, pp 283–301.

Correspondence to: Bengt Linderoth, MD, PhD, Department of Neurosurgery, Karolinska Hospital, SE-171 76 Stockholm, Sweden. Tel: 46 8 5177 2592; Fax: 46 8 30 70 91; email: bengt.linderoth@ks.se.

Neuropathic Pain: Pathophysiology and Treatment,
Progress in Pain Research and Management, Vol. 21,
edited by Per T. Hansson, Howard L. Fields, Raymond G.
Hill, and Paolo Marchettini, IASP Press, Seattle, © 2001.

14

Neuropathic Pain: The Near and Far Horizon

Howard L. Fields[a] and Raymond G. Hill[b]

[a]Department of Neurology, University of California, San Francisco, California, USA; [b]The Neuroscience Research Centre, Merck Sharp and Dohme, Terlings Park, Essex, United Kingdom

The treatment of patients with neuropathic pain has improved significantly over the past decade. However, many patients continue to suffer despite the best efforts of the medical profession, and the most effective medications often produce undesirable side effects. These patients represent a major unmet therapeutic need and they are the primary motivation for the work presented in this volume. Furthermore, while the expanded interest in this problem among scientists and clinicians is gratifying, it is clear that we still have much ground to cover. In terms of treatment development, the gaps in our understanding are significant. All of our current treatments are serendipitous and empirically based. The ultimate goal is to devise a rational approach to developing satisfactory, reliable treatment. An important means to attain this end will be to obtain an understanding of the mechanisms of action of current empirical treatments so that effectiveness can be optimized and side effects minimized in the next generation of drugs used for the treatment of neuropathic pain.

Despite these significant gaps, the progress documented in this volume is significant and encouraging. This progress is a direct result of the expansion of interest in the problem in both the scientific and clinical communities. Progress is undeniable, but it is also obvious that the clinical and basic science advances have been made along two largely independent tracks. In the laboratory, a variety of new neuropathic pain models have been developed, mostly of partial nerve injury. New molecular, cellular, and genetic approaches have been exploited in the quest for understanding (e.g., Seltzer et al. 2001). Clinically, microneurography, skin biopsies, quantitative sensory testing, functional imaging, and randomized controlled clinical trials are beginning to replace speculation with observation. Although the work along these two paths is to be encouraged, significant progress toward the goal of rational treatment development will only begin to bear fruit when these two tracks converge.

THE NEAR HORIZON

One clear advance in our understanding of neuropathic pain that has derived from a convergence of basic and clinical research is the discovery that, in many patients, partial nerve injury or inflammation can produce a state of enhanced irritability of primary afferent nociceptors. Twenty years ago, the terms *neuropathic* and *deafferentation* were used interchangeably, but we now know, from extensive human studies (see Chapters 4 and 8) and animal studies (Chapters 2, 3, and 7) that various insults to the peripheral nerves can produce phenotypic changes in primary afferent nociceptors that lead to a hyperexcitable state.

This advance is encouraging from two points of view. First, to the degree that neuropathic pain depends on input from primary afferent nociceptors, it is like other types of pain and can be expected to respond to a relatively broad range of analgesic agents with established efficacy. Second, our expanding knowledge of the neurobiology of the primary afferent nociceptor will enhance our ability to design drugs or other approaches that selectively target these nerve cells in the periphery. For example, the vanilloid receptor and the tetrodotoxin-resistant voltage-dependent sodium channel are molecules that are apparently unique to nociceptors. The interactions between these and other components of nociceptive signaling are complex (see, for example, Kwak et al. 2000; Hill 2001; Paukert et al. 2001), and it is still unclear whether there is a single nociceptive "lowest common denominator" or "final common pathway" that would be the obvious primary target for a novel treatment for neuropathic pain.

To the extent that neuropathic pain is nociceptor driven, the shibboleth that all neuropathic pains are opioid resistant can be discarded (see Chapter 11). In addition, we can hope that some of the analgesic agents currently in development may offer hope to patients with neuropathic pain. One such approach, antagonism of the N-methyl D-aspartate receptor, is available, although its clinical value has not yet been established for neuropathic pain. Furthermore, while it seems to help some patients, unless efficacy for subtype-selective NMDA antagonism can be established (see Chapter 5), the side-effect profile of this class of agent is likely to limit its use. Several pharmaceutical companies are reportedly investigating the potential of agents acting at the glycine site of the NMDA-receptor complex for the treatment of neuropathic pain (see Boyce and Rupniak 2001). The most promising approach seems to be to avoid a universal block of all NMDA receptors, focusing on the subtypes of NMDA receptor that are most likely to be involved in nociceptive processing. Much evidence now points to the NR2B subunit-containing receptor as the preferential target (see Boyce et al. 1999). This receptor is absent from the cerebellum and has a more restricted distribution than the NR2A subunit-containing receptor, having an intense expression in superficial laminae of the dorsal horn of the spinal cord and some forebrain areas concerned with sensory transmission and cognition. Transgenic mice overexpressing NR2B-containing receptors have improved cognitive performance but also show enhanced nociceptive responses to peripheral injection of either formalin or complete Freund's adjuvant (Wei et al. 2001). These changes are accompanied by greater expression of *c-fos* in the nociceptive path from the spinal dorsal horn to the brainstem and thalamus to the cortex in NR2B-overexpressing mice injected with formalin to one hindpaw (Wei et al. 2001). Studies with the NR2B-selective antagonist CP101,606 (Pfizer), aimed at treating traumatic brain injury, have shown that this compound is well tolerated in phase I volunteers and in patients in phase II (Menniti et al. 1998), but no data from pain studies are yet in the public domain. No new NMDA-receptor subunits have been discovered recently, and it is likely that we now know them all, but further novel interventions targeting this receptor complex may emerge as we understand more about its intrinsic transduction machinery (see, for example, Husi et al. 2000; Hill 2001).

N-type Ca^{2+} channel blockers may also be seen as potential therapy on the near horizon, and early reports indicate clinical efficacy with the peptidergic blocker ziconotide given intrathecally (Atanassoff et al. 2000; Matthews and Dickenson 2001). However, this target is still most challenging given that, in addition to primary afferent nociceptors, these channels are present on a variety of other nerve terminals. Obtaining agents selective for nociceptive transmission and whose use does not depend on invasive routes of administration will hinge on the existence of channel subtypes with a distinct pharmacology and appropriate regional distribution. Progress in this direction includes reports of several central and peripheral splice variants of the N-type channel and evidence that new conotoxins, typified by conotoxin VI-D (CVID), can distinguish between N-type channel splice variants and have little action at P/Q-type channels (Lewis et al. 2000). It is still, however, a major task to go from a knowledge of the pharmacology of peptide toxins to the design of small-molecule, orally bioavailable selective blocking drugs.

Of particular note in the context of calcium channels is gabapentin, for although it is not a perfect agent it is considered by many to have the best separation between wanted and unwanted effects of any currently available drug useful for treating neuropathic pain. The mechanism of action of this drug is still not fully understood but when its binding site was purified from pig brain it was found to be the $\alpha_2\delta$ subunit of the high-voltage-gated calcium channels. Both the $\alpha_2\delta$ subunit protein and ^{3}H-gabapentin binding are upregulated in the dorsal horn of the spinal cord after sciatic nerve ligature in rats. Furthermore, the antinociceptive activities of a range of gabapentin analogues correlate well with their potency at binding to the $\alpha_2\delta$ subunit (see Snutch et al. 2001 for review). The finding that there are three subtypes of $\alpha_2\delta$ subunits opens the possibility of pharmacological selectivity and may explain the differences in experimental results obtained with this compound in different brain areas.

The current gold standard of medications for the treatment of neuropathic pain is the tricyclic antidepressants (TCAs). Tricyclics have helped millions of patients with chronic pain. In addition to their effect on most types of neuropathic pain, they have established efficacy across a broad range of indications, including tension and migraine headache, cancer, and low back pain. Because of their broad range of efficacy and the unpredictability of a given patient's response, we do not know what it is about neuropathic pain that makes it susceptible to TCAs. Perhaps it has something to do with chronicity per se, rather than the specific etiology or pathophysiology of the pain. These agents' mechanisms of analgesic action for any human painful condition remain unclear. For this reason, we do not know whether drugs of this class having higher efficacy for neuropathic pain can be developed. The same point applies to anticonvulsants. As new molecular targets emerge from our knowledge of the human genome it is important that these mainstay drugs are screened for activity against each target in order to determine their site of action and thus facilitate the design of new and better drugs.

On the other hand, improvement over existing drugs may not require a fundamental molecular insight into mechanisms but may be achieved by removing some of the more obvious unwanted activities in existing agents, for example the interactions with polymorphic drug-metabolizing enzymes seen with the tricyclics (see Chapter 9).

The last decade has seen increasing interest in the interplay between the nervous and immune systems, especially with regard to pain and inflammation. One of the more promising areas of research into the mechanisms and management of neuropathic pain involves cytokines. The explosive growth in this research area and the implications for pain management are very exciting. Chapter 3 gives an excellent overview of the field. The evidence is compelling that cytokines can contribute to sensitization of primary afferent nociceptors and that they are dramatically increased in peripheral nerve following partial injury. Even more intriguing is the evidence that nerve injury is associated with widespread increases in production of cytokines in the central nervous system (CNS). The recent availability of selective cytokine inhibitors for use in human subjects creates an exciting opportunity to directly test the relevance of cytokines to human neuropathic pain and has stimulated much research activity. Recently a proteinase-activated receptor, PAR2, thought to be important in inflammation, was found to be expressed on nociceptive afferent terminals. Activation of this receptor causes rapid calcium entry and release of substance P and calcitonin gene-related peptide from both central and peripheral terminals (Vergnolle et al. 2001) and causes behavioral hyperalgesia. In mice deficient in the PAR2 receptor, stimuli causing hyperalgesia in wild-type mice were without effect. Surprisingly, activation of PAR2 also failed to cause hyperalgesia in NK_1-receptor-deficient mice, suggesting an obligatory role for the substance P signaling system.

THE HYPEREXCITABLE STATE

Clearly, primary afferent nociceptor hyperexcitability is well established as a significant contributor to certain types of neuropathic pain. To the extent that this is the case, our understanding of the underlying pathophysiology is well advanced and we have a variety of potential approaches to rational development of treatment. For these patients, the near and far horizons have a rosy glow. Furthermore, we have every reason to believe that such patients will benefit from the development of any broad-spectrum, centrally acting analgesics. Research to produce novel analgesic drugs has been only partially successful in the recent past. Some agents shown to have interesting antinociceptive profiles in animal nociception assays, including models of neuropathic pain, were ineffective when tested in humans or had an unacceptable incidence of side effects at analgesic doses. We need both more predictive animal tests and a great deal more clinical data on novel approaches in order to unlock this dilemma. One useful example from the recent past is the evaluation of NK_1-receptor antagonists, which block the action of substance P, a major neuropeptide released from nociceptive primary afferents. This area has recently been reviewed (Boyce and Hill 2000; Hill 2000). One difficulty encountered in this research is the extreme species selectivity of most of the agents optimized for activity at the human

NK_1 receptor, especially as rats and mice were the least sensitive species. This problem necessitated the development of antinociceptive assays in animals that are not normally used for this purpose and where there is a distinct lack of baseline data with standard analgesic compounds. Nevertheless, several independent research groups using a variety of species and tests were able to show that brain-penetrant NK_1 antagonists were antinociceptive, especially in the presence of inflammation, and had a profile similar to the nonsteroidal anti-inflammatory drugs (Boyce and Hill 2000). Additionally, they were active against hyperalgesia and against the expansion of dorsal horn neuron receptive fields in rats with chronic constriction injury to one sciatic nerve (Cumberbatch et al. 1999). The phenotype of mutant mice with NK_1-receptor gene deletion also indicated that pharmacological blockade of this receptor would be likely to have an antinociceptive effect. It was clear from all of the studies where artefactual efficacy (e.g., by ancillary blockade of ion channels) could be excluded that NK_1-receptor antagonists had no effect on baseline nociception and were ineffective in tests such as tail-flick and hotplate, and thus were not opioid-like analgesics. In extensive clinical trial data published to date, only a single study, with the Pfizer compound CP-99,994 given intravenously in postoperative dental pain, has shown any analgesic efficacy (Dionne et al. 1999). Other agents such as MK-869 and CP-122,271, given orally at doses known to be effective in humans against emesis, were ineffective in the same dental pain paradigm or against the pain of postherpetic neuralgia or diabetic neuropathy (reviewed in Boyce and Hill 2000). The implied risk with novel approaches to the treatment of pain, especially in the case of neuropathic pain, is that data obtained in animal tests may not always be predictive of analgesic efficacy in humans. Almost all clinical trials of NK_1 antagonists have failed to show any efficacy for pain or migraine, even though the same agents are effective against emesis induced by cancer chemotherapy or against depression. This failure is unexplained other than by species differences in physiology and pharmacology. Clinical syndromes with more inflammatory components might be suitable for demonstrating clinical efficacy with these agents, or they may be effective in combination with existing analgesics. It is noteworthy in this context that pain treatment cannot yet be said to be mechanism based. Max (2000) recently reported that he had been unable to differentiate between relief of allodynia and relief of ongoing pain in neuropathic pain patients by a range of drugs including opioids, antidepressants, adrenergic agonists, and NMDA-receptor blockers. Although the effects of drugs used were frequently suboptimal, when a particular drug was effective in a particular patient then most of the distressing symptoms were relieved. This finding suggests that the real mechanistic differences in pain symptoms may be less important than is suggested by our current repertoire of animal tests (see Chapter 1 for further discussion).

REORGANIZATION OF THE CENTRAL NERVOUS SYSTEM: THE DARK HEART OF THE NEUROPATHIC PAIN PROBLEM

In contrast to the encouraging advances in our understanding of the pathophysiology of peripherally generated neuropathic pain, progress has been dauntingly slow regarding CNS mechanisms. Unfortunately, clinical observations suggest that, to the extent that the pain is due to CNS reorganization, it may be largely refractory to current treatment regimens (see, e.g., Galer et al. 1996). Although these observations are anecdotal, they correspond to our clinical experience. It is a sad irony that our mechanistic understanding is most lacking precisely for those patients who suffer the most.

Patients with central post-stroke pain and spinal cord injury pain are among the most resistant to any currently available therapeutic approach. Although the issue has not been studied systematically, it is our impression that some patients with peripheral nervous system injury, particularly those whose condition involves profound deafferentation (anesthesia dolorosa), also fall into the category of those highly resistant to treatment.

It is difficult to be sanguine about the opportunities to improve the lot of these patients. First, there are few widely accepted animal models for centrally generated neuropathic pain, partly because there are no lesions of the human nervous system that reliably produce pain. Another problem is that most current animal models of neuropathic pain depend on stimulus-evoked behaviors. How does one know whether an experimental animal has developed constant pain in an area where peripheral stimuli no longer evoke a response? Second, once the brain has been rewired, one can question the relevance to pain generation of our knowledge about the normal anatomy and physiology of pain and pain-modulating pathways. It is also important to point out our ignorance of the extent to which central reorganization contributes to the most common forms of neuropathic pain: diabetic neuropathy, postherpetic neuralgia, and traumatic mononeuropathies. Our lack of knowledge in this basic clinical area prevents us from even guessing at the magnitude of the clinical problem, let alone its mechanism.

When one starts from a position of such profound ignorance, the options for developing new rational treatments are few. One can appeal to serendipity by trying everything available. So far this approach has yielded only marginal benefits. A few patients respond to TCAs, some to opioids or antiepileptic drugs. Neurosurgical approaches such as motor cortex or thalamic stimulation help some patients (see Chapter 13). However, we are unaware of any recent chance discoveries that would mitigate the expectation of a poor prognosis for most patients in this category. While the occasional patient has a good result, usually from a combination of treatments, most get marginal or no benefit.

Has research provided any clues to the pathophysiology of this devastating condition? There is a long history of studying animals with experimental deafferentation. Two findings in deafferented spinal cord neurons are consistent across studies and suggest mechanisms that could contribute to pain and to resistance to traditional analgesic approaches: the formation of aberrant connections to and the development of increased firing in putative pain transmission neurons.

CENTRAL NERVOUS SYSTEM MECHANISMS BY WHICH DEAFFERENTATION COULD LEAD TO PAIN

In patients with peripheral nervous system injury who have an area of maximal pain that is spatially coextensive with areas of profound sensory loss (e.g., Rowbotham and Fields 1989), primary afferent nociceptor activity is unlikely to contribute much to the pain. In such cases it is more likely the deafferentation that initiates long-term changes in the CNS, leading to pain and hyperalgesia. Furthermore, because nociceptors are normally not spontaneously active, it is unlikely that they contribute to the steady pain that develops after CNS injury. Below we will discuss experimental evidence for several mechanisms by which loss of primary afferent function or central connectivity of pain transmission neurons could lead to CNS changes that result in pain and allodynia.

Following peripheral deafferentation, there is well-documented sprouting of the central processes of surviving dorsal root ganglion neurons and development of aberrant connections in the spinal cord. Surviving dorsal root axons make functional contact with spinal cord neurons that have been deprived of their normal input (Devor and Wall 1981a,b; LaMotte et al. 1989). The small neurons in lamina II (substantia gelatinosa) of the spinal cord dorsal horn normally receive direct input from small-diameter (Aδ- and C-fiber) primary afferent nociceptors and presumably relay this message to projection neurons in laminae I and V (Light and Kavookjian 1988). Peripheral nerve damage produces substantial degeneration of C-fiber primary afferent terminals in lamina II (Jänig and McLachlan 1984; Lisney 1989). When the normal synaptic contacts made by these C-fiber afferents onto lamina II neurons is lost, the central terminals of Aβ mechanoreceptive afferents, which normally terminate only in deeper laminae (III and IV), grow into lamina II and directly contact the deafferented cells (Woolf et al. 1992; Shortland and Woolf 1993). After such reorganization, large-diameter primary afferents, including those that respond best to innocuous stimuli (Aβ), provide a major direct input to spinal neurons that normally have input exclusively from unmyelinated primary afferents. In fact, recording from dorsal horn neurons in rats with partial peripheral nerve injuries reveals a marked increase in responses to light tactile stimulation (Laird and Bennett 1993). It is of possible therapeutic interest that application of the neurotrophin nerve growth factor (NGF) prevents C fibers from degenerating and central Aβ-fibers from sprouting (Bennett et al. 1996).

In fact, clinical evidence supports this idea. Some postherpetic neuralgia (PHN) patients have profound loss of small-fiber sensory function and spatially coextensive dynamic allodynia in their region of greatest pain. In these patients, preserved Aβ primary afferents may form abnormal connections with central pain transmission neurons. Consistent with this idea, Baron and Saguer (1993, 1995) reported patients in whom the histamine-evoked axon reflex vasodilatation and flare size was impaired or abolished in skin regions with intense dynamic allodynia. Quantitative thermal sensory testing to assess C- and Aδ-fiber function confirms that some herpes zoster patients have extremely high thermal thresholds in areas with marked dynamic allodynia (Choi and Rowbotham 1997). Thus, a subset of PHN patients have pain and loss of cutaneous C-nociceptor function in a region that is coextensive with allodynic skin. In such patients, the simplest explanation consistent with animal data is that degeneration of the central terminals of unmyelinated primary afferents induces a synaptic reorganization within the dorsal horn leading to aberrant direct connections between Aβ mechanoreceptive fibers and dorsal horn neurons that have lost their normal nociceptor input.

While this is an attractive idea, there are alternative explanations for the clinical findings. There might be ongoing C-nociceptor activity from tiny sub- or intracutaneous microneuromas (Bennett 1994). In this case the peripheral terminals remain deep to the surface, resulting in elevated sensory thresholds. Another possibility is that the nociceptive C fibers may degenerate exclusively in the peripheral branch, leaving the dorsal root ganglion soma and the central axon branch intact. The cell bodies of these injured neurons could then generate ectopic impulse activity that would maintain pathological central sensitization in the presence of analgesic skin (Devor et al. 1992). In theory, because most tests have only studied the function of cutaneous C fibers, ongoing activity might originate in nociceptors of deep somatic tissues (e.g., muscle and ligaments; Wall and Woolf 1984). In all of these possible mechanisms, pain and allodynia would be due to activity in primary afferent nociceptors and thus should respond to opioids and other centrally acting analgesics.

Some patients with peripheral nerve damage or CNS damage (i.e., spinal cord transection) have virtually complete loss of sensory input to CNS regions essential for generating the perception of pain. In such patients, neuropathic pain must be the result of intrinsic CNS changes. Following primary afferent loss of a spinal segment, many dorsal horn cells begin to fire spontaneously at high frequencies (Lombard and Larabi 1983; Laird and Bennett 1993). There is some evidence that a similar process may underlie the pain that follows extensive denervating injuries in humans. For example, pain is a characteristic sequela of the deafferentation produced by brachial plexus avulsion (Wynn Parry 1980, 1984). Recordings of spinal neuron activity in a pain patient whose dorsal roots were injured by trauma to the cauda equina revealed high-frequency regular and paroxysmal bursting discharges (Loeser et al. 1967). That patient complained of spontaneous burning pain in a region rendered anesthetic by the lesion (anesthesia dolorosa).

Another potentially relevant finding is that nerve injury causes loss of spinal cord inhibitory interneurons. Many of the dorsal horn neurons that contain inhibitory neurotransmitters such as γ-aminobutyric acid (GABA) and enkephalin are located in lamina II of the dorsal horn, which is the target of most unmyelinated primary afferents (Hunt et al. 1981). Injury to peripheral nerve leads to cell death in dorsal horn laminae I–II and hyperalgesia, and both cell loss and pain behaviors can be prevented with an NMDA-receptor antagonist (Whiteside and Munglani 2001). If some of the degenerated neurons were inhibitory, one would expect disinhibition of dorsal horn neurons (Wall and Devor 1981; Woolf and Wall 1982; Laird and Bennett 1992; Blomqvist and Craig 2000). This situation could contribute to the observed increase in spontaneous activity of dorsal horn nociceptive neurons.

Although most animal research to date concerns changes produced in the dorsal horn following peripheral nerve damage, this is largely because pain researchers have traditionally focused their efforts on primary afferent neurons and the dorsal horn. In fact, there is no compelling evidence that these spinal cord changes contribute in any way to clinically significant neuropathic pain. This evidentiary gap poses a challenge to the relevance of the vast body of animal research on neuropathic pain. We must directly address the problem of the relevance of this work in human studies. Functional imaging is a possible avenue to bridge the animal and human studies. However, whereas most CNS pain research in animals concerns the primary afferent and dorsal horn, human functional imaging studies have focused almost exclusively on the forebrain, where the anatomical resolution is best. In fact, evidence from functional imaging studies indicates that neuropathic injury results in synaptic reorganization in supraspinal somatosensory relay nuclei, such as the brainstem, thalamus, and cortex (Tasker et al. 1987; Mao et al. 1993; Hsieh et al. 1995; Iadarola et al. 1995; Karl et al. 2001). If we are ever to fully understand the pathophysiology of neuropathic pain, it is essential that we begin to make sense of this evidence of supraspinal neural reorganization.

THE FAR HORIZON

This volume illustrates the current state of affairs for patients with neuropathic pain. It is a mixed bag of disappointment and hope. Clearly, we have made major strides in our understanding of the pathophysiology of pain in general, and especially of peripheral mechanisms of neuropathic pain. We have also made progress in understanding the mechanisms of action of some serendipitously discovered drugs that are effective in neuropathic pain. In addition, it is reasonable to hope that the information contained in the human genome sequence will provide a way to identify patients with a genetic predisposition to neuropathic pain, but this area of study is in its infancy. Although single gene mutations have been associated with congenital insensitivity to pain (Indo et al. 1996) and with familial hemiplegic migraine (Ophoff et al. 1998), as yet there are few clues as to the genetic basis of more common pain disorders.

Finally, when all is said and done, there is a significant population of patients who have pain subsequent to CNS reorganization. While there are some promising clues to mechanisms, we have no idea of their relevance to any human condition. Furthermore, because these patients are so often completely resistant to current therapies, the route of improving current drugs is closed off. Help for these patients will require close cooperation among clinicians, clinical scientists, and basic scientists. We hope that this volume will serve as an impetus for others to join the effort to understand and treat these patients.

REFERENCES

Atanassoff PG, Hartmannsgruber MW, Thrasher J, et al. Ziconotide, a new N-type calcium channel blocker, administered intrathecally for acute postoperative pain. *Reg Anesth Pain Med* 2000; 25:274–278.

Baron R, Saguer M. Postherpetic neuralgia. Are C-nociceptors involved in signalling and maintenance of tactile allodynia? *Brain* 1993; 116:1477–1496.

Baron R, Saguer M. Mechanical allodynia in postherpetic neuralgia: evidence for central mechanisms depending on nociceptive C-fiber degeneration. *Neurology* 1995; 45:S63–65.

Bennett GJ. Neuropathic pain. In: Wall PD, Melzack R (Eds). *Textbook of Pain*. Edinburgh: Churchill Livingstone, 1994, pp 201–224.

Bennett DL, French J, Priestley JV, McMahon SB. NGF but not NT-3 or BDNF prevents the A fiber sprouting into lamina II of the spinal cord that occurs following axotomy. *Mol Cell Neurosci* 1996; 8:211–220.

Blomqvist A, Craig AD. Is neuropathic pain caused by the activation of nociceptive specific neurons due to anatomic sprouting in the dorsal horn? *J Comp Neurol* 2000; 428:1–4.

Boyce S, Hill RG. Discrepant results from preclinical and clinical studies on the potential of substance-P receptor antagonist compounds as analgesics. In: Devor M, Rowbotham MC, Wiesenfeld-Hallin Z (Eds). *Proceedings of the 9th World Congress on Pain, Progress in Pain Research and Management*, Vol. 16. Seattle: IASP Press, 2000, pp 313-324.

Boyce S, Rupniak NMJ. Behavioural antinociception studies on NMDA receptor antagonists. In: Sirinathsinghji DJS, Hill RG (Eds). *NMDA Antagonists as Potential Analgesic Drugs*. Basel: Birkhauser, 2001, in press.

Boyce S, Wyatt A, Webb JK, et al. Selective NMDA NR2B antagonists induce antinociception without motor dysfunction: correlation with restricted localisation of NR2B subunit in dorsal horn. *Neuropharmacology* 1999; 38:611–623.

Choi B, Rowbotham MC. Effect of adrenergic receptor activation on post-herpetic neuralgia pain and sensory disturbances. *Pain* 1997; 69:55–63.

Cumberbatch MJ, Carlson E, Wyatt A, et al. Reversal of behavioural and electrophysiological correlates of experimental peripheral neuropathy by the NK_1 receptor antagonist GR205,171 in rats. *Neuropharmacology* 1999; 37:1535–1543.

Devor M, Wall PD. Effect of peripheral nerve injury on receptive fields of cells in the cat spinal cord. *J Comp Neurol* 1981a; 199:277–291.

Devor M, Wall PD. Plasticity in the spinal cord sensory map following peripheral nerve injury in rats. *J Neurosci* 1981b; 1:679–684.

Devor M, Wall PD, Catalan N. Systemic lidocaine silences ectopic neuroma and DRG discharge without blocking nerve conduction. *Pain* 1992; 48:261–268.

Dionne RA. Clinical analgesic trials of NK_1 antagonists. *Curr Opin CPNS Invest Drugs* 1999; 1:82–85.

Galer BS, Harle J, Rowbotham MC. Response to intravenous lidocaine infusion predicts subsequent response to oral mexiletine: a prospective study. *J Pain Symptom Manage* 1996; 12:161–167.

Hill RG. NK1 (substance P) receptor antagonists—why are they not analgesic in humans? *Trends Pharmacol Sci* 2000; 21:244–246.

Hill RG. Molecular basis for the perception of pain. *Neuroscientist* 2001; 7:279–292.

Hsieh JC, Belfrage M, Stone-Elander S, Hansson P, Ingvar M. Central representation of chronic ongoing neuropathic pain studied by positron emission tomography. *Pain* 1995; 63:225–236.

Hunt SP, Kelly JS, Emson PC. An immunohistochemical study of neuronal populations containing neuropeptides or gamma-aminobutyrate within the superficial layers of the rat dorsal horn. *Neuroscience* 1981; 6:1883–1898.

Husi H, Ward MA, Choudhary JS, Blackstock WP, Grant SGN. Proteomic analysis of NMDA-receptor–adhesion protein signalling complexes. *Nature Neurosci* 2000; 3:661–669.

Iadarola MJ, Max MB, Berman KF. Unilateral decrease in thalamic activity observed with positron emission tomography in patients with chronic neuropathic pain. *Pain* 1995; 63:55–64.

Indo Y, Tsuruta M, Hayashida Y, et al. Mutations in the TRKA/NGF receptor gene in patients with congenital insensitivity to pain with anhidrosis. *Nat Genet* 1996; 13:485–488.

Jänig W, McLachlan E. On the fate of sympathetic and sensory neurons projecting into a neuroma of the superficial peroneal nerve in the cat. *J Comp Neurol* 1984; 225:302–311.

Karl A, Birbaumer N, Lutzenberger W, Cohen LG, Flor H. Reorganization of motor and somatosensory cortex in upper extremity amputees with phantom limb pain. *J Neurosci* 2001; 21:3609–3618.

Light AR, Kavookjian AM. Morphology and ultrastructure of physiologically identified substantia gelatinosa (lamina II) neurons with axons that terminate in deeper dorsal horn laminae (III–V). *J Comp Neurol* 1988; 267:172–189.

Kwak J, Wang MH, Hwang SW. Intracellular ATP increases capsaicin-activated channel activity by interacting with nucleotide binding domains. *J Neurosci* 2000; 20:8298–8304.

Laird JM, Bennett GJ. Dorsal root potentials and afferent input to the spinal cord in rats with an experimental peripheral neuropathy. *Brain Res* 1992; 584:181–190.

Laird JM, Bennett GJ. An electrophysiological study of dorsal horn neurons in the spinal cord of rats with an experimental peripheral neuropathy. *J Neurophysiol* 1993; 69:2072–2085.

LaMotte CC, Kapadia SE, Kocol CM. Deafferentation-induced expansion of saphenous terminal field labelling in the adult rat dorsal horn following pronase injection of the sciatic nerve. *J Comp Neurol* 1989; 288:311–325.

Lewis RJ, Nielsen KJ, Craik DJ, et al. Novel ω–conotoxins from *Conus catus* discriminate among neuronal calcium channel subtypes. *J Biol Chem* 2000; 275:35335–35344.

Lisney SJ. Regeneration of unmyelinated axons after injury of mammalian peripheral nerve. *Q J Exp Physiol* 1989; 74:757–784.

Loeser JD, Ward AA, White LE. Chronic deafferentation of human spinal cord neurons. *J Neurosurg* 1967; 29:48–50.

Lombard MC, Larabi Y. Electrophysiological study of cervical dorsal horn cells in partially deafferented rats. In: Bonica JJ, Lindblom U, Iggo A (Eds). *Proceedings of the Third World Congress on Pain,* Advances in Pain Research and Therapy, Vol. 5. New York: Raven Press, 1983, pp 147–154.

Mao J, Mayer DJ, Price DD. Patterns of increased brain activity indicative of pain in a rat model of peripheral mononeuropathy. *J Neurosci* 1993; 13:2689–2702.

Matthews EA, Dickenson AH. Effects of spinally delivered N- and P-type voltage-dependent calcium channel antagonists on dorsal horn neuronal responses in a rat model of neuropathy. *Pain* 2001; 92:235–246.

Max MB. Is mechanism-based pain treatment attainable? Clinical trial issues. *J Pain* 2000; 1(Suppl 1):2–9.

Menniti FS, Shah AK, Williams SA. CP-101,606: an NR2B-selective NMDA receptor antagonist. *CNS Drug Rev* 1998; 4:306–322.

Ophoff RA, Terwindt GM, Frants RR, Ferrari MD. P/Q-type Ca^{2+} channel defects in migraine, ataxia and epilepsy. *Trends Pharmacol Sci* 1998; 19:121–127.

Paukert M, Osteroth R, Giesler HS, et al. Inflammatory mediators potentiate ATP-gated channels through the $P2X_3$ subunit. *J Biol Chem* 2001; 276:21077–21082.

Rowbotham MC, Fields HL. Post-herpetic neuralgia: the relation of pain complaint, sensory disturbance, and skin temperature. *Pain* 1989; 39:129–144.

Seltzer Z, Wu T, Max MB, Diehl SR. Mapping a gene for neuropathic pain-related behavior following peripheral neurectomy in the mouse. *Pain* 2001; 93:101–106.

Shortland P, Woolf CJ. Chronic peripheral nerve section results in a rearrangement of the central axonal arborizations of axotomized A beta primary afferent neurons in the rat spinal cord. *J Comp Neurol* 1993; 330:65–82.

Snutch TP, Sutton KG, Zamponi GW. Voltage dependent calcium channels—beyond dihydropyridine antagonists. *Curr Opin Pharmacol* 2001; 1:11–16.

Tasker RR, Gorecki J, Lenz FA, Hirayama T, Dostrovsky JO. Thalamic microelectrode recording and microstimulation in central and deafferentation pain. *Appl Neurophysiol* 1987; 50:414–417.

Vergnolle N, Bunnett NW, Sharkey KA, et al. Proteinase-activated receptor 2 and hyperalgesia: a novel pain pathway. *Nature Med* 2001; 7:821–826.

Wall PD, Devor M. The effect of peripheral nerve injury on dorsal root potentials and on transmission of afferent signals into the spinal cord. *Brain Res* 1981; 209:95–111.

Wall PD, Woolf CJ. Muscle but not cutaneous C-afferent input produces prolonged increases in the excitability of the flexion reflex in the rat. *J Physiol* 1984; 356:443–458.

Wei F, Wang G-D, Kerchner GA, et al. Genetic enhancement of inflammatory pain by forebrain NR2B over-expression. *Nat Neurosci* 2001; 4:164–169.

Whiteside GT, Munglani R. Cell death in the superficial dorsal horn in a model of neuropathic pain. *J Neurosci Res* 2001; 64:168–173.

Woolf CJ, Wall PD. Chronic peripheral nerve section diminishes the primary afferent A-fibre mediated inhibition of rat dorsal horn neurones. *Brain Res* 1982; 242:77–85.

Woolf CJ, Shortland P, Coggeshall RE. Peripheral nerve injury triggers central sprouting of myelinated afferents. *Nature* 1992; 355:75–78.

Wynn Parry CB. Pain in avulsion lesions of the brachial plexus. *Pain* 1980; 9:41–53.

Wynn Parry CB. Brachial plexus injuries. *Br J Hosp Med* 1984; 32:130–132, 134–139.

Correspondence to: Howard L. Fields, MD, PhD, Department of Neurology, Box 0453, University of California, San Francisco, CA 94143-0453, USA. Fax: 415-476-9386; email: hlf@itsa.ucsf.edu.

Index